AF616259

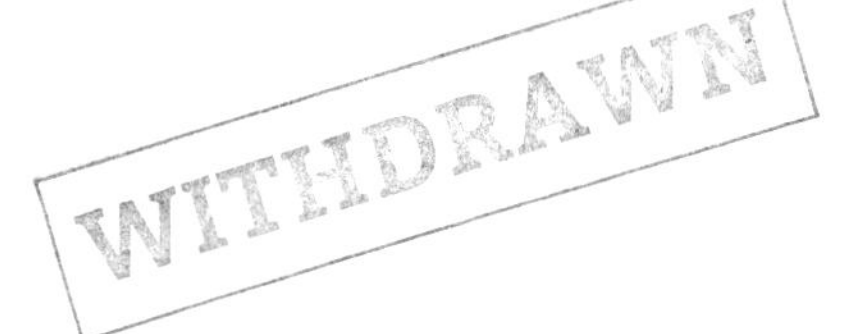
WITHDRAWN

HUMAN IMMUNITY
TO VIRUSES

Academic Press Rapid Manuscript Reproduction

Proceedings of a Symposium on Human
Immune Responses to Viruses: Recent Developments
Sponsored by the World Health Organization
Held at Wolfson College, Cambridge University
June 27–July 2, 1982

HUMAN IMMUNITY TO VIRUSES

Edited by

FRANCIS A. ENNIS

Departments of Medicine,
Molecular Genetics, and Microbiology
University of Massachusetts Medical School
Worcester, Massachusetts

1983

ACADEMIC PRESS
A Subsidiary of Harcourt Brace Jovanovich, Publishers

New York London
Paris San Diego San Francisco São Paulo Sydney Tokyo Toronto

ACADEMIC PRESS, INC.
111 Fifth Avenue, New York, New York 10003

United Kingdom Edition published by
ACADEMIC PRESS, INC. (LONDON) LTD.
24/28 Oval Road, London NW1 7DX

Main entry under title:

Human immunity to viruses.

Proceedings of a symposium sponsored by the World Health Organization, held at Wolfson College, Cambridge University, June 27-July 2, 1982.
Includes index.
1. Virus diseases--Immunological aspects--Congresses.
I. Ennis, Francis A. II. World Health Organization.
[DNLM: 1. Virus diseases--Immunology. 2. Viruses--Immunology--Congresses. QW 160 S988h 1982]
RC114.5.H87 1983 616.9'2079 83-12299
ISBN 0-12-239980-3 (alk. paper)

PRINTED IN THE UNITED STATES OF AMERICA

83 84 85 86 9 8 7 6 5 4 3 2 1

CONTENTS

II INFLUENZA

III HERPES SIMPLEX VIRUS

IV CYTOMEGALOVIRUS

V OTHER VIRUSES

CONTRIBUTORS

Numbers in parentheses indicate the pages on which the authors' contributions begin.

Charles A. Alford (219), *Departments of Pediatrics and Microbiology, University of Alabama School of Medicine, Birmingham, Alabama 35294*

Brigitte A. Askonas (137), *National Institute for Medical Research, Mill Hill, London NW7 1AA, United Kingdom*

C. Barker (257), *Department of Surgery, Hospital of the University of Pennsylvania, Philadelphia, Pennsylvania 19104*

Christine A. Biron (21), *Department of Pathology, University of Massachusetts Medical School, Worcester, Massachusetts 01605*

Neil R. Blacklow (319), *Division of Infectious Diseases, University of Massachusetts Medical School, Worcester, Massachusetts 01605*

Jack F. Bukowski (21), *Department of Pathology, University of Massachusetts Medical School, Worcester, Massachusetts 01605*

William H. Burns (203), *The Johns Hopkins Oncology Center, The Johns Hopkins School of Medicine, Baltimore, Maryland 21205*

George Cukor (319), *Division of Infectious Diseases, University of Massachusetts Medical School, Worcester, Massachusetts 01605*

Meyer E. Dworsky (219), *Departments of Pediatrics and Microbiology, University of Alabama School of Medicine, Birmingham, Alabama 35294*

Francis A. Ennis (151), *Departments of Medicine, Molecular Genetics, and Microbiology, University of Massachusetts Medical School, Worcester, Massachusetts 01605*

Morag Ferguson (335), *National Institute for Biological Standards and Control, Holly Hill, Hampstead, London NW3 6RB, United Kingdom*

H. M. Friedman (257), *Departments of Pediatrics and Medicine, Hospital of the University of Pennsylvania, Philadelphia, Pennsylvania 19104*

R. G. Grossman (257), *Department of Medicine, Hospital of the University of Pennsylvania, Philadelphia, Pennsylvania 19104*

Sonoku Habu (21), *Department of Pathology, Tokai University, Ishera, Kanagawa, Japan*

Martin V. Haspel (21), *Laboratory of Oral Medicine, National Institute of Dental Research, National Institutes of Health, Bethesda, Maryland 20205*

James E. K. Hildreth* (3), *Nuffield Department of Clinical Medicine, John Radcliffe Hospital, Headington, Oxford OX3 9DU, United Kingdom*

Kathryn V. Holmes (21), *Department of Pathology, Uniformed Services University for Health Sciences, Bethesda, Maryland 20814*

R. Husseini (133), *Department of Microbiology, University of Birmingham, Birmingham B15 2TT, United Kingdom*

David T. Karzon (111), *Department of Pediatrics, School of Medicine, Vanderbilt University, Nashville, Tennessee 37232*

F. Y. Liew (163), *Department of Experimental Immunobiology, The Wellcome Research Laboratories, Beckenham, Kent BR3 3BS, United Kingdom*

Carlos Lopez (193), *Sloan-Kettering Institute for Cancer Research, New York, New York 10021*

Cornelis J. Lucas (293), *Central Laboratory, Netherlands Red Cross Blood Transfusion Service, Laboratory of Experimental and Clinical Immunology, University of Amsterdam, Amsterdam, The Netherlands*

Henry F. McFarland (293), *Neuroimmunology Branch, National Institute of Neurological and Communicative Diseases and Stroke, National Institutes of Health, Bethesda, Maryland 20205*

Andrew McMichael† (3), *Nuffield Department of Clinical Medicine, John Radcliffe Hospital, Headington Oxford OX3 9DU, United Kingdom*

David I. Magrath (335), *National Institute for Biological Standards and Control, Holly Hill, Hampstead, London NW3 6RB, United Kingdom*

Anthony Meager (43), *Division of Viral Products, National Institute for Biological Standards and Control, Holly Hill, Hampstead, London NW3 6RB, United Kingdom*

Philip D. Minor (335), *National Institute for Biological Standards and Control, Holly Hill, Hampstead, London NW3 6RB, United Kingdom*

A. A. Nash (179), *Department of Pathology, University of Cambridge, Cambridge, United Kingdom*

Pearay L. Ogra (81), *Division of Infectious Diseases, Children's Hospital, Buffalo, New York 14222*

Ko Okumura (21), *Department of Immunology, University of Tokyo, Tokyo, Japan*

David C. Parker (21), *Department of Pathology, University of Massachusetts Medical School, Worcester, Massachusetts 01605*

Robert F. Pass (219), *Departments of Pediatrics and Microbiology, University of Alabama School of Medicine, Birmingham, Alabama 35294*

*Present address: The Johns Hopkins Medical School, Baltimore, Maryland 21205.

†Present address: The Johns Hopkins Medical School, Baltimore, Maryland 21205.

S. A. Plotkin (257), *Departments of Pediatrics and Medicine, Hospital of the University of Pennsylvania, Philadelphia, Pennsylvania 19104*

Gerald V. Quinnan, Jr. (241), *Division of Virology, Office of Biologics, National Center for Drugs and Biologics, Food and Drug Administration, Bethesda, Maryland 20205*

Marie Riepenhoff-Talty (81), *Department of Pediatrics and Microbiology, School of Medicine, State University of New York at Buffalo, and Division of Infectious Diseases, Children's Hospital, Buffalo, New York 14222*

Alain H. Rook (241), *Division of Virology, Office of Biologics, National Center for Drugs and Biologics, Food and Drug Administration, Bethesda, Maryland 20205*

Philip K. Russell (311), *Walter Reed Army Institute for Research, Division of Communicable Diseases, Washington, D.C. 20012*

Rein Saral (203), *The Johns Hopkins Oncology Center, The Johns Hopkins School of Medicine, Baltimore, Maryland 21205*

Geoffrey C. Schild (335), *National Institute for Biological Standards and Control, Holly Hill, Hampstead, London NW3 6RB, United Kingdom*

J. G. P. Sissons (101), *Departments of Medicine and Virology, Royal Postgraduate Medical School, London W12 0HS, United Kingdom*

M. L. Smiley (257), *Departments of Pediatrics and Medicine, Hospital of the University of Pennsylvania, Philadelphia, Pennsylvania 19104*

H. Smith (133), *Department of Microbiology, University of Birmingham, Birmingham B15 2TT, United Kingdom*

Moses Spitz (335), *National Institute for Biological Standards and Control, Holly Hill, Hampstead, London NW3 6RB, United Kingdom*

Sergio Stagno (219), *Departments of Pediatrics and Microbiology, University of Alabama School of Medicine, Birmingham, Alabama 35294*

S. E. Starr (257), *Departments of Pediatrics and Medicine, Hospital of the University of Pennsylvania, Philadelphia, Pennsylvania 19104*

John L. Sullivan (279), *Department of Pediatrics, University of Massachusetts Medical School, Worcester, Massachusetts 01605*

C. Sweet (133), *Department of Microbiology, University of Birmingham, Birmingham B15 2TT, United Kingdom*

Patricia M. Taylor (137), *National Institute for Medical Research, Mill Hill, London NW7 1AA, United Kingdom*

Jean-Louis Virelizier (71), *Unite d'Immunologie et de Rhumatologie Pediatriques, Hôpital Necker-Enfants Malades, Paris, France*

Robert C. Welliver (81), *Department of Pediatrics and Microbiology, School of Medicine, State University of New York at Buffalo, Buffalo, New York 14222*

Martha A. Wells (151), *Division of Virology, Bureau of Biologics, Food and Drug Administration, Bethesda, Maryland 20205*

Raymond M. Welsh (21), *Department of Pathology, University of Massachusetts Medical School, Worcester, Massachusetts 01605*

P. Wildy (179), *Department of Pathology, University of Cambridge, Cambridge, United Kingdom*

PREFACE

Effective control of many infectious diseases is now possible through the use of vaccines. Pioneering work by Pasteur and Jenner led to early prevention of, respectively, rabies and smallpox. In more modern times the breakthrough in tissue culture growth of human viruses by Enders led to the successful developments of effective viral vaccines against poliomyelitis, measles, mumps, and rubella.

These successes were accomplished with little appreciation of the immune responses of the host to the pathogen or to the vaccine. Gradually, evidence was developed that antibodies capable of blocking infection by the virus *in vitro* were associated with resistance against certain viral infections. Little information, however, was available on the contribution of cell-mediated mechanisms to the pathology of, recovery from, or protection against viral infections.

This situation is now changing dramatically because of several major developments. The observation that virus-specified killer T lymphocytes need to recognize both self and viral antigens on virus-infected cells in order to kill them was made by Zinkernagel and Doherty in 1974. Subsequently, another set of lymphocytes, called natural killer lymphocytes, which killed virus-infected cells, was described by Welsh and Zinkernagel. These results provided *in vitro* markers for detecting the presence and activity of these lymphocytes in virus infections.

With the simultaneous development of hybridomas and the production of monoclonal antibodies by Kohler and Milstein, it has become possible to separate these killer lymphocytes from lymphocytes with other functions, such as helping or suppressing antibody formation. It has also become possible to assess the effects of treatment with specifically separated lymphocytes in animal experiments, some of which have demonstrated key roles for killer T lymphocytes in recovery from influenza.

At the same time, less detailed but promising data are being developed in human studies. McMichael *et al.* reported that influenza-specific cytotoxic T lymphocytes were also restricted by viral and HLA antigens. Recently, induction of these cells by vaccines has been reported by Ennis *et al.*, and Quinnan has demonstrated that these cells are important in recovery from serious cytomegalovirus infections observed after bone marrow transplantation.

The purpose of this book is to help provide a bridge between these exciting basic laboratory observations and their contributions to a variety of serious viral diseases of humans. Our selection of viral infections to include in this book relied in large part on diseases currently under investigation with varying degrees of progress.

The authors were asked to use their expertise to help the reader become aware of research progress and opportunities in their specialized field of interest. The first portion of the book describes developments in measuring immune responses to viruses, emphasizing areas of recent progress. These general reviews are followed by detailed papers on the application of these techniques to a number of human viral diseases. The pathogenesis and natural biology of the infection is described initially, followed by a review of the immune response to the infection.

We have included a number of serious viral infections being investigated: influenza, herpes simplex, cytomegalovirus, Epstein–Barr virus, measles, dengue, and polio are included. We did not include other suggested viruses, e.g., rubella, hepatitis, because there was little new information available regarding cellular immune responses.

Ultimately, the reason for understanding the immune responses to viral infections is to be able to prevent illness and death. It is essential to apply these new techniques as much as possible to improving our understanding of human immune responses, whether antibody, lymphocyte, or lymphokine-mediated, to viruses and to viral vaccines. It is obvious that much more basic laboratory work needs to be performed in this research area, but the time has come to apply these techniques to clinical investigations of viral infections and vaccines.

ACKNOWLEDGMENTS

The papers presented in this book were presented at a conference held at Wolfson College, Cambridge University. The purpose of the small informal conference was to promote a dialogue between basic immunologists and virologists, clinical investigators, and public health authorities interested in viral diseases and their prevention. Dr. G. C. Schild, London, and Dr. Fakhry Assaad, Geneva, were very helpful in supporting the conference. We wish to thank the Fellows of Wolfson College, the World Health Organization, the International Association for Biological Standardization, Burroughs-Wellcome Company, Glaxo Operations, United Kingdom, Smith-Kline-RIT, Institut Merieux, Institute-Sieroterapico e Vaccinogeno Toscano, and Merck Sharp and Dohme for providing support for the conference. A special thanks to Josephine Pavini who typed the manuscript and dealt very patiently with the editor and contributors.

I

IMMUNE RESPONSES TO VIRUSES — OVERVIEWS

CHAPTER 1

VIRUS SPECIFIC CYTOTOXIC T CELLS

Andrew McMichael

James E.K. Hildreth

Nuffield Department of Medicine*
John Radcliffe Hospital
Oxford, England

INTRODUCTION

Cytotoxic T lymphocytes were first recognised as cells which kill foreign cells in vitro. They were thought to mediate graft rejection in vivo, but this function is now not certain (1) and cannot be their normal biological role. Their ability to kill virus infected cells was first demonstrated about ten years ago (2). These findings indicated that cytotoxic T cells could have a role in real life. Since these first experiments a wealth of information has accumulated on the function of cytotoxic T cells, particularly with regard to their recognition of infected cells and the involvement of histocompatability antigens (reviewed in 3). In this short review we shall concentrate on work with human cells which has proceeded in parallel with the more well known work on the mouse.

Virus specific cytotoxic T lymphocytes have been demonstrated for a number of viruses which infect humans. These include Influenza A and B, (4,5) Epstein-Barr (6), measles (7), mumps (8), cytomegalo (9) and herpes simplex (9) viruses. As cellular immunity to many of these viruses is discussed in this volume, we shall concentrate on cytotoxic T lymphocytes specific for influenza, which in many ways form the prototype for studies with other viruses.

*Present address: John Hopkins Medical School, Baltimore, Maryland 21205, USA.

ISBN 0-12-239980-3

INDUCTION

Cytotoxic T lymphocytes can be induced in vitro from immune volunteers. As all adults have been infected with influenza virus, the reaction measured in vitro is normally a secondary immune response. Cytotoxic T cells specific for influenza have been demonstrated in vivo during the course of influenza and after vaccination with live virus (10); similar cells specific for measles and mumps viruses have been reported as being present during the course of these diseases (7,8). Studies have indicated that induction of cytotoxic T cells from peripheral blood lymphocytes of immune volunteers requires virus antigen (11). This is normally presented as virus infected cells or live virus, but UV inactivated virus (11) and membrane fragments (12) are sufficient. Viruses are normally presented on autologous infected cells but we have found that allogeneic cells or allogeneic membrane fragments from infected cells will stimulate induction of cytotoxic T cells provided that HLA Class I histocompatability antigens are shared (12). Thus, cytotoxic precursor cells see both HLA glycoproteins of self and virus antigens on the stimulating cell.

TABLE 1. HLA Restricted Induction of Influenza Virus Specific Cytotoxic T Cells

Effector	Stimulus"	HLA Match'	%Lysis MN-A**	WT-A*	JM-A*
MN	MN-A(c)	1,8,40	21	3	
	JR-A(c)	none	6	0	
	AR-A(c)	1,8	20	0	
	AR-A(mem)	1,8	27		
	JM-A(mem)	none	3		
JM	JM-A(c)	2,15,51	2		27
	JM-A(mem)	2,15,51	2		30
	AR-A(mem)	none	0		0

"Effector lymphocytes were induced by incubation with influenza A virus infected cells (c) or membranes (mem) prepared from influenza virus infected cells.

'HLA type of MN was A1,1,B8,40; JM was A2,2B15,51; AR shared A1 and B8 with MN and no antigen with JM.WT shared no HLA antigens with MN.

*Target cells were infected with influenza A virus.

The responding cells are T lymphocytes that bear glycoproteins shared by cytotoxic and suppressor cells. Induction requires both adherent cells and helper T lymphocytes (13). A period of culture is required which must exceed 3 days. Cytotoxic T cells can be grown in media containing interleukin 2 and we have maintained influenza specific cytotoxic T cell lines for up to two months. At the end of the induction period, cytotoxic effector cells which carry the cytotoxic/suppressor (T8) and T (T3) markers (14,15), are present in the culture. The normal targets used for assay are not sensitive to natural killer cells, but if NK sensitive cell lines, such as Daudi or K562, are tested, this kind of cytolytic activity can be demonstrated (11).

Cytolytic activity is demonstrated using a chromium release assay where freshly prepared lymphocyte target cells are labelled with ^{51}chromium, infected with influenza virus and then cultured for 4 hours to allow expression of influenza virus antigens. Killing is demonstrated in a five hour chromium release assay, where effectors and target cells are mixed at varying ratios. It should be noted that maximum killing is normally in the range of 30-40%. We have found this correlates with the number of cells expressing detectable amounts of haemagglutinin on the surface after infection, using a monoclonal antihaemagglutinin antibody in the cytofluorograph (unpublished results).

VIRUS SPECIFICITY

Cytotoxic T cells stimulated by influenza virus have been shown to be specific for the influenza virus type (4,5,11). T cells induced with influenza A fail to lyse target cells infected with influenza B and vice versa (Table 2). Occasionally, however, a low degree of cross reactivity is observed which remains unexplained. Provided natural killer cell activity is excluded, influenza specific cytotoxic T cells do not lyse EBV transformed cell lines (unpublished results).

A particularly interesting finding has been the observation that there is full cross rectivity between different influenza A viruses. This was first observed in the mouse and has been confirmed in several laboratories working with both mouse and man (17,18,5,11). In the secondary induction system described above, this cross reactivity is universal. In certain situations such as a primary immune response in vivo and secondary induction in mice, with purified haemagglutinin, a degree of influenza A subtype specificity has been observed (16,19). It is likely therefore that both crossreactive and haemagglutinin specific subpopulations are present in the normal response, but the former are more numerous.

TABLE 2. Specificity of Cytotoxic T Lymphocytes

Effector Cells' (HLA type)	Virus	Target Cells* RD	NH	NG
RD (A2,10,B18,44)	AUSSR:H1N1	36.0	36.4	0.6
	A/X31:H3N2	36.0		
	B/HK	0.6		
NH (A2,32,B40,44)	A/USSR:H1N1	31.7	27.9	0.4
	A1X31:H3N2		22.5	
	B/HK		1.0	
NG (A1,24,B8,37)	A/USSR	5.2		23.3

'Effector cells were sensitised with influenza A/USSR virus infected autologous cells.
*Results are shown as per cent lysis.

The nature of the influenza virus antigen seen on infected cells by cytotoxic T cells is uncertain. We have used a number of monoclonal antibodies specific for influenza virus haemagglutinin to inhibit cytotoxic T cell mediated lysis of infected cells but have found only partial inhibition with one antibody. The experience of others in murine systems is similar (20,21). Recent results examining the specificity of cloned cytotoxic T cell lines derived from the mouse, yield interesting results. Some clones appear to be specific for haemagglutinin, but Bennink et al (22) have shown that one clone was specific for either the product of the polymerase gene or a surface antigen modified by its action. These and more recent studies are described in a later chapter in this volume.

SPECIFICITY FOR HLA

Zinkernagel and Doherty (3) have demonstrated that virus specific cytotoxic T cells recognise both virus and histocompatability antigens on the surface of infected cells, possibly because of some interaction between the two. The specificity of human influenza specific cytotoxic T cells for HLA antigens was demonstrated by testing the ability of induced killer cells to lyse virus infected target cells from different individuals (4,5). It was found that effector and target had to share HLA A or B antigens (Table 1). This has been found with other human virus systems and indeed is used as evidence that cytotoxic T cell responses are being measured. Recently clones of human cytotoxic T cells specific for EBV viral antigens have been described and are restricted to either an HLA A or B antigen of self (23). That the HLA antigen itself is being recognised was demonstrated by blocking HLA restricted killing with monoclonal antibodies that identify monomorphic determinants, β-2 microblobulin and polymorphic determinants (24).

Lysis of target cells that is not restricted by HLA is observed only exceptionally. We have seen only three donors, in more than two hundred, whose effector cells lyse HLA mismatched, virus infected, target cells. One of these was studied in detail and it was found that the effector cell carried T cell antigens T3 and T8 but lysed allogeneic lymphocytes whether virus infected or not (15). Unlike cytotoxic T cell activity, killing was not inhibited by antibodies specific for the T3 and T8 antigens (see below) and it was concluded that it was more closely related to natural killer cell activity than cytotoxic T cell killing.

Apparent exceptions where target cells are not lysed despite HLA antigen sharing are more frequent. This was first apparent to us as a phenomenon associated with HLA A2 (25), but more recent results have indicated that this is found frequently with other HLA antigens as well. Biddison et al (26) described a similar phenomenon and indicated that the HLA A2 antigen of one of their donors was different. This donor's cytotoxic T cell did not lyse any other HLA A2 bearing cell, infected with virus; as a target cell this donor's cell was not lysed by any other effector cell. Biochemical characterisation of the HLA A2 antigen has revealed that it was slightly different, although no serological difference could be detected with alloantisera or monoclonal antibodies. Biddison et al have recently described three other HLA A2 'variants' (27). We have also identified three in our laboratory although no biochemical characterisation has yet been done. The reaction patterns seen with two such donors AM and DH are shown in Table 3. It is of interest that the AM A2 also appears different in EBV specific killing (H. Gaston and A.Rickinson, personal communication) and Y antigen specific killing (28).

TABLE 3. Definition of HLA A2 Subtypes by Influenza Virus Specific Cytotoxic T Cells.

	Influenza A virus infected target cells.					
	JF	JR	Nc	AT	AM'	DH'
JF	100"	125	*	91	0	*
JR	59	100	n.t.	47	15	9
Nc	*	n.t.	100	n.t.	0	*
AT	n.t.	85	58	100	15	2
AM'	n.t.	33	31	55	100	16
DH'	*	28	*	15	9	100

"Results are expressed as relative lysis where killing of autologous target cells is corrected to 100 and lysis of other target cells is related to this value. (This allows data from several different experiments to be compared).

*All effector cell target cell combinations share only HLA A2 unless marked with an asterisk when another antigen was shared and the result is omitted for clarity.

'Because the cells are not recognised as targets and kill HLA A2 matched cells poorly AM and DH are considered to carry HLA A2 variant antigens (see text).

These findings and results from Holland (E.Goulmy & J.Van Rood, personal communication) indicate that 10% of HLA A2 antigens are variant and can be distinguished by cytotoxic T cells. It remains to be seen whether the variants are all of one, or two types or whether each are unique HLA mutations. Biochemical characterisation of the variants and ultimately gene nucleotide sequencing should indicate how these variants have arisen and which part of the molecule they alter. These studies should give insight into how cytotoxic T cells recognise HLA antigen. This exquisite specificity for A2, where minor variations are distinguished, contrasts sharply with the broad cross reactivity of the cytotoxic T cells for different influenza A viruses.

Another reason for apparent nonrecognition of virus infected target cells is the phenomenon of haplotype preference. Biddison et al (29) and McMichael (30) have described individuals whose cytotoxic T cells lyse target cells of one parental haplotype but not the other, in family studies. The explanation for this finding is not understood, but Biddison et al have suggested that it has a genetic basis because HLA identical siblings responded in the same way in a large family study (29). If virus and HLA antigens have to associate on the cell surface it is possible that some antigens interact better than others with particular antigens. Another possibility is that the failure of recognition as is at the level of antigen presentation to the helper T cell necessary for cytotoxic T cell induction, a typical Ir gene phenomenon.

These above findings raise the possibility that HLA type influences the cytotoxic T cell response to influenza virus infection. It should be pointed out however that all of these individuals respond to autologous target cells infected with the virus. Non responders have been observed, but we cannot exclude the possibility that these are poorly immune individuals (see below).

VIRUS-HLA INTERACTION

Various explanations for H-2 or HLA restriction have been proposed, but none is entirely satisfactory. There are two principal schools of thought, (1) that there is a single receptor seeing a combination antigen formed by HLA and virus or (2) that there are a pair of receptors, one specific for virus and one specific for HLA antigen. In both models a possible explanation for that haplotype preference or Ir gene like results would revolve around the possible interaction between HLA and virus. We have therefore attempted to demonstrate a virus-HLA interaction in influenza A infected human lymphocytes.

Mice were immunised with human cells or human-mouse hybrid cells infected with influenza virus and monoclonal antibodies specific for infected cells were sought. Thirty-seven fusion experiments of this type were carried out and culture supernatents were screened against virus, virus infected cells and uninfected cells. A number of culture supernatents were observed which appeared to react only with infected cells. However, on cloning these cell lines, and preparing either high titre supernatants or ascitic fluids, this pattern of reactivity was lost and all antibodies reacted with normal uninfected cells. An explanation for these findings was found when the antibodies were purified, radio-labelled and their binding characteristics on infected lymphocytes were measured by Scatchard analysis. We found, as Liberti et al (31) had found, that the affinity binding was greater on infected than uninfected cells (32). Further experiments revealed that binding affinity increased when neuraminidase treated cells were used instead of influenza virus infected cells. The phenomenon was not limited to anti HLA antibodies, but the only changes in affinity observed were increases, and not all antibodies showed this effect. At the first sight, this result appears to indicate a conformational change in the HLA molecule as a result of virus infection or neuraminidase treatment. However, it is possible that by removing charged sialic acid residues from the cell surface, the neuraminidase merely allows better access of the antibody to the cell surface glycoproteins. These findings could also offer an explanation for the recent report from Wylie et al (33) of monoclonal antibodies specific for virus infected cells. Their antibodies were produced by splenic fragment cultures in very low concentrations and high titre hybridoma antibodies were obtained.

We have also failed to co-precipitate influenza virus and HLA antigens from infected cells. In addition HLA antigens and anti HLA monoclonal antibodies failed to block haemagglutinin binding to cells or influenza virus infection of cells. Similarly, monoclonal antihaemagglutinin antibody had no effect on monoclonal anti HLA antibody binding to infected cells.

We can find no evidence therefore for virus-HLA interactions on the cell surface. Other groups have reported similar negative findings using co-precipitation and co-capping techniques (see 3).

THE CYTOTOXIC T CELL RECEPTOR

The nature of the T cell receptor is currently under investigation in many laboratories. One approach has been to generate anti-idiotype antibodies in the hope of defining unique structures on cloned T cells which could be the receptor. The second general approach has been to characterise factors secreted by T cells, usually suppressor T cells, which show antigen binding function and which modulate the function of target cells. Despite intense effort however, the answer remains elusive.

An approach which is particularly appropriate to the study of human T cells is to study the T cell specific antigens recognised by monoclonal antibodies made in the mouse. The argument behind this approach is that the T cell receptor must be expressed on the cell surface, it is likely to be different in small but immunogenic detail between the two species and some antibodies which bind to the structure should interfere with antigen recognition. Monoclonal antibodies made in the mouse, have identified six surface markers specific for human T lymphocytes (34).

We and others (13,15,35,36) have tested the capacity of antibodies specific for each of these antigens to inhibit cytotoxic T cell function. Two antibodies recognising the T3 antigen and the T8 antigen block killing. It should be noted however that not all antibodies to the T8 antigen inhibit lysis possibly because either the antigen itself is heterogenous or only certain parts of the structure are involved.

Figure 1 gives a typical result where one of the antibodies Leu 2a (anti T8) was added, in the absence of complement, when the killer and target cells were mixed. Inhibition by this antibody and anti T3 requires saturating amounts of monoclonal antibody to be present.

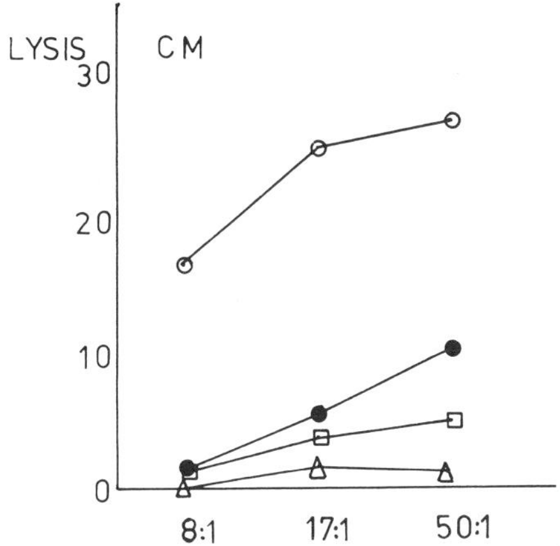

FIGURE 1. Inhibition of cytotoxic T cell mediated lysis by an anti T cell monoclonal antibody. Influenza A/USSR virus specific CM T cells were tested on autologous cells infected with homologous virus at killer: target ratios of 8:1, 17:1 and 50:1 in the absence (o) and presence (●) of anti Leu 2a monoclonal antibody (without complement). Effector cells were also tested on influenza A/USSR HLA mismatched target cells (□) and influenza B/Hong Kong infected autologous target cells (△).

Hildreth et al (37) have recently defined another monoclonal antibody which inhibits killing at subsaturating concentrations. This antibody also blocks natural killer cell activity unlike T3 and T8 specific reagents, and is therefore unlikely to be involved in a specific recognition process. The T3 and T8 antigens could be good candidates for a part of the T cell receptor. This is not necessarily so however and the antiT3 antibodies for instance, which are mitogenic to T lymphocytes at great dilution (38), could affect cell function in some nonspecific way. The T8 antigen is similar to the Ly2, 3 antigen of the mouse and it is known that this type of antibody blocks mouse cytotoxic T cell function. Furthermore, cytotoxic T cell clones that lack the T8 (Lyt2/3) antigen can kill but not recognise target specifically (39).

TABLE 4. Human T Cell Antigens

Antigen*	Defined by	Distribution	Mwtx10^{-3}	CTL Function"
T1	OKT1 Leu1	pan T	69	no effect
T3	OKT3 Leu4	pan T	19	blocks
T4	OKT4 Leu3a	Helper T	62	no effect
T8	OKT 8 Leu2a	cytotoxic T and suppressor T	32 30	Leu2a blocks
T11	OKT11	pan T	50	no effect
MHM23	MHM23	T>B	180 94	blocks

*Provisional nomenclature

"Effect on influenza virus specific HLA restricted cytotoxicity when antibody is added to the effector and target cells (without complement).

These experiments offer an approach to identifying the T cell receptor, but the problem is not yet solved.

FUNCTION OF VIRUS SPECIFIC CYTOTOXIC T CELLS IN VIVO

Our experiments have indicated that cytotoxic T lymphocytes specific for influenza virus can be induced from the peripheral blood of healthy human volunteers. Because activation in vitro is necessary, the circulating cells must be regarded as T memory cells. We are not able to induce a response from all individuals; there has been a decline such that now only 25% of donors give a response compared to 60% in 1978. A decline in the response has been observed in several individuals.

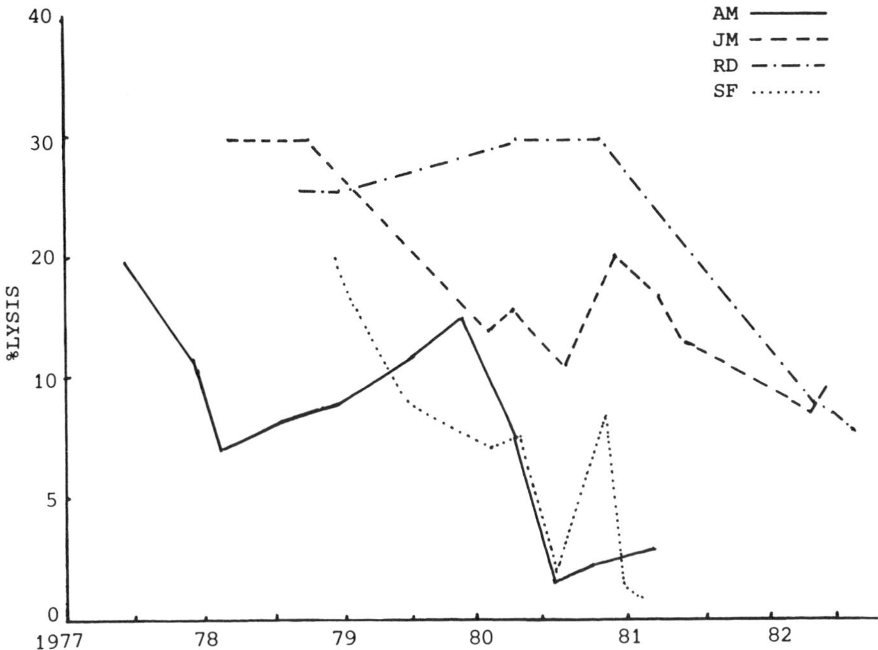

FIGURE 2. Declining cytotoxic T cell immunity to influenza. Lysis of autologous influenza A virus infected target cells by cytotoxic T cells induced from peripheral blood lymphocytes, at a killer:target cell ratio of 50:1 is plotted against time for four representative individuals.None of these volunteers (Figure 2) had influenza during the time of the investigation and we assume therefore their last natural attack was before 1977. Experiments of this type, (which are not wholly satisfactory, because this decline was not anticipated) indicate therefore that T cell memory after presumed natural infection fades with time, lasting approximately six years.

We have been able to boost cytotoxic T cell memory by vaccination (49). Ennis et al (10) carried out a larger study and showed that memory was very short lived, less than six months. Experiments in the mouse have also indicated that memory induced after natural infection is longer lasting than memory induced by vaccination (41).

We have attempted to correlate cytotoxic T memory levels

with protection against influenza virus infection. Sixty-three volunteers attending the MRC Common Cold Research Unit were inoculated with live influenza A/Munich and their course followed over a week. It was found that those with measurable cytotoxic T memory responses at the time of entry to the study shed no more than trace amounts of virus. About half of those with no measurable levels of cytotoxic T memory failed to shed virus, but the remaining shed significant quantities of virus. This effect was independent of the pre-existing levels of serum antibody (42).

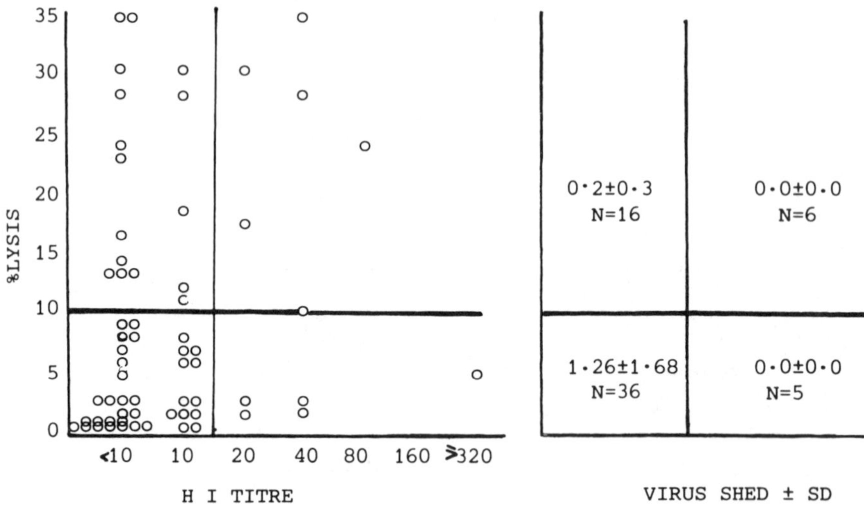

FIGURE 3. Protection by Cytotoxic T Lymphocytes. Lysis of autologous influenza A/USSR virus infected target cells at a killer:target cell ratio of 50:1 by 63 volunteers, is plotted against their serum antiheamagglutinin antibody titre. In the right hand panel the mean virus shed (EID_{50}) for volunteers in each quadrant is shown, indicating that either HI antibody or cytotoxic T cell memory is protective.

These results indicate that cytotoxic T memory correlates with protection against influenza in terms of clearing the virus rapidly and hence lack of virus shedding. It cannot however be conclusively proved that the cytotoxic T cells themselves are responsible, or that they mediate the effect by lysis of infected cells. There are indications that cytotoxic T cells can release interferon (43) on contact with infected cells and this would be an equally efficient method of terminating a virus infection.

The role of cytotoxic T cells in natural influenza infection is of crucial importance. We would like to advance a hypothesis that they are involved in clearing the virus infection. Because of the two to three days taken for induction, and the nature of the cells' function, they would not be able to prevent infection and therefore could not prevent a stimulus to the memory B cells. Because cytotoxic T cell recognition of the virus is crossreactive, there should be a cross protective effect. This will not be manifest as heterotypic immunity in terms of protection against a serum antibody rise or indeed virus shedding in the very early stages of the illness. It should be apparent as a more rapid clearing of the virus and therefore less severe illness. It is pertinent therefore that during the 1968 pandemic it was observed that half the cases recorded in which there was an antibody rise did not report clinical illness (44).

CONCLUSIONS

Humans that have been infected with influenza virus can develop memory cytotoxic T lymphocytes. These show a cross reactive virus specificity and HLA restriction. There is a possibility that the HLA type may influence the quality of these cells function. A role for cytotoxic T lymphocytes in influenza has been outlined. It is possible that HLA type may in some subtle way affect recovery from this virus illness. We have been unable to identify nonresponders consequent to their HLA type, but unless we challenge with an efficient vaccine we cannot exclude the possibility that they exist. If our argument is correct however, HLA types associated with poor immune responses could have been eliminated during previous pandemics, such as the 1919 outbreak, when mortality from influenza has been very high. Cytotoxic T lymphocytes probably have been an important role in controlling other virus infections such as Epstein Barr virus infection, measles, mumps (8) and cytomegalo virus infections, which are discussed elsewhere in this volume.

Vaccination protocols that boost cytotoxic T cell immunity may offer the advantage of cross protection, although the benefits are likely to be less severe illness rather than complete protection. Prophylactic antibody therefore still has an extremely important role to play and the ideal vaccine would anticipate the haemagglutinin subtype of the virus so as to offer complete protection, yet at the same time boost cytotoxic T cell immunity to offer some benefit against unexpected variants.

ACKNOWLEDGMENTS

We are grateful to our colleagues Frances Gotch and Gary Noble who contributed to the work in press that is described. This work was supported by a grant from the Medical Research Council to A.J. McM. and from the Rhodes Trust to J.E.K.H.

REFERENCES

1. Loveland, B.E. and McKenzie, F.C. 1982. Which T cells cause graft rejection? Transplantation 33, 217.
2. Marker, O. and Volkert, M. 1973. Studies on cell mediated immunity for lymphocytic choriomeningitis virus in vivo. J. Exp. Med. 137, 1511.
3. Zinkernagel, R.M. and Doherty,P.C. 1979. MHC restricted cytotoxic T cells: Studies on the biological role of polymorphic antigens determining T cell restriction specificity, function and responsiveness. Adv. Immunol. 27,51.
4. McMichael, A.J., Ting, A., Zweerink, H.J. and Askonas, B.A. 1977. HLA restriction of cell-mediated lysis of influenza virus infected human cells. Nature (Lond). 270,524.
5. Biddison,W.E., Shaw, S. and Nelson,D.L. 1979. Virus specificity of human influenza virus-immune cytotoxic T cells. J. Immunol. 122,660.
6. Rickinson,A.B., Wallace, L.C. and Epstein,M.A. 1980. HLA restricted T-cell recognition of Epstein-Barr virus-infected B cells. Nature. 283,865.
7. Kreth,H.W., terMeulen,V. and Eckert,G. 1982. Demonstration of HLA restricted killer cells in patients with acute measles. Med. Microbiol. Immunol. 165,203.
8. Kreth,H.W., Kress,H.G., Ott,H.F. and Eckert, G. 1982. Demonstration of primary cytotoxic T cells in venous blood and cerebrospinal fluid of children with mumps meningitis. J. Immunol. 128,241.
9. Sethi,K.K., Stroehmann,I. and Brandis,H. 1980. Human T cell cultures from virus specific and HLA restricted cell lysis. Nature 286,718.
10. Ennis,F.A., Rook,A.H., YiHua,Q., Schild,G.C., Riley,D., Pratt,R. and Potter,C.W. 1981. HLA restricted virus specific cytotoxic T-lymphocyte responses to live and in inactivated influenza vaccines. Lancet ii. 887.
11. McMichael,A.J. and Askonas,B.A. 1978. Influenza virus specific cytotoxic T cells in man: induction and

properties of the cytotoxic cell. European Journal of Immunology. 8,705.

12. Hildreth,J.E.K., Gotch,F.M. and McMichael,A.J. 1982. Plasma membranes from influenza virus-infected cells induce human secondary virus-specific CTL responses. Submitted for publication.
13. Biddison,W.E., Sharrow,S.O. and Shearer, G.M. 1981. T cell subpopulations required for the human cytotoxic T lymphocyte response to influenza virus: evidence for T cell help. J. Immunol. 127,487.
14. Zhang,Y., Nelson,D.L. and Biddison,W.E. 1981. Ia positive accessory cells are required for the induction of human influenza virus-immune cytotoxic T lymphocytes in mechanisms of lymphocyte activation. Ed. K. Resch & H.Kirchner, Elseview,North Holland p.388.
15. McMichael,A.J., Gotch,F.M. and Hildreth,J.E.K. Dissection of HLA restricted and unrestricted cell mediated cytotoxicity with monoclonal antibodies. Eur. J. Immun., in press.
16. Zweerink,H.J., Askonas,B.A., Millican,D., Courtneidge, S.A. and Skehel,J.J. 1977. Cytotoxic T cells to type A influenza virus; viral heamagglutinin induces A strain specificity while infected cells confer cross-reactive cytotoxicity. Eur. J. Immunol. 7, 630.
17. Braciale, T.J. 1977. Immunologic recognition of influenza virus infected cells. I generation of a virus strain specific and a cross reactive population of cytotoxic T cells in responses to type A influenza viruses of different subtypes. Cell Immunol. 33, 423.
18. Effros, R.B., Doherty,P.C., Gerhard,W. and Bennink, J. 1977. Generation of both crossreactive and virus specific T cell populations after immunisation with serologically distinct influenza A viruses. J. Exp. Med. 145,557.
19. Ennis, F.A., Martin,W.J. and Verbonitz, M.W. 1977. Haemagglutinin specific cytotoxic T cell response during influenza infection. J. Exp. Med. 145, 893.
20. Askonas,B.A. and Webster, R.G. 1980. Monoclonal antibodies to haemagglutinin and H-2 inhibit the crossreactive cytotoxic T cell populations induced by influenza. Eur. J. Immunol. 10,151.
21. Effros,R.B. Frankel,M.E. Gerhard,W. and Doherty,P.C. 1979. Inhibition of influenza immune T cell effector function by virus specific hybridoma antibody. J.Immunol. 123,1343.
22. Bennink,J.R., Yewdell,J.W. and Gerhard,W. 1982. A viral polymerase involved in recognition of influenza virus infected cells by a cytotoxic T cell clone. Nature 296,306.

23. Wallace,L.E., Rickinson,A.R., Rowe,M. and Epstein,M.A. 1982. Epstein-Barr virus specific cytotoxic T cell clones restricted through a single HLA antigen. Nature.
24. McMichael,A.J., Parham,P. Brodsky,F.M. and Pilch,J.R. 1980. Influenza virus specific T lymphocytes recognise HLA molecules; HLA molecules; blocking by monoclonal anti HLA antibodies. J. Exp. Med. 152, 195.
25. McMichael,A.J. 1978. HLA restriction of human cytotoxic T lymphocytes specific for influenza virus. Poor recognition of virus associated with HLA A2. Journal of Experimental Medicine. 148,1458.
26. Biddison,W.E., Krangel,M.S., Strominger,J.L., Ward,F.E., Shearer,G.M. and Shaw,S. 1980. Virus-immune cytotoxic T cells recognise structural differences between serologically indistinguishable HLA-A2 molecules. Human Immunol. 3,225.
27. Biddison,W.E., Kostyn,D.D., Strominger,J.L. and Krangel,M.S. 1982. Delineation of immunologically and biochemically distinct HLA-A2 antigens. J. Immunol. In press.
28. Pfeffer,P.F. and Thorsby,E. 1982. HLA restricted cytotoxicity against male specific (H-Y) antigen after acute rejection of an HLA-identical sibling kidney. Clonal distribution of the cytotoxic cells. Transplantation in press.
29. Shaw,S. and Biddison,W.E. 1979. HLA-linked genetic control of the specificity of human cytotoxic T cell responses to influenza virus. J. Exp. Med. 149,565.
30. McMichael, A.J. 1980. HLA restriction of human cytotoxic T cells. Springer. Semin. Immunopathol. 3,3.
31. Liberti,P.A., Hackett,C.J. and Askonas,B.A. 1979. Virus infection of lymphoblasts alters the binding affinity of anti H-2. Eur. J. Immunol. 9, 751.
32. Hildreth,J.E.K. and McMichael,A.J. 1981. "Interaction between influenza A virus and HLA-DR antigens". In Resch., K. and Kircher,H. (eds.) Mechanisms of Lymphocyte Activation. Elsevier North Holland, Amsterdam. 599.
33. Wylie,D.E. and Klinmann,N.R. 1981. The murine B cell repetoire responsive to an influenza-infected syngeneic cell line. J.Immunol. 127,194.
34. Reinherz,E.L. and Schlossman,S.F. 1981. The characterisation and function of human immunoregulatory T lymphocyte subsets. Immunology Today. 2,69.
35. Ledbetter,J.A., Evans, R.L., Lipinski,M., Cunningham-Ruddles C., Good, R.A. and Herzenberg,L.A. 1981. Evolutionary conversation of surface molecules that distinguish T lymphocyte helper/inducer and

cytotoxic suppressor subpopulations in mouse and man. J. Exp. Med. 153,310.
36. Plastoucas,C.D. and Good,R.A. 1981. Inhibition of specific cell mediated cytotoxicity by monoclonal antibodies to human T cell antigens in the absence of complement. In Resch, K. and Kirchner, H. (eds.) Mechanisms of Lymphocyte Activation. Elsevier/North Holland, Amsterdam. 461.
37. Hildreth,J.E.K., Gotch,F.M., Hildreth,P.K. and McMichael, A.J. 1982. A human lymphocyte function associated antigen involved in cell mediated lympholysis. Eur. J. Immunol., in press.
38. VanWauwe,J.P., deMey, J.R. and Gossens, J.G. 1980. OKT3: a monoclonal anti-human T lymphocyte antibody with potent mitogenic properties. J. Immunol. 124, 2708.
39. Glasebrook,A.L., Sarmiento, M., Loken, M., Dialynas, D.P. Quintas, J., Eisenberg, L., Lutz, C.Y., Wilde, D. and Fitch, F.U. 1981. Murine T lymphocyte clones with distinct immunological functions. Immunol. Rev. 54, 225.
40. McMichael,A.J., Gotch, F.M., Cullen, P., Askonas, B.A. and Webster, R.E. 1981. The human cytotoxic T cell response to influenza A vaccination. Clin. Exp. Immunol. 43,276.
41. Webster,R.G. and Askonas,B.A. 1980. Cross protection and crossreactive cytotoxic T cells induced by influenza virus vaccines in mice. Eur. J. Immunol. 10,396.
42. McMichael,A.J., Gotch,F.M., Noble,G.R. and Beare,A.S. 1982. The role of cytotoxic T lymphocytes in human influenza. Submitted for publication.
43. Morris,A.G., Lin,Y.L. and Askonas,B.A. 1982. Immune interferon release when a cloned T cell line meets its correct influenza infected target cell. Nature. 295,150.
44. Foy,H.M., Cooney, M.K. and Allen, I. 1976. Longitudinal studies of Types A and B influenza among Seattle school children. J. Inf. Dis. 134, 362.

CHAPTER 2

REGULATION AND ROLE OF NATURAL CELL-MEDIATED IMMUNITY DURING VIRUS INFECTIONS[6]

Raymond M. Welsh, Christine A. Biron, David C. Parker, Jack F. Bukowski[1]

[1]Department of Pathology
University of Massachusetts Medical School
Worcester, Massachusetts

Sonoku Habu[2]

[2]Department of Pathology
Tokai University
Ishera, Kanagawa, Japan

Ko Okumura[3]

[3]Department of Immunology
University of Tokyo
Tokyo, Japan

Martin V. Haspel[4]

[4] Laboratory of Oral Medicine
National Institute of Dental Research, NIH
Bethesda, MD

Kathryn V. Holmes[5]

[5]Department of Pathology
USUHS
Bethesda, MD

[6]ACKNOWLEDGEMENTS: Supported by USPHS Research Grant AI17672, AI00432, and Grant #R07403 from the Uniform Services, University of the Health Sciences

ISBN 0-12-239980-3

A. INTRODUCTION

Viral diseases are commonly self-limiting and of short duration, frequently abating before a substantial virus-specific immune response is mounted. Viral infections are often subclinical, somehow being controlled in early stages in a way that prevents disseminated disease. The body has non-immune natural resistance barriers which probably play a major role in controlling infections. The mechanisms of natural resistance fall into two classes, inducible and noninducible. The noninducible barriers include serum factors such as natural antibody, complement and antiviral lipoproteins, which may act independently or coordinately to inactivate viruses (1). A host may have cells genetically resistant to virus infection. Of significance in this regard is the ability of viruses to replicate in macrophages, which assimilate many of the viral particles entering the body (2). Other factors such as body temperature and tissue acidity may likewise confine and eventually abort an infection before it becomes disseminated The second class of natural immunity mechanisms are those which get induced during the course of infection. Of utmost importance in this regard is the virus-induced synthesis of interferon (IFN), which can directly protect cells from virus replication (3). IFN alone may be responsible for the self-limiting features of many virus infections, but IFN can also act to induce other host defense mechanisms. Included among these is the activation of natural killer (NK) cells and of macrophages (4,5). These cells, particularly the NK cells, may exert a nonspecific cell mediated cytotoxicity against virus-infected targets. In this paper we will examine the regulation of NK cell activity during virus infection and make an assessment of which cytotoxic cells might mediate non immune lysis of virus-infected targets.

B. NATURE OF THE NK CELLS

NK cells are cytotoxic lymphocytes found in all tested vertebrates (6,7,8). They normally lyse a restricted number of targets, usually T cell lymphomas, but their cytotoxicity can be augmented and their target range expanded by IFN treatment (9). These we call "activated", as opposed to "endogenous" NK cells (9). In several tested species NK cells are characterized as nonadherent, nonphagocytic, immunoglobulin-negative, Fe-receptor-positive lymphocytes expressing some T cell antigens and the glycosphingolipid

Asialo Gm_1 (6,7,8). Specific alloantisera and monoclonal antibodies further define NK cells in each species. NK cells are large lymphocytes containing azurophilic granules (10,11,12). Most of these large granular lymphocytes (LGL) probably are NK cells at different states of differentiation (13).

The current data on the mechanisms of NK cell-mediated lysis are consistent with an activation-secretion hypothesis. Binding of NK cells to targets requires Mg^{++} and occurs at 4°C (14). After binding microvilli from the NK cell project into lacunae of the target cell. At this time point inhibitors of proteases, phospholipase A2, and transmethylation are active, suggesting the processing of membrane determinants (15,16,17). There is next a Ca^{++} - dependent step, which can be blocked by strontium or inhibitors of calmodulin (17). It is thought that after membrane processing there is a Ca^{++} flux across the membrane, perhaps followed by a respiratory burst since inhibitors of respiration block at that stage (17,18,19). By electron microscopy, lysosome-like granules can be seen emanating from the golgi and collecting under the NK cell membrane contiguous with the target cell (20). Inhibitors of microtubule-dependent lysosomal discharges block cytotoxicity (18,19). Some investigators have reported the isolation from stimulated lymphocytes of lymphotoxins which lyse NK-sensitive targets (21,22). Others have hypothesized that this toxin binds to a hexose-phosphate receptor on the target cell (23). Once this putative lethal element has been delivered onto the target cell, the NK cell and target may be separated, but the target will go on to die.

Interferon activates NK cells to lyse sensitive targets more rapidly and greatly expands their target range (24,13). IFN may augment cytotoxicity by increasing the ability of NK cells to bind to targets via expression of receptors (25) or by enhancing the lytic activity, perhaps via a new phospholipase A2 (26) or cyclic nucleotide dependent activation of the NK cell (27). IFN-treated NK cells have a much greater capacity than endogenous cells to recycle after a lethal hit and go on to kill again (13,24,28). In virus infections, IFN may also act to induce the proliferation of NK cells and, paradoxically, to protect target cells from NK cell-mediated lysis. These phenomena are discussed below.

C. NK CELL ACTIVATION AND PROLIFERATION DURING VIRUS INFECTION

NK cells become activated during the early stages of most virus infections (29,30,31,32,33,34). In mice injected with 2 $X10^4$ plaque forming units (PFU) of lymphocytic choriomeningitis virus (LCMV), IFN titers and NK cell activity peak at day 2-3 post infection, while virus-specific cytotoxic T cells peak at 7-8 days postinfection (33,35). These activated NK cells differ from endogenous NK cells in characteristics in addition to cytotoxic activity. They are more adherent to nylon wool (36), have increased Fc receptor-mediated adherence (36), display increased sensitivity to lysis by anti-thy antibody plus complement (C) (36,37) and decreased sensitivity to lysis by antibody to NK alloantigen (38) or to asialo GM_1 plus C (Welsh, unpublished). While endogenous NK cells when separated by centrifugal elutriation consist chiefly of small to medium sized lymphocytes, the LCMV-activated NK cells consist of a population of large blast-size cells (36). These cells are indeed blasts, as we have shown by labeling the lymphocytes with ^{3}H-Thymidine and examining their ability to lyse targets in a single cell agarose cytotoxicity assay that includes autoradiography. While less than 1% of the total lysis is mediated by blast NK cells from control mice, at least 20% of the augmented levels of lysis by NK cells from LCMV-infected mice is mediated by blasts (39,40,41). Thus, the augmented NK cell activity seen during a virus infection is a product of both NK cell cytolytic activity and induction of NK cell blastogenesis. The difference in the phenotype of activated vs endogenous NK cells may reflect the difference between resting and proliferative NK cell populations. Subsequent work has shown that blast NK cells get induced by LCMV to high levels in athymic nude mice, suggesting that T cell factors are not involved in the blastogenesis (41). In fact, purified IFN type B, when injected into mice, induces NK cell blastogenesis, as indicated in the elutriation profile shown in figure 1. The mechanism by which IFN stimulates blastogenesis of NK cells in vivo is not known.

At later stages of viral infection, the IFN levels decrease, along with NK cell activation and blastogenesis (35,39). It could be predicted at this time that in areas in the body where virus-specific T cells are located, T cell dependent IFN-γ production may serve to locally activate NK cells. Spleen cells isolated from mice 6 days post-LCMV infection contain viral antigen plus an expanding population of virus-specific T cells. When cultured, these cells produce high levels of IFN-γ and concomitent high levels of activated NK cells (42).

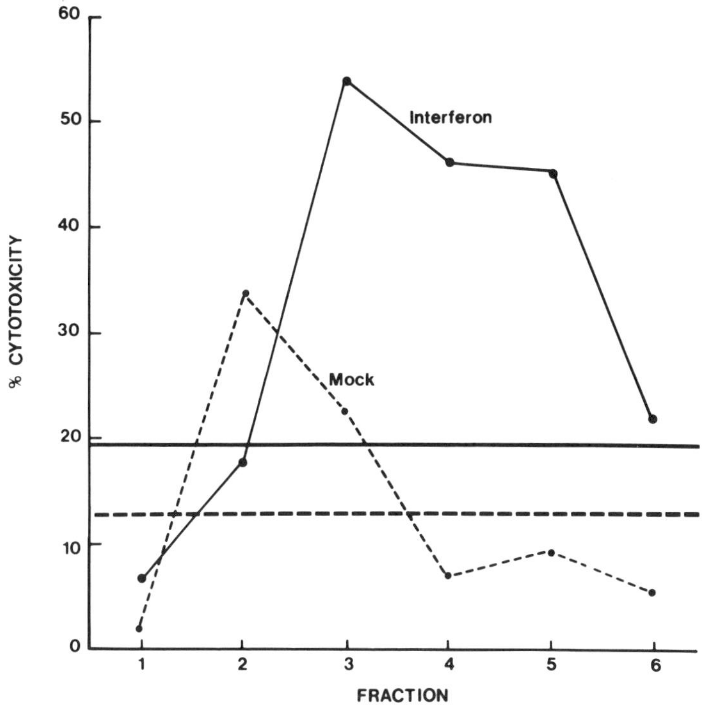

FIGURE 1. Size distribution of effector cells after treatment with either IFN or a mock IFN preparation. Mice (C3H/St) were injected intravenously with either 10^5 U of β type IFN having a specific activity of 10^7 U/mg protein (——) or an equivalent protein concentration prepared from mock-infected cells (---). Spleen cells were isolated after 16H and separated by centrifugal elutriation. Cytotoxicity against YAC-1 target cells was determined in a ^{51}Cr release assay. Blast cells are contained in fractions 4, 5 and 6.

D. INTERFERON PROTECTION OF TARGET CELLS

While IFN induces the activation and blastogenesis of NK cells, it paradoxically will induce target cells to become resistant to NK cell mediated lysis (43,44,45,46,47). Protection does not occur if cells are treated with inhibitors of RNA or protein synthesis before IFN treatment (45,47). All tested murine cells sensitive to the antiviral effects of IFN were protected from NK cells, while cells resistant to the antiviral effects (xenogeneic cells, teratocarcinomas, IFN-resistant variants) do not become protected (47).

The mechanism of this target cell protection is not known. IFN-treated target cells bind to NK cells but fail to inhibit the lysis of sensitive cells in cold target competition assays (43,45,46,47,48). It has been suggested that NK cells become inactivated after lysing a target and that this is the basis for competition. Since they do not lyse IFN-treated targets, those targets do not compete (28,48). Others have suggested that NK cells release a lymphotoxin when exposed to target cells, and if targets are first treated with IFN less lymphotoxin is released (22). This may indicate that IFN-treated targets have receptors for NK cells but lack membrane elements involved in the triggering of the NK cell lymphotoxins.

The biochemical basis of IFN protection is likewise unclear, though IFN induces a number of changes on the cell surface such as an increase in the expression of glycoproteins, glycosphingolipids, and sialic acid (49). The high sialic acid phenotypoe has been linked to resistance to NK cell mediated lysis in other systems (49,50). Protection of target cells from NK cell mediated lysis occurs in vivo after administration of IFN or virus infection. Thymocytes and tumor cells isolated from LCMV-infected mice resist lysis by activated NK cells in assays in vitro (43,47). Tumor cells treated with IFN radiolabelled with ^{125}IUDR,and injected into syngeneic mice by the intravenous route are rejected from these mice less rapidly than untreated tumor cells (47). Since the effector causing tumor cell rejection in this type of assay is thought to be an NK cell (51,52), it appears that IFN-treated cells resist NK cells mediated lysis in vivo.

When assessing the potential damage due to target cells by activated NK cells during a virus infection, one must therefore take into account that the virus-induced IFN is protecting target cells as it activates NK cells. It has been postulated that virus-infected cells may resist IFN-protection, perhaps because cellular RNA and protein synthesis required for IFN-induced effects, may be inhibited (53). This would allow IFN-activated NK cells to lyse virus-infected cells but not IFN-protected uninfected cells in vivo. This phenomenon would of course only occur with cyto-pathic virus infections. IFN does protect LCMV-infected L-929 cells from NK cell mediated lysis, but the LCMV infec-tion under these conditions is relatively non cytopathic (unpublished data). Interestingly, the virus systems which have provided the best data linking NK cells to resistence involve cytopathic viruses (this is discussed later in the text).

E. LYSIS OF VIRUS INFECTED CELLS BY NK CELLS

Several investigators, using a number of viruses, have shown that leukocytes mediate greater lysis of cultures containing virus-infected as compared to uninfected cells (40,53,54,55,56,59,60,61,62,63).

This is actually a complex phenomenon that varies with the virus and the target cell and is often misinterpreted. Enhanced sensitivity of virus-infected targets to NK cells could be due to: 1. virus-induced impairment of a cell's ability to repair its membrane (64), 2. to enhanced adhesion of NK cells to virus-infected targets due either to viral glycoproteins or to virus-induced cellular receptors (46,56), 3. to an in situ activation of NK cells via viral glycoproteins, which have been shown to be able to activate NK-like cells directly (57,65,66), or 4. to the activation of NK cells by virus-induced IFN (62). This latter (IFN) mechanism is a prominent cause of enhanced lysis when cytotoxicity assays are run for periods longer than 8 hours. Santoli et al (62,63) originally documented that human fibroblasts infected with a variety of viruses were lysed by NK cells in human peripheral blood leukocytes in overnight assays. The generation of virus-induced IFN correlated with the cytotoxicity, and the IFN was shown to activate NK cells. Thus, in these systems, which included influenza, herpes simplex, paramyxo, vaccinia, and mumps viruses, the increased lysis was actually due to activation of effector cells rather than to increased sensitivity of target cells. We confirmed this result in the mouse system and then specifically asked the question: are virus-infected targets innately more sensitive to NK cell mediated lysis (46). This was done by exposing already activated NK cells to virus-infected targets in short term (4 hours) assays in order to preclude further NK cell activation. The results of those experiments indicated that virus infections had varied effects on target cells, rendering them either unaltered, more resistant, or more sensitive to NK cell mediated lysis (46).

The virus-induced resistance to NK cell-mediated lysis in some cases may have been mediated by IFN, as discussed above. Interestingly, Sendai virus-infected L-929 cells bound to NK cells with enhanced efficiency but were lysed poorly by them. In contrast, HSV-infected Vero cells neither bound to nor were lysed by NK cells. Thus, the mechanisms for resistance may differ (46).

We presented a report examining enhanced lysis of virus infected cells by activated NK cells in very short assays (46). Sendai virus infected Vero cells were preferentially lysed by activated NK cells in assays as short as 1 hour. These targets bound to NK cells with higher than normal efficiency, and this may be the cause of this sensitivity, along with the fact that Vero cells do not produce IFN, which could protect the targets. Using non-activated cells as effectors, preferential killing against virus-infected targets in short-term assays has been reported for a few other virus infections, including measles (57), Epstein-Barr (56) and mouse hepatitis virus (MHV) (60).

F. VIRUS KILLER (VK) CELLS

We have recently undertaken an investigation of the effector cell which lysis MHV-infected 3T3 cells and have found that, at least in this virus infection, natural cytotoxicity is mediated by a cell other than an NK cell. We operationally define this cell as a virus killer, or "VK" cell. In this assay, 3T3 cells are infected with MHV, radiolabeled with ^{51}chromium, and plated into microtiter wells at 1×10^4 cells in 200μl medium per well. Twenty-four hours later, the medium is aspirated, and spleen leukocytes from normal, uninfected mice are added to each well in a total of 200μl. The assay period is from 3-4 hours, though some lysis can be detected by 1 hour. The proportion (P) of radiolabel released is computed for each well: P=supernatant/(supernatant + NP40-extracted pellet). The percent specific ^{51}chromium release (lysis) is calculated by the formula 100x (Ptest-Pmem control)-(1-Pmem control). Under these conditions MHV-infected but not unfected cells are lysed to significant levels. The amount of lysis is proportional to the concentration of effector cells and is suggestive of single hit kinetics.

Lysis is mediated by cells from C3H/St,BALB/C, BALB/C athymic nude, DBA/2, C57BL/6 normal and C57BL/6 mice carrying the beige mutation conferring NK cell deficiency. Among the organs, cytotoxicity is highest by spleen leukocytes and intermediate by bone marrow cells. Peritoneal cells or thymocytes kill poorly.

Some properties of the VK cell are listed in tables 1 and 2.

TABLE 1. Characterization of Cell which Lyses MHV-Infected 3T3 Cells

Exp.	Effector	^{51}Chromium Release (lysis) 3T3 (MHV)*	YAC-1
1.	C3H/St Untreated	33.0	39.0
	Nylon Adherent	31.0	7.8
	Nylon Nonadherent	6.6	30.0
2.	C3H/St Untreated	19.0	22.0
	Complement (C')	16.0	19.0
	Anti Asialo GM_1 + C'	21.0	5.9
	Anti Thy + C'	19.0	17.0
3.	C3H/St Untreated	39.0	13.0
	Anti-Asialo GM_1 in vivo	36.0	0.3
4.	DBA/2 Untreated	28.0	14.0
	$F(ab')_2$-Anti-Fab Rosettes	28.0	3.2
	Non Rosettes	8.1	29.0
	RBC (control) NonRosettes	27.0	14.0

Spleen leukocytes were isolated and examined for cytotoxicity against 3T3 cells infected with the A-59 strain of MHV or against the highly NK-sensitive YAC-1 cells. Assays were for 4H at effector to target ratios of 100:1. Exp. 1: Nylon wool column, Exp 2: leukocytes were treated with antibodies and complement to deplete certain cell types before assay. Exp 3: mice were injected with 20 ul rabbit anti asialo GM_1 antiserum to deplete NK cell activity in vivo. Exp 4: leukocytes were exposed to sheep erythrocytes (RBC) or to RBC conjugated to $F(ab')_2$ fragments from a antiserum. Rosetting cells were pelleted through ficoll gradients to separate them from non rosetting (immunoglobulin-negative) cells.

*Uninfected 3T3 cells were not lysed in these short-term assays.

It is clear that this belongs to a class of cells distinct from the NK cell. The VK cell is predominantly nylon wool adherent, Ia positive, and is not depleted by in vitro or in vivo treatment with anti-asialo GM_1. In contrast, the NK cell is predominantely nylon wool non adherent, Ia and asialo GM_1-positive. The VK cell reacts with antibodies to light chain, indicating that it is surface immunoglobulin positive. It rosettes with erythrocytes bearing an $F(ab')_2$ directed against immunoglobulin light chain, and the VK cell

Table 2. Comparison of NK and "VK" Cells

	NK	VK
Lymphocyte morphology	+	+
Phagocytic	–	–
Thy antigen	±	–
Ia antigen	–	+
Asialo GM_1 Antigen	+	–
Surface immunoglobulin	–	+
Nylon adherence	–	+
In nude mice	+	+
In beige mice	±	+
H-2 restriction	–	
Rapid (<4H) killing	+	+
Lability in culture	+	+

is also depleted by this antibody using panning techniques. Similar panning techniques with $F(ab')_2$ directed against IgD or IgM did not deplete VK cell activity. This suggests that the VK cell is not a B cell, most of whom bear these antigens. More likely, the VK cell has cytophilic antibody binding, perhaps, to Fc receptors. $F(ab')_2$ to light chain, when incorporated into assays, does not inhibit killing of targets by the VK cell, suggestive that the antibody present is not required for lysis. NK cell assays run in parallel with these cell separations show clear distinction between the VK and NK cells, as the NK cells, though expressing Fc receptors, are enriched after depletion of Ig-bearing cells.

The VK cell is similar to the NK cell in that it is Thy-negative, phagocytosis-negative, plastic non-adherent, and labile in culture. Lysis of MHV-targets can be elicited by small sized cells fractionated by centrifugal elutriation, that is, cell populations lacking any detectable granulocytes and containing only 2% macrophages as measured by histological staining technique. One tested anti-macrophage antiserum plus complement did not eliminate activity. The short term lysis assay and single hit kinetics of lysis are also features of NK cell-mediated lysis. It could be argued that virus-induced IFN is activating cells in this short term MHV assay, but this seems unlikely since lysis occurs in presence of actinomycin D and antibody to IFN.

The most likely candidate of potentially cytotoxic effector cells with properties compatible with this long list of characteristics seems to us to be a subclass of small monocytes. This has not yet been proven, and at this point in time, we will continue to functionally define the cell which lyses-MHV-infected targets as the VK cell.

The question that next arises is whether the VK cell is unique only to the MHV system, or does it participate in the preferential natural cytotoxicity against other virus infected targets. We thus far have investigated only one other system, that of LCMV infection of 3T3 or L-929 cells. In this system, under certain conditions of infection, preferential lysis of virus infected cells can be demonstrated. Treatment of effector cells with antibody to asialo GM_1 plus complement eliminates virtually all the cytotoxic activity against the NK-sensitive YAC-1 cells but only about half of the activity against LCMV-infected cells. Passage of cells through nylon wool columns greatly enriches for cytotoxic activity against YAC-1 cells, but cells from both nylon adherent and nonadherent fractions lyse LCMV-infected targets. Thus, lysis in this system is mediated both by NK cells and cells of another type. Another interesting feature of the LCMV system is that interleukin-2, a lymphocyte mitogen produced by T helper cells, greatly augments the natural killing of virus infected cells, when compared to uninfected cells (Table 3).

It has previously been reported that 1L-2 augments NK cell mediated lysis against very sensitive YAC-1 cells (67). In our system, the augmentation of lysis appears somewhat greater (in total amount of lysis) against LCMV-infected targets than uninfected targets. The effector cell causing 1L-2-dependent augmented lysis in our system has not yet been characterized, mainly because of the contamination with other cytotoxic cells types. This is, however, a functionally interesting phenomenon, since natural cytotoxic cells with tendencies to preferentially lyse virus-infected targets may be produced as a byproduct of T cell mediated immune reactions.

TABLE 3. IL-2-Induced Augmented Lysis of Virus-Infected Cells

		%Specific ^{51}Cr Release	
Exp.	Target Cell	Spleen Cells	Spleen Cells + IL-2
1.	3T3 + LCMV	42	58
	3T3	12	15
2.	L-929 + LCMV	12	44
	L-929	2	5
3.	L-929 + LCMV	25	39
	L-929	7	10

Spleen cells from 4 week old C3H mice (exp. 1 and 3) or 6 week old BALB/c mice (exp.2) were exposed to infected or uninfected target cells in a 16 hour ^{51}Cr release assay at an effector to target ratio of 100:1. Rat interleukin-2 (IL-2) obtained from Collaborative Research, Inc., Waltham, Mass., was included at 20 U/ml in the medium in some of the assays. Spontaneous release ranged from 21-37% for uninfected cells and 29-38% for LCMV-infected cells.

G. NATURAL CELL MEDIATED CYTOTOXICITY AGAINST VIRUS-INFECTED TARGET CELLS IN VIVO

The measurement of clearance of ^{125}IUDR-labeled tumor cells injected intravenously into mice has been accepted as a method for measuring NK cell mediated cytotoxicity in vivo (51,52). Work by several groups has shown that NK-sensitive target cells are rejected more rapidly than NK-resistant targets, and that mice with genetically high levels of NK cells reject targets more efficiently than do mice with low NK cell levels (51,52,68,69). Further, rejection is enhanced when mice are treated with agents such as poly I:C or LCMV, which augment NK cell activity, and rejection is inhibited when mice are treated with NK-depressing agents, such as cyclophosphamide and silica (52,69).

We have shown that L-929 cells infected with any of a variety of viruses (LCMV, herpes simplex virus, cytomegalovirus, Sindbis virus) and tested in this assay are rejected from mice more rapidly than are uninfected cells (39). Rejection of LCMV infected cells occurs at 2-3 times the levels of uninfected cells. The rejection is blocked if the mice are treated with cyclophosphamide or hydrocortisone acetate but not with cobra venom factor, which destroys complement. These data indicate that a cell mediated host response causes lysis of these implanted cells. Mice infected 3 days previously with LCMV or poly I:C had activated NK cells and rejected both the virus-infected and the uninfected cells very rapidly. Under these conditions of high NK cell activation, no preferential lysis of virus-infected targets was observed. In short term in vivo assays, implanted virus-infected cells did not enhance the rejection of uninfected cells. These results were all consistent with the hypothesis that 1. NK cells become locally activated in the vicinity of virus-infected cells and lyse them preferentially and 2. with time the infection becomes more systemic, activating many NK cells, which then lyse the infected and uninfected cells without preference.

Recent work in our laboratory has challenged and refuted hypothesis number one. Mice were injected with antibody to asialo Gm_1, and this depleted the NK cell activity measured in vitro as shown previously (70). These NK cell-depleted mice rejected implanted YAC-1 cells very poorly, that is about 15 times less efficiently than controls (Table 4). In contrast, this antibody treatment had no effect on the rejection of either uninfected or LCMV-infected L-929 cells. This indicates that the effector cell mediating natural in vivo lysis or natural cytotoxicity against LCMV-infected cells was not a typical NK cell. Whether the VK cell or other natural cytotoxic cells, such as macrophages or NC cells, mediate this rejection is not known. The augmented and nonpreferential lysis of L-929 cells seen in mice experiencing acute (Day 3) LCMV infection was, however, partially inhibited by treatment with antibody to asialo GM_1 (Table 3). This suggests that NK cells, when activated by virus infection, will lyse L-929 cells. However, the preferential rejection of virus infected cells at early stages of the infection is unlikely caused by NK cells.

H. EVIDENCE FOR A ROLE OF NK CELLS IN VIRUS INFECTIONS IN VIVO.

The evidence linking NK cells to resistance against virus infections is for the most part indirect and unconvincing. NK cells could function to impede the progress of the infection either by lysing virus-infected cells or by being major producers of IFN. Several laboratories have reported on both of these possibilities using in vitro systems.

It is possible that NK cells may be important in some virus systems but not others. Our investigations with the LCMV system fail to support the hypothesis that NK cells play a role in that infection. The levels of NK activity in various mouse strains is a genetic trait, but there is no apparent relationship between high-vs-low-NK strains and susceptibility to LCMV. Mice carrying the beige mutation, which confers a deficiency in the ability of NK cells to mediate lysis, synthesize normal levels of LCMV (71) and have an LD50 comparable to normal mice. Mice treated with silica, which decreases NK cell function, are killed by LCMV at levels compatible to normal mice, and the T cell-dependent clearance of virus in adoptively immunized mice is not impeded by silica (Bukowski and Welsh, unpublished). Further, depletion of the NK cell activity in LCMV persistently infected mice with antibody to Asialo Gm_1 does not appreciably influence the titer of the virus. A far more convincing series of experiments links NK cells with resistance to herpes virus infections. NK cells are derived from bone marrow and appear to be related to bone marrow cells which exert a genetically determined resistance to bone marrow allographs and certain tumor cell implants (72).

The genetics of resistance to HSV-1 correlates with this system and is mediated by a bone marrow cell (73,74). Mice with a genetically determined high NK cell activity are more resistant to cytomegalovirus (CMV) than those with low NK activity (75). NK cell-deficient beige mice are particularly sensitive to CMV. If beige mice receive bone marrow transplants from beige/+ mouse littermates, their NK cell activity and resistance to CMV are both restored (76). These results suggest but do not conclusively demonstrate that NK cells may play a role in certain virus infections. Depletion of NK cell activity in vivo with immunological reagents such as antibody to Asialo Gm_1 should now allow for careful dissection of this phenomenon. Our preliminary results indicate that mice depleted of NK cells with antibody to Asialo GM_1 synthesize more CMV, MHV, and vaccine virus (but not LCMV) than do normal mice.

I. DISCUSSION AND CONCLUSION

While NK cells become activated and are induced to proliferate during virus infection, their role in contributing to the pathology of, or resistance to, virus infections remains unclear. By various mechanisms NK cells or a newly described "VK" cell may preferentially lyse virus-infected targets in vitro are rejected by some natural cytotoxicity mechanism that is not an NK cell. Whether this type of in vivo cytotoxicity would occur against virus-infected normal tissue is not known. One factor that may inhibit autotoxicity by NK cells during virus infections is, paradoxically IFN. IFN protects target cells from lysis by activated NK cells, and this phenomenon can be demonstrated in vivo. Certain virus infected cells may resist the IFN-protection effects, but even then it is not clear whether lysis of virus-infected targets by NK cells inhibits spread of infection or augments it by liberating infectious virus from the lysing cell.

NK cells could, however, contribute to resistance to virus infections by other mechanisms. NK cells produce IFN in response to virus infections, and this could directly inhibit virus infection and spread. At later times in the infection, NK cells could specifically lyse virus-infected targets binding antiviral antibody. The effector cell of antibody-dependent cell cytotoxicity (ADCC) is called a "K", or killer cell, but most laboratories agree that the NK and K lymphocytes are indistinguishable (77). NK/K cells have Fc receptors which allow them to bind to antibody coated targets. We have shown that virus-infected targets remain sensitive to ADCC even when they resist natural killing (46).

In several virus systems in mice there is evidence that NK cells may contribute to resistance, while in others NK cells appear to play no significant role. Thus far, the most convincing experiments suggesting that they play a role have been with CMV. With the recent availability of reagents which selectively reduce NK cell activity in vivo, the contribution of NK cells to the pathogenesis of virus infections in laboratory animals should soon be dissected.

REFERENCES

1. Cooper, N.R., and R.M. Welsh. 1979. Antibody and complement-dependent viral neutralization. Springer Seminars in Immunopathology. 2:285
2. Mims, C.A. 1964. Aspects of the pathogenesis of virus diseases. Bacteriol. Rev. 28:30.
3. Isaacs, A., and J. Lindenmann. 1957. Virus interference. I. The interferon. Proc. Roy. Soc. B. 147:258.
4. Welsh, R.M. 1981. Natural cell mediated immunity during virus infections. In Natural Resistance to Tumors and Viruses. Edited by O. Haller. Springer-Verlag, Berlin, p.83.
5. Schultz, R.M., and M.A. Chirigos. 1979. Selective neutralization by anti interferon of macrophage activation by L-cell interferon, Brucella abortus ether extract, Salmonella typhimurium lypopolysaccharide, and polyanions. Cell Immunol. 48:52.
6. Kiessling, R., and H. Wigzell. 1979. An analysis of the murine NK cell as to structure, function, and biological relevance. Immunolog. Rev. 44:165.
7. Herberman, R.B., J.Y. Djeu, H.D. Kay, J.R. Ortaldo, C. Riccardi, G.D. Bonnard, H.T. Holden, R. Fagnani, A.

Santoni, and P. Puccetti. 1979. Natural killer cells: characteristics and regulation of activity. Immunol. Rev. 44-43.
8. Welsh, R.M. Natural killer cells and interferon. CRC Critical Reviews in Immunology. (In Press).
9. Welsh, R.M. 1978. Mouse natural killer cells: Induction, specificity, and function. J. Immunol. 121:1631.
10. Luini, W., D. Boraschi, S. Alberti, A. Aleotti, and A. Tagliabue. 1981. Morphological characterization of a cell population responsible for natural killer activity. Immunology 43:663.
11. Reynolds, C.W., T. Timonen, and R.B. Herberman. 1981. Natural killer (NK) cell activity in the rat. I. Isolation and characterization of the effector cells. J. Immunol. 127:282.
12. Timonen, J., A. Ranki, E. Saxsula, and P. Hayry. 1979. Human natural cell-mediated cytotoxicity against fetal fibroblasts. III. Morphological and functional characterization of the effector cells. Cell Immunol. 48:121.
13. Timonen, T., J.R. Ortaldo, and R.B. Herberman. 1982. Analysis by a single cell cytotoxicity assay of natural killer (NK) cell frequencies among human large granular lymphocytes and of the effects of interferon on their activity. J. Immunol. 128:2514.
14. Roder, J.C., R. Kiessling, P. Biberfold, and B. Andersson. 1978. Target-effector interactions in the natural killer (NK) cell system. II. Isolation and characterization of the effector cells. J. Immunol. 121:2509.
15. Hoffman, T., F. Hirata, P. Bougnoux, B.A. Fraser, R.H. Goldfarb, R.B. Herberman, and J. Axelrod. 1981. Phospholipid methylation and phospholipase A activation in cytotoxicity by human natural killer cells. Proc. Natl Acad. Sci. 78:3839.
16. Hudig, D., J. Haverty, C. Fulcher, D. Redelman, and J. Mendelsohn. 1981. Inhibition of human natural cytotoxicity by macromolecular antiproteases. J. Immunol. 126:1569.
17. Quan, P.C., J. Ishizaka, and B.R. Bloom. 1982. Studies on the mechanism of NK cell lysis. J. Immunol. 128:1786.
18. Roder, J.C., S. Argov, M. Klein, C. Pettersson, R. Kiessling, K. Andersson, and M. Hansson. 1980. Target-effector interaction in the natural killer cell system. V. Energy requirements, membrane integrity and the possible role of lysosomal enzymes. Immunology 40:107.

19. Roder, J.C., and T. Haliotis. 1980. A comparative analysis of the NK cytolytic mechanism and regulatory genes. In Natural Cell-Mediated Immunity Against Tumors. Edited by R.B. Herberman. Academic Press, NY, p.379.
20. Carpen, O., I. Virtanen, and E. Saksela. 1981. The cytotoxic activity of human natural killer cells requires an intact secretory apparatus. Cell. Immunol. 58:97.
21. Wright, S.C., and B. Bonavida. 1981. Selective lysis of NK-sensitive target cells by a soluble mediator released from murine spleen cells and human peripheral blood lymphocytes. J. Immunol. 126:1516.
22. Wright, S.C., and B. Bonavida. 1982. Lysis of NK targets by natural killer cytotoxic factors (NKCF): Dual effects of interferon-treatment of effector on target cells. Fed. Proc. 41:476.
23. Forbes, J.T., R.K. Bretthauer, and T.N. Oeltmann. 1981. Mannose 6-, and fructose 6-phosphates inhibit human natural cell-mediated cytotoxicity. Proc. Natl. Acad. Sci. 78:5797.
24. Silva, A., B. Bonavida, and S. Targan. 1980. Mode of action of interferon-mediated modulation of natural killer cytotoxic activity: Recruitment of pre-NK cells and enhanced kinetics of lysis. J. Immunol. 125:479.
25. Minato, N., L. Reid, H. Cantor, P. Lengyel, and B. Bloom. 1980. Mode of regulation of natural killer activity by interferon. J. Exp. Med. 152:137.
26. Bougnoux, P.F., Hirata, T., Timonen, and J. Hoffman. 1981. Effects of interferon (IFN) on phospholipid metabolism in human peripheral blood cells. Proc. 14th International Leukocyte Culture Conf.
27. Tovey, M.G., and C. Rochette-Egly. 1980. The effect of interferon on cyclic nucleotides. Ann. New York Acad. Sci. 350:266.
28. Perussia, B., and G. Trichieri. 1981. Inactivation of natural killer cell cytotoxic activity after interaction with target cells. J. Immunol. 126:754.
29. Gidlund, M., A. Orn, H. Wigzell, A. Senik, and I. Gresser. 1978. Enhanced NK activity in mice injected with interferon and interferon inducers. Nature 273:759.
30. Herberman, R.B., M.E. Nunn, H.T. Holden, S. Staaz, and J.Y. Djeu. 1977. Augmentation of natural cytotoxic reactivity of mouse lymphoid cells against syngenic and allogeneic target cells. Int. J. Cancer 19:564.
31. MacFarlan, R.I., W.H. Burns, and D.O. White. 1977. Two cytotoxic cells in peritoneal cavity of virus-infected mice: antibody-dependent macrophages and non specific killer cells. J. Immunol. 119:1566.

32. Quinnan, G.V., and J.E. Manischewitz. 1979. The role of natural killer cells and antibody-dependent cell-mediated cytotoxicity during murine cytomegalo-virus infection. J. Exp. Med. 150:1549.
33. Welsh, R.M., and R.M. Zinkernagel. 1977. Hetero-specific cytotoxic cell activity induced during the first three days of acute lymphocytic choriomeningitis virus infection in mice. Nature 268:646.
34. Wong, C.Y., J.J. Woodruff, and J.F. Woodruff. 1977. Generation of cytotoxic T lymphocytes during Coxsackie virus B-3 infection III. Role of sex. J. Immunol. 119:591.
35. Welsh, R.M. 1978. Cytotoxic cells induced during lymphocytic choriomeningitis virus infection of mice. I. Characterization of natural killer cell induction. J. Exp. Med. 148:163.
36. Kiessling, R., E. Eriksson, L.A. Hallenbeck, and R.M. Welsh. 1980. A comparative analysis of the cell surface properties of activated versus endogenous mouse natural killer cells. J. Immunol. 125:1551.
37. Herberman, R.B., M.E. Nunn, and H.T. Holden. 1978. Low density of Thy 1 antigen on mouse effector cells mediating natural cytotoxicity against tumor cells. J. Immunol. 121:304.
38. Kumar, V., M.C. Barnes, M. Bennett, and R.C. Burton. 1982. Differential expression of NK 1.2 antigen on endogenous and activated natural killer cells. J. Immunol. 128:1482.
39. Biron, C.A., and R.M. Welsh. 1982. Activation and role of natural killer cells in virus infections. Medical Microbiol. Immunol. 170:155.
40. Biron, C.A., and R.M. Welsh. 1982. Proliferation and role of natural killer cells during viral infection. Edited by R.B. Herberman. Academic Press, NY (pp493-498).
41. Biron, C.A., and R.M. Welsh. 1982. Activation and blastogenesis of natural killer cells during virus infection in vivo. J.Immunol. 129:2788
42. Welsh, R.M., and W.F. Doe. 1980. Cytotoxic cells induced during lymphocytic choriomeningitis virus infection of mice. III. Natural killer cell activity in cultured spleen leukocytes concomitant with T cell dependent immune interferon production. Infect. and Immunity 30:473.
43. Hansson, M., R. Kiessling, B. Andersson, and R.M. Welsh. 1980. Effect of interferon and interferon inducers on the NK sensitivity of normal mouse thymocytes. J. Immunol. 125:2225.

44. Moore, M., W.J. White, and M.R. Potter. 1980. Modulation of target cell susceptibility to human natural killer cells by interferon. Int. J. Cancer 25:565.
45. Trichieri, G., and D. Santoli. 1978. Anti-viral activity induced by culturing lymphocytes with tumor-derived or virus-transformed cells. Enhancement of natural killer activity by interferon and antagonistic inhibition of susceptibility of target cells to lysis. J. Exp. Med. 147:1314.
46. Welsh, R.M., and L.A. Hallenbeck. 1980. Effect of virus infections on target cell susceptibility to natural killer cell mediated lysis. J. Immunol. 124:2491.
47. Welsh, R.M., K. Karre, M. Hansson, L.A. Kunkel, and R.W. Kiessling. 1981. Interferon-mediated protection of normal and tumor target cells against lysis by mouse natural killer cells. J. Immunol. 126:219.
48. Trinchieri, G., D. Granato, and B. Perussia. 1981. Interferon-induced resistance of fibroblasts to cytolysis mediated by natural killer cells: Specificity and mechanism. J. Immunol. 126:335.
49. Yogeeswaran, G., R.M. Welsh, A. Gronberg, R. Kiessling, M. Patarroyo, G. Klein, M. Gidlund, H. Wigzell, K. Nilsson. 1982. Surface sialic acid of tumor cells correlates inversely with susceptibility to natural killer cell mediated lysis NK cells and other natural effector cells. Edited by R.B.Herberman, Academic Press, NY (pp. 765).
50. Yogeeswaran, G., A. Gronberg, M. Hansson, T. Dalianis, R. Kiessling, and R.M. Welsh. 1981. Correlation of glycophingolipids and sialic acid in YAC-1 lymphoma variants with their sensitivity to natural killer cell mediated lysis. Int. J. Cancer 28:517.
51. Gorelik, E., and R.B. Herberman. 1981. Radiosotope assay for evaluation of in vivo natural cell-mediated resistance of mice to local transplantation of tumor cells. Int. J. Cancer 27:709.
52. Riccardi, C., P. Pucetti, A. Santoni, and R.B. Herberman. 1979. Rapid in vivo assay of mouse natural killer (NK) cell activity. J. of Natl. Cancer. Inst. 63:1041.
53. Santoli, D., and H. Koprowski. 1979. Mechanisms of activation of human natural killer cells against tumor and virus-infected cells. Immunol. Rev. 44:125.
54. Anderson, M.J. 1978. Innate cytotoxicity of CBA mouse spleen cells to Sendai-virus infected L cells. Infect. Immun. 20:608.
55. Ault, K.A., and H.L. Weiner. 1979. Natural killing of measles-infected cells by human lymphocytes. J. Immunol. 122:2611.

56. Blazer, B., M. Patarroyo, E. Klein, and G. Klein. 1980. Increased sensitivity of human lymphoid lines to natural killer cells after induction of the Epstein-Barr viral cycle by super-infection or sodium butyrate. J. Exp. Med. 151:614.
57. Casali, P., and M.B.A. Oldstone. Killing of measles virus infected cells by human lymphocytes: failure to demonstrate any role for extracellular interferon or specific antibody in vitro. (Submitted).
58. Ching, C., and C. Lopez. 1979. Natural killing of Herpes virus type-1 infected target cells: normal human responses and influence of antiviral antibody. Infect. Immunol. 26:48.
59. Harfast, B., J. Anderson, and P. Perlmann. 1978. Immunoglobulin-independent natural cytotoxicity of Fc receptor-bearing human blood lymphocytes to mumps virus-infected target cells. J. Immunol. 121:755.
60. Haspel, M., K.V. Holmes, and R.M. Welsh. 1981. Natural cell-mediated cytotoxicity against mouse hepatitis virus (MHV) infected cells. Abstracts of the Amer. Soc. for Microbiol.
61. Lee, G.D., and R. Keller. 1982. Natural cytotoxicity to murine cytomegalovirus-infected cells mediated by mouse lymphoid cells: role of interferon in the endogenous natural cytotoxicity reaction. Infection and Immunity 35:5.
62. Santoli, D., G. Trinchieri, and H. Koprowski. 1978. Cell-mediated cytotoxicity against virus-infected target cells in humans. II. Interferon induction and activation of natural killer cells. J. Immunol. 121:532.
63. Santoli, D., G. Trinchieri, and F.S. Lief. 1978. Cell-mediated cytotoxicity against virus-infected target cells in humans. I. Characterization of the effector lymphocyte. J. Immunol. 121:526.
64. Kunkel, L.A., and R.M. Welsh. 1981. Metabolic inhibitors render "resistant" target cells sensitive to natural killer cell mediated lysis. Int. J. Cancer 27:73.
65. Casali, P., J.G.P. Sissons, M.J. Buchmeier, and M.B.A. Oldstone. 1981. In vitro generation of human cytotoxic lymphocytes by virus. Viral glycoproteins induce non specific cell mediated cytotoxicity without release of interferon. J. Exp. Med. 154:840.
66. Harfast, B., C. Orvelc, A. Alsheikhzy, T. Andersson, P. Perlmann, and E. Norrby. 1980. The role of viral glycoproteins in mumps virus-dependent lymphocyte mediated cytotoxicity in vitro. Scand. J. Immunol. 11:391.

67. Kuribayashi, K., S. Gillis, D.E. Kern, and C.S. Henney. 1981. Murine NK cell cultures: Effects of interleukin-2 and interferon on cell growth and cytotoxic reactivity. J. Immunol. 126:2321.
68. Karre, K., G.O. Klein, R. Kiessling, G. Klein, and J.C. Roder. 1980. Low natural in vivo resistance to syngeneic leukemias in natural killer-deficient mice. Nature 284:624.
69. Talmadge, J.E., K.M. Meyers, D.J. Prieur, and J.R. Starkey. 1980. Role of natural killer cells in tumor growth and metastasis: Normal and beige mice. J. Natl. Cancer Inst. 65:929.
70. Habu, S., H. Fukui, K. Shimamtura, M. Kasai, Y. Nagai, K. Okumura, and N. Tamaoki. 1981. In vivo effects of anti-asialo GM_1. Reduction of NK activity and enhancement of transplanted tumor growth in nude mice. J. Immunol. 127:34.
71. Welsh, R.M., and R.W. Kiessling. 1980. Natural killer cell response to lymphocytic choriomeningitis virus in beige mice. Scand. J. Immunol. 11:363.
72. Kiessling, R., P.S. Hochman, O. Haller, G.M. Shearer, H. Wigzell, and G. Cudkowicz. 1977. Evidence for a similar or common mechanism for natural killer cell activity and resistance to hemopoietic grafts. Eur. J. Immunol. 7:655.
73. Lopez, C. 1975. Genetics of natural resistance to Herpes virus infections in mice. Nature 258:152.
74. Lopez, C., and M. Bennett. 1978. Genetic resistance to HSV-1 in the mouse is mediated by a marrow (M)-dependent cell. Fourth International Congress for Virology, p.82.
75. Bancroft, G.J., G.R. Shellam, and J.E. Chalmer. 1981. Genetic influences on the augmentation of natural killer (NK) cells during murine cytomegalovirus infection: correlation with patterns of resistance. J. Immunol. 126:988.
76. Shellam, G.R., J.E. Allan, J.M. Papiditrio, and G.J. Bancroft. 1981. Increased susceptibility to cytomegalovirus infection in beige mutant mice. Proc. Nat. Acad. Sci. (USA) 78:5104.
77. Ojo, E., and H. Wigzell. 1978. Natural killer cells may be the only cells in normal mouse lymphoid populations endowed with cytolytic ability for antibody-coated tumour target cells. Scand. J. Immunol. 7:297.

CHAPTER 3

INTERFERONS: THEIR ROLE IN NATURAL RESISTANCE TO VIRUS INFECTIONS

Anthony Meager

Division of Viral Products
National Institute for Biological Standards and Control
Holly Hill, Hampstead
London NW3, England

INTRODUCTION

Interferon (IFN) was discovered by Isaacs and Lindenmann (1) in 1957, but it has taken the 25 years since then to inravel the complexity of the interferon system and to partially evaluate its clinical potential. The main stumbling block to the understanding of the IFN system has been, until recently, the very small quantities of IFN that could be obtained from stimulated human cells which were insufficient for molecular studies. It was however recognised from physicochemical and antigenic properties of IFN that there must exist more than one type of IFN (2). Three different types of human IFN have been described and were originally named Leukocyte, Fibroblast and Immune IFN to indicate the source of cells producing each individual type. In 1978 a nomenclature committee (3) changed the designation of these three interferon types to α (Leukocyte), β (fibroblast) and γ (immune) (Table 1). These are abbreviated HuIFNα, HuIFNβ and HuIFNγ and these terms will be used throughout this review. Similarly the mouse IFNs are abbreviated MuIFNγ, β and γ.

All HuIFNs so far identified are inducible, secreted proteins or glycoproteins with monomeric molecular weights of about 20,000 (48,165) and sharing the common property of eliciting an antiviral state in homologous cells to which they come into contact. They are extremely potent; only a few nanograms of IFN are required to trigger the antiviral state (2). The biological activity of IFNs has thus been most conveniently estimated in terms of the antiviral activity in in vitro virus-cell bioassay systems. Hence, the

ISBN 0-12-239980-3

unit of IFN antiviral activity has been arbitrarily defined as the reciprocal of the dilution of an IFN preparation which inhibits virus growth by fifty per cent. Many different virus-cell bioassays have been designed, but it is possible to compare results from different laboratories by the use of WHO international reference preparations of IFNs. The specific activities of pure HuIFNγ and HuIFNβ have been estimated to be in the range of 10^8 - 10^9 International Units (IU)/mg protein on this basis (2).

CELL SOURCES OF NATURAL IFNs

The major producer cell types and the main stimuli for the three different types of IFN are given in Table 1. However, this is a simplified view of IFN induction and production since most cell types will respond to inducers by producing a mixture of IFNs.

TABLE 1. Different Types of Human Interferon

Interferon Type	Old Name	Stimulus for Production	Major Producer Cells
Alpha (α)	Leucocyte	Viruses, Bacteria, Xenogeneic or allogeneic tumor cells Virus Infected Cells, B-cell mitogens	Null lymphocytes B Lymphocytes Macrophages
Beta (β)	Fibroblast	Viruses, Polynucleotides	Fibroblasts Epithelial cells
Gamma (γ)	Immune	Allogeneic cells or virus infected syngeneic cells Foreign antigens, T cell mitogens	T lymphocytes

For example, Newcastle disease virus (NDV) induced human fibroblasts will produce HuIFNβ as the major IFN type but also will produce a small amount of HuIFNγ (4). Cells of the lymphoid system can produce IFNα, β or γ depending on the inducing circumstances (5). For example, IFNα is the major type produced by virus infected null cells and macrophages (6,7), by B lymphocytes in response to xenogeneic or allogeneic tumour cells (8) and by natural killer (NK) cells in contact with their tumor or virus infected targets (9-12). On the other hand, T-lymphocytes produce primarily IFNγ in response to allogeneic or virus-infected cells (13-16). It is probable that more than one subset of T-lymphocytes including T-gamma cells produce IFNγ (5,17,18,104) and that macrophage/monocyte involvement is required for induction (19,20) whilst T-suppressor lymphocytes regulate the amount of IFNγ production (21). Macrophages and monocytes produce interleukin 1 (IL-1), a lymphokine necessary for the T-cell production of interleukin 2 (IL-2) which in turn has been postulated to be required for IFNγ synthesis (22-24,99). Such requirements for IFNγ production do not apparently appertain to the recent demonstrations of the release of IFNγ from a human T cell line (25) and a number of murine T-cell clones (26) after T-cell mitogen induction. These cells however lacked any functional T cell characteristics. Much more conclusive evidence for the T-cell nature of the IFNγ producing cell has been provided by the recent findings that clones of murine antigen-specific, H-2 restricted cytotoxic T-lymphocytes (CTL), which are dependent on 1L-2 for growth, release IFNγ on co-culture with influenza infected, matched target cells (27) or with allogeneic cells presenting antigen (28). Finally, Hooks et al (29) have demonstrated that T cells with Fc receptors for IgG (Tg) from a patient with a proliferative disorder of these cells spontaneously produced IFNγ when cultured in vitro. Thus at present the IFNγ producing cells appear to be restricted to the T-cell lineage, although it is possible that in future other cell types may be shown to produce it. IFNγ may therefore be regarded as immune specific, and its production in vitro from peripheral blood lymphocytes may reflect the degree of T-cell sensiti zation to any particular antigen and thus act as a barometer of cell mediated immunity (30).

BIOCHEMISTRY OF DIFFERENT INTERFERON TYPES AND SUBTYPES

The recent upsurge in interest in IFN has led to the rapid and successful cloning of several different IFNmRNAs from stimulated human cells. Sequencing studies of the DNA copies inserted into bacterial plasmids has given predicted amino acid sequences for the individual HuIFN types which agree with the partial amino acid sequences worked out for

HuIFNγ and β with small amounts of these proteins purified to homogeneity (31-34). These studies have put the antigenic differences previously noted for HuIFNγ and β and γ (2) on a firm molecular basis.

A major discovery from the IFNmRNA cloning work was the existence of substantial molecular heterogeneity within the HuIFNγ type. There are at least eight and probably as many as fourteen HuIFNγ subtypes (35-38). From their cDNA sequences they have been predicted to contain 165 - 166 amino acids (a signal polypeptide of 23 amino acids precedes the amino acid sequence of the HuIFNγ protein), are probably non-glycosylated, and have molecular weights of approximately 19,500. All the HuIFNγ subtypes share a high degree (~80%) of amino acid sequence homology (36,38). For example, there are only 28 (17%) amino acid differences between the $\gamma 1(d)$ and $\gamma 2(A)$ subtypes. Both these subtypes have been expressed in bacteria and the products shown to be biologically active (35,39,40).

HuIFNβ, of which only one subtype β_1 has been cloned and fully characterised (41 for refs), shows only 29% homology with HuIFN γ at the amino acid sequence level (42), ie 118 (71%) differences out of 166 amino acids. However, the γ and β subtypes are clearly related and appear to have diverged from a common ancestral gene (42), HuIFN β_1 is, unlike the γ subtypes, a glycoprotein, the glycosylation occurring at ASN p 80, and has a molecular weight of 21-23000 (41). A recent report by Skup et al (43) indicates that there are two MuIFNβ subtypes, and studies on the HuIFNβ mRNA (44) are suggestive that more than one human β subtype exists.

HuIFNγ has been shown to be a smaller protein than either HuIFNα or β. It contains only 146 amino acids and has a calculated molecular weight of 17,110 (45,46) without taking into account probable glycosylation at ASN p28 and ASN p100. Epstein (47) noted a definitive pattern of single amino acid homology if the amino acid sequences of IFNα and $IFN\gamma_2$ were compared although at first glance little homology was apparent between IFNα and IFNγ or β. However, greater homology than suggested by Epstein (47) ie 12% can be demonstrated if the amino acid sequence of IFNα is compared to that of $IFN\gamma_1$ if certain sequence deletions are allowed. In this case there could be up to 29 positions (20% homology) of identical amino acids or most conservative replacements (ASP for ASN; ILE for LEU, etc) if the GLU-GLU p 40-41 for both γ and γ_1 are included. There is less homology with HuIFNβ, but there are 14 positions in the sequences of γ_1, γ_2, β and γ where there are identical or similar amino acids, suggesting conservation at these positions may be important for biological function (s). For example one interesting structural similarity occurs at p 137-140 in the γ subtypes, p 139 - 142 in β and p 124-127 in γ. Purified HuIFNγ prepared from mitogen induced peripheral blood lymphocytes shows some heterogeneity when separated on polycrylamide gels (48) suggesting the possibility of multiple subtypes. On the other hand this could be due to differences in the degree oif glycosylation of HuIFNγ. No evidence has yet been found for heterogeneity in the mRNA coding for HuIFNγ (49-51,58) or MuIFNγ (52).

The cellular genes for HuIFNγ subtypes and HuIFNγ have been shown to be located on chromosome 9 (53-55) and are unusual in that they contain no introns (35,36,38,41). The gene for HuIFNγ does however contain introns (45,46) suggesting that it has a different ancestral origin to the common ancestral gene from which the present day HuIFNγ and β genes have evolved.

TABLE 2. Biological Activities of Human Interferons

1. Antiviral effects
2. Effects on cell mediated immunity
   (a) enhancement of cytotoxicity of macrophages and lymphocytes
   (b) enhancement of histocompatibility antigen expression
   (c) inhibition of suppressor T-cell activity
   (d) enhancement of lymphocyte migration
3. Effects on antibody production by B-lymphocytes
4. Enhancement (priming) of subsequent interferon production
5. Inhibition of tumor cell growth
6. Pyrogenic effect in vivo

BIOLOGICAL ACTIVITIES OF HUMAN INTERFERONS

Interferons display diverse biological actions (Table 2) the range of which is astonishing (see refs 2,5,56,57). All three types of HuIFN (α,β and γ) appear to have many of the biological actions listed (Table 2) in common, and this is surprising in view of the now known primary structure differences. However, the conservation of single amino acids in precise sequence order observed among the three types of IFN may point to some degree of tertiary structure similarities which underly the common biological activities of IFNs. The effectiveness (potency) of each IFN type and subtype then remains to be answered, and this almost certainly relates to (i) the target-cell specificity of each individual interferon molecule, (ii) the binding affinity of different IFNs to cell surface receptors, and (iii) the antiviral mechanisms induced.

Expression of human IFN genes in E. coli has been achieved for a number of HuIFNα subtypes (35,39,40,40), HuIFNβ_1 (41, 60-62) and HuIFNγ (45). The HuIFNs produced by E. coli have been shown to have antiviral action which is similar to the respective HuIFNs produced by human cells, despite the lack of glycosylation of HuIFN β_1 and γ by E. coli. Some of the bacterially produced HuFINα subtypes have also since been shown to enhance antibody dependent cell-mediated cytotoxicity (ADCC), to enhance natural killer (NK) activity of lymphocytes, to enhance monocyte-mediated cytotoxic activities, to inhibit the growth of tumour cells and to suppress antigen and mitogen induced inhibition of leukocyte migration (63-66). Moreover, these studies and recent ones carried out with HuIFNs produced by human cells (67,68) have used essentially homogeneous, pure IFN types and subtypes and clearly demonstrate that the biological actions are associated with the IFN molecule and are not due to impurities.

Whilst no unique biological action has been yet attributed to any of the different HuIFN types, clear differences in host cell range have been demonstrated (2). The HuIFNα type (normally a mixture of α subtypes) exhibits a far greater degree of heterologous activity than either HuIFNβ or γ. (2) For example, HuIFNα will protect bovine and feline cells against virus challenge, whereas the β and γ types are much less effective (2). With the advent of bacterially produced HuIFNα subtypes, it has also been possible to show that the individual subtypes exhibit different target-cell specificities (35,59,69) and that the products of hybrid interferon genes (α_1 - α_2 recominants) have different specificities again from their parental subtypes (70,71). It has also been found that the different α subtypes elicit different degrees of antiviral resistance against several viruses (69,71,91) suggesting the interaction of IFNs with host target cells is complex.

All IFNs interact with host cell surface receptors to trigger the antiviral state. For HuIFNα β and γ, these receptors are the products of genes located on chromosome 21 (5 for refs) and it has been reproducibly found that human fibroblasts which are trisomic for chromosome 21 (Downs syndrome) are more sensitive to HuIFNs. However, whilst the receptors for IFNα and β are probably the same, there is growing evidence that those for IFNα are different from the α/β receptors (72,73). Following interaction with HuIFNα or β, human lymphocytes (74) or fibroblasts (75) synthesize 8 or 10 new polypeptides respectively. A similar pattern of induced polypeptides has also been observed in fibroblasts following IFNγ treatment (76) despite receptor differences and probable different induction pathway (88). However, qualitative and quantitative differences in the polypeptides induced by HuIFNα/β on the one hand and HuIFNγ on the other have been observed (77) and some donor lymphocytes are refractory to a purified IFNα subtype in this respect (74). These differences suggest the individual HuIFNs activate differing antiviral mechanisms which may account for the empirically observed variable degrees of antiviral resistance to different viruses (69,71,77,91) and offers a possible explanation for the heterogeneity of the HuIFNα type; a single component of the usual mixture may exhibit a limited range of donor or cell-type specificities. They may also account for the potentiation effects found for antiviral activity when cells are simultaneously treated with IFNα/β and IFNγ (78) and the differential potencies of IFNα/β compared to IFNγ observed for the non-antiviral actions of IFNs (see 76 for refs). It must be stressed that the HuIFNγ preparations used in all studies to date have been only partially purified from lymphokine-rich culture fluids, and that any differences in the biological actions of IFN α/β and IFNγ can only unequivocally be proven when homogeneous, pure IFNγ is available.

Besides the induction of specific polypeptides by interferon, a number of enzymatic activities have also been shown to be induced. Principle among these are (2'p5'A)n synthetase, an endoribonuclease and a protein kinase (see 56 for Review). Although all three IFN types induce these enzymes (79,80) it is as yet uncertain whether the antiviral effects observed can be attributed to these enzymatic activities alone (81-80) it is as yet uncertain whether the antiviral effects observed can be attributed to these enzymatic activities alone (81-85,91,92) or whether other mechanisms inhibit virus replication (eg 86,87). Again some quantitative differences have been observed in the levels of (2'p5'A)n synthetase induced by IFN α/β and impure IFNγ preparations (77) and its appearance is relatively late when induced by IFNγ compared to IFN α/β induction (88). No correlation between the induction of (2'p5'A)n synthetase by IFN α, β or γ and their ability to inhibit the growth of certain cell lines has been shown (89,90).

In addition to the above effects, IFNs also initiate complex changes in the plasma membranes of cells (93). These changes often parallel the decreased proliferative activity of cells treated with IFN (2). Tamm and co-workers (94) have suggested that coordinate changes in the plasma membrane leading to its increased rigidity involve increases in abundance of underlying actin-containing microfilaments. Such plasma membrane changes would be expected to influence virus budding or maturation and cell-cell recognition events involved in the immune response (93). More importantly however, it has been found that IFN treatment increases the amount of histocompatibility antigens (HLA-A, B, C. and β_2 microglobulin) expressed at the cell surface (95,96). These increases in histocompatibility antigen expression are directly related to an IFN induced increase in HLAmRNA level (97) which is comparable in its kinetics and dose-response to the induction of (2'p5'A)n synthetase mRNA by IFNs, and as such correlates better with the antiviral function of interferon than its antiproliferative action (98). Increased HLA expression in the cells of a virally infected host probably aids the elimination of HLA-matched infected cells by cytotoxic lymphocytes.

Cell-mediated lysis is a major arm of the host defense against viral infection. Three kinds of cytolytic effectors play a role at one point or another in thus protecting the host: natural killer (NK) cells, cells active in antibody (Ab) dependent cell-mediated cytotoxicity (ADCC) and cytotoxic T lymphocytes. Macrophages may also be included in this category of cytotoxic cells. IFNs have been shown to enhance NK activity (9), ADCC (100), to activate macrophages (101) and to increase CTLs possibly by inhibiting the generation of suppressor T-lymphocytes (102). (Many of these aspects of cell-mediated immunity are more adequately reviewed by other authors in this volume). NK activity and ADCC are possibly mediated by a common subset of lymphocytes, but there is considerable heterogeneity within the NK, ADCC and CTL populations with respect to cell surface phenotype (103). Recent findings (105,106) also indicate that besides IFN, interleukin 2 (IL2) and possibly other lymphokines play a role in augmenting the activity of cytotoxic lymphocytes.

IFN has also been shown to suppress leukocyte migration inhibition, to enhance or suppress antibody formation and to inhibit the development of delayed type hypersensitivity (DTH) reactions (see 107,108 for refs) further illustrating the complexity and diversity of immune reactions apparently triggered by IFN. It is as yet unclear whether IFN is directly responsible for these changes in immune function or whether such changes reflect adjustments made within the immune system as a consequence of IFNs direct action elsewhere. For example, Harfast et al (109) have reported that IFN acted directly on human B lymphocytes to modulate immunoglobulin synthesis, but did not rule out the possibility that IFN caused this indirectly by inhibiting the action of suppressor cells.

Cells pre-treated with interferon, and thus in the antiviral state, respond to IFN inducers by producing increased amounts of IFNα/β compared to untreated cells (2) and this phenomenon is called "priming." Such priming could occur in vivo and lead to amplification of the biological actions of IFNs. In an analogous fashion, sensitization of host lymphocytes by vaccination or injection of foreign antigens leads to enhanced levels of IFNγ being produced on secondary stimulation in vitro (15,28,110). Unfractionated lymphocytes from sensitized individuals or mice produce both IFNα and IFNγ when rechallenged with a virus (15,111,112) and this combination may lead to a potentiation of antiviral action (78).

Finally HuIFNα has demonstrable pyrogeneity in vivo (113) and elevation of body temperative may inhibit virus replication.

Therefore, in theory, the interferon system could play a crucial role in host resistance to and recovery from virus infections. The sequence of events following a hypothetical virus infection in vivo may be as follows:

(i) localised production of IFN α/β and immediate protection of surrounding cells through the induction of antiviral mechanisms eg indicated by (2'p5'A)n synthetase and endonuclease activities (114). Concommitantly priming of IFN production and enhanced expression of histocompatibility antigens would also occur in these cells.

(ii) systemic spread of IFN via the blood to simultaneously induce the antiviral state in lymphocytes and macrophages (115) and activate cytotoxic lymphocytes and macrophages.

(iii) further production of IFNα and IFNγ by cytotoxic cells on contact with virus infected target cells and amplification or re-inforcement of antiviral action.

Individuals previously exposed to the virus or recently vaccinated against the virus could be expected to resist the virus infection more strongly because of increased production of IFNs from primed or sensitized lymphocytes, the presence of greater numbers of specific CTL, and the possibility of ADCC.

ROLE OF INTERFERONS IN HOST RESISTANCE TO VIRAL INFECTIONS

Despite this barrage of defense mechanisms triggered by IFNs, and despite more than twenty years of intensive experimentation, the evidence for a role of IFN in the resolution of acute viral infection is predominantly inferential. However, there is growing evidence derived largely from clinical trials in which purified IFN has been used therapeutically against a number of viral infections that IFN can be of some benefit, and hence suggesting IFN is required by the host to mount an effective immune response to infection.

There are several indications that IFN is important to the

host to counter viral infections. Firstly, no IFN is detected in the sera of healthy individuals, but is nearly always found in the sera of patients with acute viral disease. Levin and Hahn (115) have also demonstrated the peripheral blood mononuclear cells (PBMC) to be in the antiviral state when derived from patients showing clinical symptoms of viral infections. In the case of persistent infections the PBMC can often be shown to be spontaneously releasing IFN when cultured in vitro (115). If the illness is very severe, the IFN system can sometimes be demonstrated to be deficient by stimulating PBMCs for IFN production; low yields of IFN are derived compared to healthy controls.

Some children are peculiarly susceptible to rhinovirus (common cold) infections and Isaacs et al (116) have shown the IFN production system to be deficient in this group. IFNα is present in the amniotic fluid of pregnant women from the 16th week until the end of pregnancy (117) and it probably protects the embryo from virus infection. It is noteworthy that the first trimester, when no IFN is present, represents the period when the foetus is most susceptible to viral infection eg. by rubella. IFN is produced before any humoral response and often coincides with the period of virus shedding eg influenza A infections (131) and is associated with an increased NK cell activity (118).

Patients undergoing immunosuppressive therapy following organ transplants or cancer patients who become immunosuppressed following the administration of chemotoxic drugs are very susceptible to external virus infections, eg. measles, and internal virus reactivations eg cytomegalovirus (CMV) and herpes zoster. In immunosuppressed patients with progressive herpes zoster no IFN was found in the sores/vesicles, but resolution of the lesions was accompanied by IFN in the vesicle fluid (119). However, in herpes labialis the vesicles contain large amounts of IFN from an early stage of infection, and the amount increases with the age of the vesicle in parallel to the growth of the virus (herpes simplex virus - HSV) (120). There was no apparent correlation between IFN titre and the severity of the disease.

Respiratory syncytial virus (RSV) which is the most common cause of lower respiratory tract disease in infants and young children (121,122) and which probably is an important cause of respiratory illness in adults (123,124) poses an interesting case regarding the role of IFN in the resolution of acute infection. Re-infection by RSV is common in spite of the presence of virus-specific antibody (125) and attempts to prevent the infection by vaccination have been unsuccessful (126,127). Data from clinical studies indicate that most children infected with RSV had no IFN in their sera and nasal washings (128-130) in contrast to the situation in influenza A infections (131), and Chonmaitree et al (132) have shown that RSV is a relatively poor inducer of IFN in isolated PBMC. Thus, the resistance and recovery mechanisms for RSV infection remain unclear, but it is suggested that the poor IFN inducing ability of RSV is the reason for the lack of adequate cell-mediated immunity. As such, and because RSV has been shown to be sensitive to IFN in vitro (133-136), RSV infection may be a prime candidate for IFN therapy. As an interesting footnote, lifelong recurrent RSV infections may lead to persistent low level RSV genome expression (137) and whilst RSV is not known to become a generalised virus infection, there is one report (138) which demonstrates the presence of RSV antigens in the abnormal bone osteoclasts from each of twelve Paget disease patients: Paget disease is a slowly progressive, painful, deformity-inducing disease of bone that afflicts as many as 3 percent of adults worldwide.

Viruses do not become resistant to interferon as such, but some appear to have evolved almost diabolical ways of avoiding interferon-mediated host defense mechanisms. One example is rabies virus. Rabies virus is a known inducer of IFN in vitro (see 2 for refs), but its replication at the bite wound and later as it spreads towards the brain is so low that too little IFN is produced for the progrss of the disease to be halted. And yet it has been convincingly demonstrated that IFN administered to rabies infected animals before the appearance of clinical symptoms has a protective effect (eg. 139) and thus is a clear indication that IFN is important for the prevention of this disease.

In animals, in particular in mice, a role for IFN in resistance to viral disease is more readily demonstrable. For example, treatment of mice with anti-mouse IFN antibody markedly enhances susceptibility to a number of virus infections (140). Mice that are genetically susceptible to HSV infection produce very low levels of IFN on HSV challenge, whereas genetically resistant mice produce high levels of serum IFN (141). However, in contrast A/J mice which are genetically resistant to mouse hepatitis virus type 3 (MHV3) produce comparatively little IFN and have only low NK cell activity when contrasted to the susceptible C57 BL/6 strain suggesting that IFN and NK cell activity are less important in the defense of mice against MHV3 (142).

Based on the evidence presented, viruses may be grouped into three categories: (i) viruses which induce IFN and for which IFN probably plays a role in the natural resistance to infection eg influenza virus, herpes zoster; (ii) viruses that induce IFN and for which IFN is apparently less important in the natural resistance to infection, eg. HSV-herpes labialis in man, MHV3 in mice; (iii) viruses which induce IFN poorly, but for which IFN could be a prime determinant in the prevention of establishment of the infection eg RSV, rabies virus, adenovirus. However, it is uncertain that such categorization is relevant in deciding which virus infections will respond best to exogenous IFN therapy because of the large number of biological variables encountered eg clinical status of patients, and the relative inexperience in the administration of this new and powerfully bioilogically active group of proteins. For instance, it is often not known when to commence treatment, what dose of IFN is required, what type of IFN is required, by what route it should be administered, and how long treatment should be maintained. Despite these problems, some beneficial prophylactic and therapeutic treatments of virus infections have already been effected with IFN, thus lending more support for a role of IFN in the mediation of many such diseases.

Used topically on the eye, IFN $\alpha_{(Le)}$ and IFNβ produce beneficial results in acute herpes simplex keratitis (143) and adenovirus keratitis (144). Intralesional injection of IFN α/β into warts caused by papilloma viruses has been shown to give a small but significant suppressive effect on the size of the warts (145,146).

An early study (147) suggested that large doses of impure IFN $\alpha_{(Le)}$ administered intranasally could lead to the amelioration of the symptoms of rhinovirus infections in volunteers. In more recent investigations Scotland and co-workers and co-workers (148,149) have found that very high doses of purified IFN $\alpha_{(le)}$ and IFN $_{\alpha\text{-}2}$ from E. coli administered intranasally and used prophylactically could prevent rhinovirus colds.

IFN has been extensively used to treat patients with herpes virus infections by intramuscular or intravenous injections of repeated doses of IFN $\alpha_{(le)}$ (1-10X10^6 Iu/dose). For instance, Merigan and coworkers (150,151) have conducted trials, to examine the efficacy of IFNα, with immunosuppressed cancer patients suffering from herpes zoster. Beneficial results have been obtained which appeared to coincide with increased levels of cell-mediated and humoral responses in these patients. Merigan (152) also reports some benefits of IFNα treatment of chickenpox in leukaemic children.

Cheeseman et al (153,154) have used IFNα to prophylactically treat renal transplant patients in order to prevent herpes virus reactivation; HSV, cytomegalovirus (CMV) and Epstein-Barr virus (EBV) reactivations were significantly inhibited, but not completely prevented. In these patients it was possible that the use of anti-lymphocyte globulin antagonised the effects of IFN. Reactivation occurred with normal frequency when IFN treatment was terminated.

IFNα appears to have little effect on herpes labialis recurrences (155), although in patients undergoing trigeminal ganglia surgery for the treatment of tic douloureux showed diminished frequency and severity of herpes labialis lesions in an IFN treated group compared to a group given a placebo (156).

Chronic hepatitis B infections have also been treated with IFNα both alone (157) and in combination with adenine arabinoside (158). In placebo controlled double-blind trials, the combination therapy has proved more effective than either the use of IFNα or adenine arabinoside by themselves (158).

Many other virus infections eg. measles in immunosuppressed patients, are now being treated with IFN as the supply position improves. However, there are problems in the use of IFNs, for example endogenous anti-IFN immunoglobulins have been found in some patients receiving IFNα or β (159,160) and in high dosage IFNs are not without side-effects (113). It has also been reported (161) that natural HuIFN subtypes may differ from those α subtypes synthesized in response to cloned IFN genes in bacteria in that the former have 10 amino acids removed from the C-terminal end when compared to the predicted amino acid sequence from the cloned gene. This difference may account for the increased immunogeneity of recombinant $HuIFN_{\alpha A}$ (159) as compared to natural $HuIFN\alpha_{(Le)}$ (162).

Virtually nothing is known about the potential of HuIFNγ for the amelioration or abrogation of the symptoms of virus infections. Although IFNγ is produced by mixed lymphocyte cultures and cytotoxic T cells on contact with virus infected targets in vitro, it is not detected in the serum following virus infections: it has only been routinely detected in the sera of patients with autoimmune disease (163,164). The precise in vivo role of IFNγ therefore remains vague, and efforts to resolve this question will depend on the results of future clinical trials using purified HuIFNγ. The overall picture remains one of guarded optimism although it will probably take several years to fully evaluate the clinical potential of IFNs.

REFERENCES

1. Isaacs, A. and Lindenmann, J. 1957. Virus interference: I. The interferon. Proc. Royal Soc. B. 147,258.
2. Stewart, W.E. II 1979. The Interferon System (Springer-Verlag, New York).
3. Stewart, W.E. II, Blalock, J.E., Burke, D.C., Chany, C., Dunnick, J.K., Falcoff, E., Friedman, R.M., Galasso, G.J., Joklik, W.K., Vilcek, J., Youngner, J.S. and Zoon, K.C. 1980. Interferon nomenclature. Nature, London 286,110.

4. Havell, E.A. Hayes, T.G. and Vilcek, J. 1978. Synthesis of two distinct interferons by human fibroblasts. Virology 89,330.
5. Epstein, L.B. 1981. Interferon-gamma, Is it really different from the other interferonsμ In "Interferon 3" pp 13-44 (Ed. I. Gresser) Academic Press, New York.
6. Peter, H.H., Dallugge, H., Zawatsky, R., Euler, S., Leibold, W. and Kirchner, H. 1980. Human peripheral null lymphocytes II Producers of type-1 interferon upon stimulation with tumor cells, Herpes simplex virus and corynebacterium parvum. Eur. J. Immunol. 10, 547.
7. Roberts, N.J., Jr., Douglas, R.G., Simons, R.M. and Diamond, M.E. 1979. Virus induced interferon production by human macrophages. J. Immunol. 123,365.
8. Weigent, D.A., Langford, M.P., Smith, E.M., Blalock, J.E., and Stanton, G.J. 1981. Human B lymphocytes produce leukocyte interferon after interaction with foreign cells. Infect. Immun. 32,508.
9. Saksela, E., 1981. Interferon and natural killer cells. In "Interferon 3" pp 43-63 (Ed I Gresser) Academic Press, N York).
10. Timonen, T., Saksela, E., Virtanen, I. and Cantell, K. 1980. Natural killer cells are responsible for the interferon production induced in human lymphocytes by tumour cell contact. Eur. J. Immunol. 10,422.
11. Trinchieri, G., Perussia, B., and Santoli, D. 1980. In Natural Cell Mediated Immunity Against Tumours (ed R Herberman) pp 655-670. Academic Press, New York.
12. Djeu, J., Timonen, T. and Herberman, R.B. 1981. Abstract-14th International Leucocyte Culture Conference Heide lberg Immunobiology 159,85.
13. Ito, F., Aoki, H., Kimura, T., Takano, M., Maeno, K. and Shimokata, K. 1980. Enumeration of immune interferon-producing cells induced by allogeneic stimulation. Infect. Immun. 28, 542.
14. Perussia, B., Mangoni, L., Engers, H.D. and Trinchieri, G. 1980. Interferon production by human and murine lymphocytes in response to alloantigens. J. Immunol. 125, 1589.
15. Ennis, F.A., and Meager, A. 1981. Immune interferon produced to high levels by antigenic stimulation of human lymphocytes with influenza virus. J. Exp. 154, 1279.
16. Green, J.A., Cooperband, S.R. and Kibrick, S. 1969. Immune specific induction of interferon production in cultures of human blood lymphocytes. Science 164, 1415.
17. Chang, T-W., Testa, D., Kung, P.C. Perry, L. Dreskin, H.J. and Goldstein, G. 1982. Cellular origin and interactions involved in γ-interferon production induced by OKT3 monoclonal antibody. J. Immunol. 128, 585.

18. Landolfo, S., Kirchner, H. and Simon, M.M. 1982. Production of immune interferon is regulated by more than one T cell subset: Lyt-1,2,3 and Qat-5 phenotypes of murine T lymphocytes involved in IFNγ production in primary and secondary mixed lymphocyte reaction. Eur. J. Immunol. 12,295.
19. Epstein, L.B. 1976. The ability of macrophages to augment in vitro mitogen-and antigen-stimulated production of interferon and other mediators of cellular immunity by lymphocytes p 201-234. In D.S.Nelson (ed). The immunobiology of the macrophage. Academic Press, Inc., New York.
20. Arbeit, R.D., Leary, P.L. and Levin, M.J. 1982. Gamma interferon production by combinations of human peripheral blood lymphocytes, monocytes and cultured macrophages. Infect. Immun. 35,383.
21. Torres, B.A., Yamamoto, J.K. and Johnson, H.M. 1982. Cellular regulation of gamma interferon production: Lyte phenotype of the suppressor cell. Infect. Immun. 35, 770.
22. Farrar, W.L., Johnson, H.M. and Farrar, J.J. 1981. Regulation of the production of immune interferon and cytotoxic T lymphocytes by interleukin 2. J. Immunol. 126,1120.
23. Yamamoto, J.K., Farrar, W.L., Johnson, H.M. 1982. Interleukin 2 regulation of mitogen induction of immune interferon (IFNγ) in spleen cells and thymocytes. Cell Immunol. 66,333.
24. Johnson, H.M. and Torres, B.A. 1982. Phorbol ester replacement of helper cell and interleukin 2 requirements in gamma interferon production. Infect. Immun. 36,911.
25. Nathan, J., Groopman, J.E., Quan, S.G., Bersch, N. and Golde, D.W. 1981. Immune (γ) interferon produced by a human T-lymphoblast cell line. Nature (Lond) 292,842.
26. Marcucci, F., Waller, M., Kirschner, H. and Krammer, P. 1981. Production of immune interferon by murine T-cell clones from longterm cultures. Nature (Lond) 291,79.
27. Morris, A.G., Lin, Y-L, Askonas, B.A. 1982. Immune interferon release when a cloned cytotoxic T cell line meets its correct influenza-infected target cell. Nature (Lond) 295,150.
28. Klein, J.R., Raulet, D.H., Pasternak, M.S. and Bevan, M.J. 1982. Cytotoxic T lymphocytes produce immune interferon in response to antigen or mitogen. J. Exp. Med. 155,1198.
29. Hooks, J.J., Haynes, B.F., Detrick-Hooks, B., Diehl, L.F., Gerrard, T.L. and Fauci, A.S. 1982. Gamma (Immune) interferon production by leukocytes from a patient with a T_G cell proliferative disease. Blood 59,198.
30. Ito, Y., Nishiyama, Y., Shimokata, K., Takeyama, H. and Kumi, A. 1979. Immune interferon produced in vitro as a

quantitative indicator of cell-mediated immunity. Microbiol. Immunol. 23,1109.

31. Zoon, K.C., Smitn, M.E., Bridgen, P.J., Anfinsen, C.B., Hunkapiller, M.W., Hood, L.E. 1980. Amino-terminal sequence of the major component of human lymphoblastoid interferon. Science 207,527.
32. Allen, G. and Fantes, K.H. 1980. A family of structural genes for human lymphoblastoid (leukocyte-type) interferon. Nature (Lond) 287,408.
33. Levy, W.P., Shively, J., Rubenstein, M., Del Valle, U. and Pestka, S. 1980. Amino-terminal amino acid sequence of human leukocyte interferon. Proc. Natl. Acad. Sci. USA. 77,5102.
34. Knight, E. Jr., Hunkapillar, M.W., Korant, B.D., Hardy, R.W.F. and Hood, L.E. 1980. Human fibroblast interferon: amino acid analysis and amino terminal amino acid sequence. Science 207,525.
35. Streuli, M., Nagata, S. and Weissmann, C. 1980. At least three human type α interferons: structure of α_2. Science 209, 1343.
36. Nagata, S., Mantei, N. and Weissmann, C. 1980. The structure of one of the eight or more distinct chromosomal genes for human interferon - α. Nature (Lond) 287,401.
37. Lawn, R.M., Adelman, J., Dull, J.J., Gross, M., Goeddel, D. V. and Ullrich, A. 1981. j DNA sequence of two closely linked human leukocyte interferon genes. Science 212, 1159.
38. Goeddel, D.V., Leung, D.W., Dull, J.J., Gross, M., Lawn, R. M., McCandliss, R. Seebury, P.H., Uullrich, A., Yelverton, E. and Gray, P.W. 1981. The structure of eight distinct cloned human leukocyte interferon cDNAs. Nature (Lond) 290,20.
39. Nagata, S., Taira, H., Hall, A., Johnsrud, L., Streuli, M., Ecsodi, J., Boll, W., Cantell, K. and Weissmann, C. 1980. Synthesis in E. coli of a polypeptide with human leukocyte interferon activity. Nature (Lond) 284,316.
40. Goeddel, D.V., Yelverton, E., Ullrich, A., Heyneker, H.L., Miozzari, G., Holmes, W., Soeburg, P.H., Dull, T., May, L., Stebbing, N. Crea, R., Maeda, S., McCandliss, R., Sloma, A. Tabor, J.M., Gross, M., Familletti, P.C. and Pestka, S. 1980. Human leukocyte interferon produced by E. coli is biologically active. Nature (Lond) 287,411.
41. Derynck, R., Devos, R., Remant, E., Saman, E., Stanssans, P., Tavernier, J., Volckaert, G., Content, J., DeClercq, E. and Fiers, W. 1981. Isolation and characterization of a human fibroblast interferon gene and its expression in Escherichia coli. Rev. Infect. Dis. 3,1186.
42. Taniguchi, T, Mantei, N., SAchwarzstein, M., Nagata, S., Muramatsu, M. and Weissmann, C. 1980. Human leukocyte and

fibroblast interferons are structurally related. Nature (Lond) 285,547.

43. Skup, D., Windass, J.D., Sor, F., George, H., Williams, B.R.G., Fukuhara, H., DeMaeyer-Guignard, J. and DeMaeyer,E. 1982. Molecular cloning of partial cDNA copies of two distinct mouse IFNβ m RNAs. Nuc Acid Res 10, 3069.
44. Sehgal, P.B., Sagar, A.D., Braude, I.A. and Smith, D. 1981. Heterogeneity of human α and β interferon mRNA species. In "The Biology of the Interferon System" (Eds E. deMaeyer, G.Galasso and H. Schellenkens) pp 43-46. Elsevier/North Holland, Amsterdam.
45. Gray, P.W. Leung, D.W., Pennica, D., Yelverton, E., Najarian, R., Simonsen, C.C., Derynek, R., Sherwood, P.J., Wallace, D.M., Berger, S.L., Levinson, A.D. and Goeddel, D.V. 1982. Expression of human immune interferon cDNA in E coli and monkey cells. Nature (Lond) 295,503.
46. Devos, R., Cheroutre, H., Taya, Y., Degrave, W., Van Heuverswyn, H. and Fiers, W. 1982. Molecular cloning of human immune interferon cDNA and its expression in eukaryotic cells. Nuc Acid Res 10,2487.
47. Epstein, L.B. 1982. Interferon-gamma: success, structure and speculation. Nature (Lond) 295,453.
48. Yip, Y.K., Barrowclough, B.S., Urban, C. and Vilcek, J. 1982. Purification of two subspecies of human γ (immune) interferon. Proc.Natl.Acad. Sci., USA 79,1820.
49. Weening, H., Fuse, A., Opdenakker, G., VanDamme, J., DeLey, M. and Billiau, A. 1982. Messenger RNA of human immune interferon: isolation and partial characterization. Biochem. Biophys. Res. Comm. 104,6.
50. Wallace, D.M., Hitchcock, M.J.M., Reber, S.B. and Berger, S.L. 1981. Translation of human immune interferon messenger RNA in xenophus laevis oocytes. Biochem. Biophys. Res. Comm. 100,865.
51. Taniguchi, T., Pang, R.H.L., Yip, Y.K., Henriksen, D. and Vilcek, J. 1981. Partial characterization of gamma (immune) interferon mRNA extracted from human lymphocytes. Proc. Natl. Acad. Sci. USA 78,3469.
52. Fuse, A., Heremans, H., Opdenakker, G. and Billian, A. 1982. Messenger RNA of mouse immune interferon (MuIFNγ) Biochem. Biophys. Res. Comm. 105,1309.
53. Meager, A., Graves, H., Burke, D.C. and Swallow, D.M. 1979. Involvement of a gene on chromosome 9 in human fibroblast interferon production. Nature (Lond) 280,493.
54. Owerbach, D., Rutter, W.J., Shows, T.B., Gray, P., Goeddel, D.V. and Lawn, R.M. 1981. Leukocyte and fibroblast interferon genes are located on human chromosome 9. Proc. Natl. Acad. Sci. USA 78,3123.

55. Slate, D.L., D'Eustachio, P., Pravtcheva, D., Cunningham, L., Nagata, S., Weissmann, L. and Ruddle, F.H. 1982. Chromosomal location of a human α interferon gene family. J. Exp. Med. 155, 1019.
56. Lengyel, P. 1982. Biochemistry of interferons and their actions pp 251-282 in Ann. Rev. Biochem. Vol. 51 (Annual Reviews Inc.).
57. Methods in Enzymology Vol. 79 1981. Interferons Part B Ed. S. Peska. (Academic Press, New York).
58. Derynck, R., Leung, D.W., Gray, P.W. and Goeddel, D.V. 1982. Human interferon γ is encoded by a single class of mRNA. Nuc Acid Res 10,3605.
59. Yelverton, E., Leung, D., Weck, P., Gray, P.W. and Goeddel, D.V. 1981. Bacvterial synthesis of a novel human leukocyte interferon. Nuc. Acid. Res. 9,731.
60. Pestka, S., Maeda, S., Hobbs, D.S., Chiang, T.R.C., Costello, L.L., Rehberg, Levy, W.P., Chang, N.T., Wainwright, N.R., Hiscott, McCandliss, R., Stein, S., Moschera, J.A. and Staehelin, T. 1982. The human interferons: The proteins and their expression in bacteria pp 51-74 in Recombinant DNA, Proceedings of the Third Cleveland Symposium on Macromolecules (Ed. A.G.Walton) Elsevier, Amsterdam.
61. Taniguchi, T., Guarente, L., Roberts, T.M. Kimelman, D., Douhan, J., III, Ptashne, M. 1980. Expression of the human fibroblast gene in Escherichia coli. Proc. Natl. Acad. Sci. USA 77,5230.
62. Goeddel, D.V., Shepard, H.M., Yelverton, E., Leung, D. and Crea, R. 1980. Synthesis of human fibroblast interferon by E. coli. Nuc. Acid. Res. 8,4057.
63. Masucci, M.G., Zigetti, R., Klein, E., Klein, G., Gruest, J., Montagnier, L., Taira, H., Hall, A., Nagata, S. and Weismann, C. 1980. Effect of interferon α_1 from E. coli on some cell functions. Science 209,1431.
64. Lee, S.H., Kelley, S., Chiu, H. and Stebbing, N. 1982. Stimulation of natural killer cell activity and inhibition of proliferation of various leukemic cells by purified human leukocyte interferon subtypes. Cancer Res. 42, 1312.
65. Herberman, R.B., Ortaldo, J.R., Mantovani, A., Hobbs, D.S., Kung, H-F and Pestka, S. 1982. Effect of human recombinant interferon on cytotoxic activity of natural killer (NK) cells and monocytes. Cell Immunol. 67,160.
66. Lotzova, E., Savary, C.A. Gutterman, J.U. and Hersh, E.M. 1982. Modulation of natural killer cell-mediated cytotoxicity by partially purified and cloned interferon -α. Cancer Res. 42,2480.
67. Attallah, A.M., Zoon, K., Folks, T., Huntington, J. and Yeatman, T.J. 1981. Multiple biological activities of

homogeneous human alpha interferon. Infect. Immun. 34,1068.
68. Claeys, H., VanDamme, J., DeLey, M., Vermylen, C. and Billiau, A. 1982. Activation of natural cytotoxicity of human peripheral blood mononuclear cells by interferon: a kinetic study and comparison of different interferon types. Brit. J. Haematol. 50,85.
69. Weck, P.K., Apperson, S., May, L. and Stebbing, N. 1981. Comparison of the antiviral activities of various cloned human interferon α - subtypes in mammalian cell cultures. J. Gen. Virol. 57, 233.
70. Streuli, M., Hall, A., Boll, W., Stewart, W.E., Nagata, S. and Weissmann, C. 1981. Target cell specificity of two species of human interferon - α produced in Escherischia coli and of hybrid molecules derived from them. Proc. Natl. Acad. Sci. USA 78, 2848.
71. Weck, P.K., Apperson, S., Stebbing, N., Gray, P.W., Leung, D., Shepard, H.M. and Goeddel, D.V. 1981. Antiviral activities of hybrids of two major human leukocyte interferons. Nuc Acid Res. 9,6153.
72. Branca, A.A. and Baglioni, C. 1981. Evidence that types I and II interferons have different receptors. Nature (Lond) 294,769.
73. Ankel, H., Krishnamurti, C., Besancon, F., Stefanos, S. and Falcoff, E. 1980. Mouse fibroblast (Type 1) and immune (type II) interferons: pronounced differences in affinity for gangliosides and in antiviral and antigrowth effects on mouse leukemia L-1210R cells. Proc. Natl. Acad. Sci. USA 77,2528.
74. Cooper, H.L. 1982. Effect of bacterially produced interferon - α_2 on synthesis of specific peptides in human peripheral lymphocytes. Febs Lett 140,109.
75. Weil, J., Epstein, L.B. and Epstein, C.J. 1980. Synthesis of interferon-induced polypeptides in normal and chromosome 21-aneuploid human fibroblasts: relationship to relative sensitivities in antiviral assays. J. Interferon Res. I, III.
76. Epstein, L.B., Weil, J. Lucas, D.O., Cox, D.R. and Epstein, D.J. 1981. In "The Biology of the Interferon System." (eds E deMaeyer, G. Galasso and H. Schellenkens) pp 247-256. Elseview/North-Holland, Amsterdam.
77. Rubin, B.T. and Gupta, S.L. 1980. Differential efficacies of human type I and type II interferons as antiviral and antiproliferative agents. Proc. Natl. Acad. Sci., USA 77, 5928.
78. Fleischman, W.R., Jr. Georgiades, J.A., Osborne, L.C. and Johnson, H.M. 1979. Potentiation of interferon activity by mixed preparations of fibroblast and immune interferon. Infect. Immun. 26, 248.

79. Hovanessian, A.G. 1979. Intracellular events in interferon-treated cells. Differentiation 15,139.
80. Hovanessian, A.G., Meurs, E., Aujean, O., Vaquero, C., Stefanos, S. and Falcoff, E. 1980. Antiviral response and induction of specific proteins in cells treated with immune T (Type II) interferon analogous to that from viral interferon (Type I) - treated cells. Virology 104,195.
81. Meurs, E., Hovanessian, A.G. and Montagnier, L. 1981. Interferon-mediated antiviral state in human MRC 5 cells in the absence of detectable levels of 2-5A synthetase and protein kinase. J. Interferon Res. 1,219.
82. Wood, J.N. and Hovanessian, A.G. 1979. Interferon enhances 2-5A synthetase in embryonal carcinoma cells. Nature (Lond) 282,74.
83. Verhaegen, M., Divizia, M., Vandenbussche, P., Kuwata, T. and Content, J. 1980. Abnormal behaviour of interferon-induced enzymatic activities in interferon-resistant cell line. Proc. Natl. Acad. Sci. USA 77,4479.
84. Silverman, R.H., Cayley, P.J., Knight, M., Gilbert, C.S. and Kerr. I.M. 1982. Control of the ppp (A2 p)nA system in Hela cells: effects of interferon and virus infection. Eur. J. Biochem. 124,131.
85. Holmes, S.L. and Gupta, S.L. 1982. Interferon action in humanfibroblasts: induction of 2'5'-oligodenylate synthetase in the absence of detectable protein kinase activity. Arch. Virol. 72,137.
86. Riggin, C.H. and Pitha, P.M. 1982. Effect of interferon on the exogenous Friend Murine Leukemia Virus infection. Virology 118,202.
87. Maheshwari, R.K., Banerjee, D.K., Waechter, C.J. Olden, K. and Friedman, R.M. 1980. Interferon treatment inhibits glycosylation of viral protein. Nature (Lond) 287,454.
88. Baglioni, C. and Maroney, P.A. 1980. Mechanisms of action of human interferons: induction of 2'5'-oligo (A) polymerase. J. Biol. Chem. 255,8390.
89. Vandenbussche, P., Divizia, M., Verhaegen-Lewalle, M., Fuse, A., Kuwata, T., DeClercq, E. and Content, J. 1981. Enzymatic activities induced by interferon in human fibroblast cell lines differing in their sensitivity to the anticellular activity of interferon. Virology, III, II.
90. Verhaegen-Lewalle, M., Kuwata, T., Zhang, Z-X, DeClercq, E., Cankell, K. and Content, J. 1982. 2-5A synthetase activity induced by interferon α, β, γ in human cell lines differing in their sensitivity to the anticellular and antiviral activities of these interferons. Virology 117,425.

91. Samuel, C.E. and Knutson, G.S. 1981. Mechanism of interferon action: cloned human leukocyte interferons induce protein kinase and inhibit vesicular stomatitis virus but not reovirus replication in human amnion cells. Virology 114,302.
92. Robbins, C.H., Kramer, G., Saneto, R., Hardesty, B. and Johnson, H.M. 1981. Dissociation of protein kinase activity and the induction of the antiviral state in a cell line responsive to the antiviral effects of interferon. Biochem. Biophys. Res. Comm. 103,103.
93. Friedman, R.M. 1979. Interferons: interaction with cell surfaces. In "Interferon I" pp 53-74 (ed I. Gresser) Academic Press, New York.
94. Wang, E., Pfeffer, L.M. and Tamm, I. 1981. Interferon increases the abundance of submembranous microfilaments in Hela-S_3 cells in suspension culture. Proc. Natl. Acad. Sci. USA 78,6281.
95. Fellous, M., Kamoun, M., Gresser, I. and Bono, R. 1979. Enhanced expression of HLA antigens and α_2-microglobulin on interferon-treated human lymphoid cells. Eur. J. Immunol. 9,446.
96. Heron, I., Hokland, M. and Berg, K. 1978. Enhanced expression of β_2-microglobulin and HLA antigens on human lymphoid cells by interferon. Proc. Natl. Acad. Sci. USA 75,6215.
97. Fellous, M., Nir., U., Wallach, D., Merlin, G., Rubenstein, M. and Revel, M. 1982. Interferon-dependent induction of mRNA for the major histocompatibility antigens in human fibroblasts and lymphoblastoid cells. Proc. Natl. Acad. Sci. USA 79,3082.
98. Basham, T.Y., Bourgeade, M.R., Creasey, A.A. and Merigan, T.C. 1982. Interferon increases HLA synthesis in melanoma cells. Interferon-resistant and sensitive cells. Proc. Natl. Acad. Sci. USA 79,3265.
99. Torres, B.A., Farrar, W.L. and Johnson, H.M. 1982. Interleukin 2 regulates immune interferon (IFNγ) production by normal and suppressor cell cultures. J. Immunol. 128,2217.
100. Hokland, P. and Berg, K. 1981. Interferon enhances the antibody-dependent cellular cytotoxicity (ADCC) of human polymorphonuclear leukocytes. J. Immunol. 127,1588.
101. Boraschi, D., Soldateschi, D. and Taliabue, A. 1982. Macrophage activation by interferon: dissociation between tumoricidal capacity and suppressive activity. Eur. J. Immunol. 12,320.
102. Fradelizi, D. and Gresser, I. 1982. Interferon inhibits the generation of allospecific suppressor T lymphocytes. J. Exp. Med. 155,1610.

103.Fast, L.D., Hansen, J.A. and Newman, W. 1981. Evidence for T cell nature and heterogeneity within natural killer (NK) and antibody-dependent cellular cytotoxicity (ADCC) effectors: a comparison with cytolytic T lymphocytes (CTL). J. Immunol. 127,448.
104.O'Malley, J.A., Nussbaum-Blumenson, A., Sheedy, D., Grossmayer, B.J. and Ozer, H. 1982. Identification of the T-cell subset that produces human γ interferon. J. Immunol. 128, 2522.
105 Grimm, E.A., Mazumber, A., Zhang, H.Z. and Rosenberg, S.A. 1982. Lymphokine-activated killer cell phenomenon. J. Exp. Med. 155,1823.
106.Thoman, M.L. and Weigle, W.O. 1982. Cell-mediated immunity in aged mice: an underlying lesion in IL2 synthesis. J. Immunol. 128,2358.
107.Szigeti, R., Masucci, M.G., Masucci, G., Klein, E., Klein, G. and Berthold, W. 1980. Interferon suppresses antigen-and mitogen-induced leukocyte migration inhibition. Nature (Lond) 288,594.
108.DeMaeyer, E. 1981. Interferon and the immune system. A review (limited to α and β interferons). In "The Biology of the Interferon System" (eds E deMaeyer, G. Galasso and H. Schellenkens) pp 203-209. Elseview/North Holland, Amsterdam.
109.Harfast, B., Huddlestone, J.R., Casali, P., Merigan, T.C. and Oldstone, M.B.A. 1981. Interferon acts directly on human B lymphocytes to modulate immunoglobulin synthesis. J. Immunol. 127,2146.
110.Havell, E.A., Spitalny, G.L. and Patel, P.J. 1982. Enhanced production of murine interferon γ by T cells generated in response to bacterial infection. J. Expr. Med. 156,112.
111.Green, J.A., Yeh, T-J, Overall, J.C., Jr. 1981. Sequential production of IFNα and immune-specific IFN-γ by human mononuclear leukocytes exposed to herpes simplex virus. J. Immunol. 127,1192.
112.Kelsey,D.K., Overall, J.C., Jr. and Glasgow, L.A. 1982. Production of alpha and gamma interferons by spleen cells from cytomegalovirus-infected mice. Infect. Immun. 36,651.
113.Scott, J.M., Secher, D.S., Flowsers, D., Bate, J., Cantell, K. and Tyrrell, D.A.J. 1981. Toxicity of interferon. Brit. Med. J. 282,1345.
114.Nilsen, T.W., Maroney, P.A. and Baglioni, C. 1982. Synthesis of (2'-5') oligoadenylate and activation of an endoribonuclease in interferon-treated HeLa cells infected with reovirus. J. Virol. 42, 1039.
115.Levin,S. and Hahn, T. 1981. Evaluation of the human interferon system in viral disease. Clin. Exp. Immunol. 46,475.

116. Isaacs, D., Clarke, J.R., Tyrrell, D.A.J., Webster, A.D.B. and Valman, H.B. 1981. Deficient production of leukocyte interferon (IFNγ) in vitro and in vivo in children with recurrent respiratory tract infections. Lancet 1981 II, 950.
117. Lebon, P., Girard, S., Thepot, F. and Chany, C. 1982. The presence of α-interferon in human amniotic fluid. J. Gen. Virol. 59,393.
118. Ennis, F.A., Meager, A., Beare, A.S., Yi-Hua, Q., Riley, D., Scharz, G., Schild, G.C. and Rook, A.H. 1981. Interferon induction and increased natural killer-cell activity in influenza infections in man. The Lancet II (1981) 891.
119. Stevens, D.A., and Merigan, T.C. 1972. Interferon, antibody, and other host factors in herpes zoster. J. Clin. Invest. 51,1170.
120. Spruance, S.L., Green, J.A., Chiu, G., Yeh, T-J., Wenerstrom, G. and Overall, J.C., Jr. 1982. Pathogenesis of herpes simples labialis: correlation of vesicle fluid interferon with lesion age and virus titer. Infect. Immun. 36,907.
121. Chanock, R.M. and Parrott, R.H. 1965. Acute respiratory disease in infancy and childhood: present understanding and prospects for prevention. Pediatrics 36,21.
122. Kim, H.W. Arrobio, J.O., Brandt, C.D., Jeffries, B.C., Pyles, G., Reid, J.L., Channock, R.M. and Parrott, R.H. 1973. Epidemiology of respiratory syncytial virus infection in Washington, D.C.: importance of the virus in different respiratory tract disease syndromes and temporal distribution of infection. Am. J. Epidemiol. 98,216.
123. Hall, W.J., Hall, C.B. and Speers, D.M. 1978. Respiratory syncytial virus infection in adults: clinical, virologic and serial pulmonary function studies. Ann Intern. Med. 88,203.
124. Mathur, U., Bentley, D.W. and Hall, C.B. 1980. Concurrent respiratory syncytial virus and influenza A infections in the institutionalized elderly and chronically ill. Ann.Intern. Med. 93,49.
125. Chanock, R.M., Kim, H.W., Brandt, C. and Parrott, R.H. 1976. Respiratory syncytial virus p365-382. In A.S.Evans (ed) Viral infections of humans: epidemiology and control. Plenum. Medical Book Co., New York and London.
126. Bellanti, J.A. 1977. Development of nonimmunologic, non-specific mechanisms and specific immunologic mechanisms in resistance to airways and pulmonary infections in infants and children. Pediatr. Res. 11,224.
127. Wright, P.F., Shinozaki, T., Fleet, W., Sell, S.H., Thompson, T. and Karzon, D.T. 1976. Evaluation of a live

attenuated respiratory syncytial virus vaccine in infants. J. Pediatr. 88,931.

128. Hall, C.B., Douglas, R.G., Jr., Simons, R.L. and Geiman, J.M. 1978. Interferon production in children with respiratory syncytial, influenza and parainfluenza virus infections. J. Pediatr. 93,28.

129. McIntosh, K. 1978. Interferon in nasal secretions from infants with viral respiratory tract infections. J. Pediatr. 93,33.

130. Ray, C.G., Gravelle, C.R. and Chin, T.D.Y. 1967. Circulating interferon in infants and children with acute respiratory illness. J. Pediatr. 71,27.

131. Jao, R.L., Wheelock, E.F. and Jackson, G.G. 1970. Production of interferon in volunteers infected with Asian influenza. J. Infect. Dis. 121,419.

132. Chonmaitree, T., Roberts, N.J., Jr. Douglas, R.G. Jr., Hall, C.B. and Simons, R.L. 1981. Interferon production by human mononuclear leukocytes: differences between respiratory syncytial virus and influenza viruses. Infect. Immun. 32,300.

133. Corbitt, G. 1971. Interferon and respiratory syncytial virus. Lancet II, 492.

134. Gardner,P.S., McGuckin, R., Beale, A.J. and Fernandes, R. 1970. Interferon and respiratory syncytial virus. Lancet I, 574.

135. Hill, D.A., Baron, S. and Channock, R.M. 1969. Sensitivity of common respiratory viruses to an interferon inducer in human cells. Lancet II, 187.

136. Moehring, J.M. and Forsyth, B.R. 1971. The role of the interferon system in respiratory syncytial virus infections. Proc. Soc. Exp. Biol. Med. 138,1009.

137. Holland, J., Spindler, K., Horodynski, F., Grabau, E., Nichol, S. and Vandepol, S. 1982. Rapid evolution of RNA genomes. Science 215,1577.

138. Mills, B.G., Singer,F.R., Weiner, L.P. and Holst, P.A. 1981. Immunohistological demonstration of respiratory syncytial virus antigens in Paget disease of bone. Proc. Natl. Acad. Sci. USA 78,1209.

139. Hilfenhaus, J., Karges, H.E., Weinmann, E. and Barth, R. 1975. Effect of administered human leukocyte interferon on experimental rabies in monkeys. Infect. Immun. 11,1156.

140. Gresser, I., Tovey, M.G. Mauoy, C. and Bandu, M-T 1976. Role of interferon in the pathogenesis of virus diseases in mice as demonstrated by the use of anti-interferon serum: II. Studies with herpes simplex, moloney sercoma, vesicular stomatitis, newcastle dsiease and influenza viruses. J. Exp. Med. 144,1316.

141. Zawatzky, R., Hilfenhaus,J., Marucci,F. and Kirchner, H. 1981. Experimental infection of inbred mice with herpes

simplex virus type 1. I Investigation of humoral and cellular immunity and of interferon induction. J. G en. Virol 53,31.
142.Schindler, L., Engler,H. and Kirchner, H. 1982. Activation of natural killer cells and induction of interferon of mouse hepatitis virus type 3 in mice. Infect. Immun. 35,869.
143.Sundmacher,R. Cantell,K. Skoda,R. Hallermann,C. and Newmann-Haefelin,D. 1978. Human leukocyte and fibroblast interferon in a combination therapy of dendritic keratitis. Albrecht Von Graefes Arch. Klin. Exp. Ophthalmol. 208,229.
144.Romano,A., Revel, M., Guariri-Rotman,D., Blumenthal, M. and Stein,R. 1980. Use of human fibroblast-derived (beta) interferon in the treatment of epidemic adenovirus kerato-conjunctivitis. J. Interferon Res. 1,95.
145.Ho,M. Pazin,G.J., White,L.T., Haverkos,H., Wechster,R.L., Breinig,M.K., Cantell,K. and Armstrong,J.A. 1981. Intralesional treatment of warts with interferon - α and its longterm effect on NK cell activity, in "The Biology of the Interferon System" pp 361-365 (eds E. deMaeyer,G. Galasso and H.Schellenkons) Elsevier/North-Holland,Amsterdam.
146.Scott,G.M. and Csonka, G.W. 1979. Effect of injections of small doses of human fibroblast interferon into genital warts. A pilot study. Br.J.Vener.Dis. 55,442.
147.Merigan,T.C. Reed, S.E., Hall,T.S. and Tyrrell, D.A.J. 1973. Inhibition of respiratory virus infection by locally applied interferon. Lancet I,563.
148.Scott,G.M., Phillpotts,R.J., Wallace,J. Secher,D.S., Cantell,K. and Tyrrell,D.A.J. 1982. Purified interferon as protection against rhinovirus infection. Br. Med. J. 284,1822.
149.Scott,G.M., Phillpotts,R.J., Wallace,J., Gauci,C.L., Tyrrell, D.A.J. and Greiner,J. 1982. Prevention of rhinovirus colds by human interferon alpha-α2 from Escherichia coli. Lancet II,186.
150.Merigan,T.C., Rand,K.H., Pollard,R.B., Abdallah,P.S., Jordan,G.W. and Fried,R.P. 1978. Human leukocyte interferon for the treatment of herpes zoster in patients with cancer. New Eng. J. Med. 298,981.
151.Merigan,T.C., Gallagher,J.G., Pollard,R.B. and Arvin,A.M. 1981. Short-course human leukocyte interferon in treatment of herpes zoster in patients with cancer. Antimicrob. Agents Chemother. 19,193.
152.Merigan,T.C. 1981. Clinical utilization of human interferons. In "Interferon 3 1981" pp 137-154. (ed I Gresser) Academic Press. New York.

153. Cheeseman,S.H., Rubin,R.H., Stewart,J.A., Tolkoff,N.E., Cosini,A.B., Cantell, K., Gilbert,J., Winkle,S., Herrin,J.T., Black, P.H., Russel, P. and Hirsch,M.S. 1979. Controlled clinical trial of prophylactic human-leukocyte interferon in renal transplantation: Effects on cytomegalovirus and herpes siplex virus. New Eng. J. Med. 300,1345.
154. Cheeseman,S.H., Henle,W., Rubin,R.H., Tolkoff-Rubin,N.E., Cosimi,G., Cantell,K., Winkle,S., Herrin,J.T., Black,P.H., Russell,P.S. and Hirsch,M.S. 1980. Epstein-Barr virus infection in renal transplant recipients. Effects of antilymphocyte globulin and interferon. Ann Intern. Med. 93,39.
155. Haverkos,H.W., Pazin,G.J., Armstrong,J.A. and Ho,M. 1980. Follow-up of interferon treatment of herpes simplex. New Eng. J. Med. 303,699.
156. Pazin,G.J., Armstrong,J.A., Lam,M.T., Tarr,G.C., Jannetta,P.J. and Ho,M. 1979. Prevention of reactivated herpes simplex infection by human leukocyte interferon after operation on the trigeminal root. New Eng. J. Med. 301,225.
157. Greenberg,H.B., Pollard,R.B., Lutwick,L.I., Gregory,P.B., Robinson,W.S. and Merigan,T.C. 1976. Effect of human leucocyte interferon on hepatitis B virus infection in patients with chronic active hepatitis. New Eng J. Med. 295,517.
158. Scullard,G.H., Pollard,R.B., Smith,J.L., Sacks,S.L., Gregory,P.B., Robinson,W.S. and Merigan,T.C. 1981. Antiviral treatment of chronic hepatitis B virus infection I. Changes in viral markers with interferon combined with adenine arabinoside. J. Infect. Dis. 143,772.
159. Gutterman,J.U. et al 1982. Recombinant human leucocyte interferon (IFNrA): a clinical study of pharmacokmetics single dose tolerance, and biologic effects in cancer patients. Ann Intern. Med. in press.
160. Vallbracht,A., Treunier,J., Flehmig,B., Joester,K-E, and Niethammer,D. 1981. Interferon-neutralising antibodies in a patient treated with human fibroblast interferon. Nature (Lond) 289,496.
161. Levy,W.P., Rubinstein,M., Shively,J., Del Valle,U., Lai,C-Y, Moschera,J., Brink,L., Gerber,L., Stein,S. and Pestka,S. 1981. Amino acid sequence of a human leukocyte interferon. Proc. Natl. Acad. Sci., USA 78,6168.
162. Ingimarsson,S., Cantell,K., Carlstrom,G., Dalton,B., Paucker,K. and Strander,H. 1981. Immune reactions and longterm therapy with human leukocyte interferon. Acta.Med. Scand. 209,17.

163. Hooks,J., Moutsopoulus,H.M., Geis,S.A., Stahl,N.I., Decker,J.L. and Notkins,A.L. 1979. Immune interferon in the circulation of patients with autoimmune disease. New Eng. J. Med. 301,5.
164. Ohno,S., Kato,F., Matsuda,H., Fuji,N. and Minagawa,T. 1982. Detection of gamma interferon in the sera of patients with Behcet's disease. Infect. Immun. 36,202.
165. Knight,E.Jr. 1980. Purification and characterization of interferons. In Interferon 2 pp 1-12. (Ed I.Gresser) Academic Press,New York.

CHAPTER 4

HUMORAL IMMUNE RESPONSE TO VIRUSES IN HUMANS

Jean-Louis Virelizier

Unite d'Immunologie et de Rhumatologie Pediatriques
Hopital Necker-Infants Malades
Paris, France

Antibody was the first antiviral host defense mechanism to be recognized. More recently, many cellular effectors of antiviral immunity have been described, leading to exciting discoveries and promoting intense research in this area. Remarkable progress in fundamental and applied cellular immunology now permits us to evaluate the role of cytotoxic cells and interferons in host defense against viruses. Many modern studies in this area have investigated the complex cellular interactions involved in the regulation of antiviral responses. It would be unwise, however, to consider that research on the mechanisms and roles of antibody response in antiviral immunity is obsolete. The aim of the present overview is not to review the huge amount of data accumulated in this area, but rather to discuss the various implications of antiviral antibody in terms of markers of immunity to viral infections, protection and immunopathology, as important areas for future research. In fact, research on humoral and cellular immunity cannot be dissociated from cellular immunology in view of the complex interactions always implicated in immune responses.

Antibody formation is the result of the collaboration between B and T lymphocytes, through various helper factors some of which are specific for the antigen and HLA restricted, whereas others are nonspecific, but essential for the amplification of the clonal response of T cells (like interleukin 2). However, macrophages are essential in such reactions, since they both present viral antigens and secrete nonspecific, amplifying factors such as interleukin 1 (1). Other T cells suppress antibody secretion, so that the expression of clones of B memory cells is regulated by helper and suppressor T lymphocytes, as shown in mice immunized with purified influenza haemagglutinin (2). On the other hand,

ISBN 0-12-239980-3

one type of cytotoxic cell acts through antibody-dependent recognition of viral antigens on the membrane of infected target cells. Finally, virus-antibody complexes are trapped by macrophages, which can either inactivate or replicate the virus, according to the type of virus considered. It would thus be artificial to envisage antibody formation independently of the various cell-types involved in immune responses to viruses (3).

VIRAL ANTIGENS RECOGNIZED BY ANTIBODY

Viruses have complex structures most components of which can be recognized as immunogens by B and T cells. In this respect, they differ from the simple antigens purposely chosen by fundamental immunologists. For example, fourteen varicella-zoster virus antigens were identified that induce antibodies during primary and recurrent infections. These antigens included the major nucleocapsid polypeptide (mol. wt 155,000) and 3 glycoproteins (mol. wt. 130,000; 88,000; and 50,000) plus a number of "minor" antigens (4). Virus antigens, moreover, are presented to the immunological system not only as viral particles with external antigens, but also as membrane neo-antigens in infected cells. Such cells may thus present internal components of the virion, like the ribonucleoprotein (5) and the matrix protein (6) in the case of influenza virus. Furthermore, non-structural antigens of the influenza virus can be exposed on the membrane of infected cells (7). Finally, recognition of such membrane antigens may be modified by the variable permissivity of cells to virus infection, and influenced by their copresentation with histocompatibility antigens to T cells.

TYPES OF ANTIBODY RESPONSES

The immune system responds to viral infections by producing a large variety of immunoglobulins of various specificities and classes. Antibody reactivity varies qualitatively during the immune response to immunogens such as poliovirus (8), influenza (9) and adenovirus (10). Antibody of the IgM class is first produced, and is thus helpful in determining how recently a viral infection occured, as shown with influenza infection for example (11). With some viruses, however, the IgM responses can be detected for a long period of time. Thus serum IgM antibody to rubella virus was found to persist for 6 months in 68% and a year in 38% vaccines (12). Looking at idiotypes of antiviral antibodies is now possible, and this new methodology will make it possible to better dissect the clonal expansion of virus-specific B lymphocytes, as shown with antibody to influenza virus hemagglutinin. Thus, studies of the idiotypes expressed during primary and secondary anti-haemagglutinin responses of mice immunized with B/Lee virus revealed persistence of some idiotypes during both primary and secondary responses, whereas others are expressed only in one or the other type of response (13).

In some types of infection, looking at serum antibody only may not be sufficient, since local responses are probably more relevant to recovery. Analysis of the bronchoalveolar lavage fluids of volunteers immunized against influenza with either subcutaneous vaccine or by aerosol showed that local antibody was best stimulated by aerosol immunization, found in the IgG as well as IgA class and was locally produced (14). Local production of mumps IgG and IgM antibodies has been observed in patients during meningitis. The ratio between mumps IgG and IgM antibodies was higher in CSF than in serum, suggesting that the synthesis of IgG antibodies in central nervous system is more efficient than that of IgM antibodies (15).

ANTIBODY PROFILE AS A TOOL FOR THE INVESTIGATION OF HOST-VIRUS RELATIONSHIP

The availability of multiple serological markers for a single virus permits us to follow the fate of a chronic infection, and thus gives indirect evidence on the ability of the host to cope with this infection. In the case of hepatitis B, looking simultaneously at circulating antigens, such as HBs and HBe, and antibody to various components of the virus, such as anti-HBe, anti-HBc and anti-HBs makes it possible to differentiate between acute hepatis, chronic carrier state, convalescence, or complete recovery (16). Similarly, the profile of antibody to VCA, EA and EBNA antigens gives a good indication of the control of Epstein-Barr virus infections (17). An abnormal profile associating high anti-VCA and anti-EA but low anti-EBNA antibody should stimulate a search for an underlying immunological defect. In such cases, defects of the interferon system have been found (18).

HOST PROTECTION BY ANTIBODY

In the mouse there is clear evidence that passive transfer of specific IgG antibody in immuno-suppressed recipients can protect against yellow fever, Coxsackie B_3 and influenza infections. Observations in patients with agammaglobulinemia also indicate that humoral immunity is essential for protection and recovery from enterovirus infections. Thus the frequency of poliomyelitis has been calculated to be 10,000 times higher than that of the normal population (19). Attenuated poliovirus vaccine can produce a chronic progressive neurologic disease in such patients (20). Similarly, agammaglobulinemia is complicated by persistent and fatal echovirus central-nervous system infections (21), sometimes associated with secondary myositis (22). The notion that enterovirus infection can be controlled by endogenous production of antibody has important therapeutic implications. Indeed, we were able to stop the progression of a meningo-encephalitis due to an attenuated poliovirus vaccine by transfer of specific antibody to a child with Bruton's type agammaglobulinemia (23).

Evidence that antibody is protective in normal people comes from the observation that maternal antibody can protect infants against respiratory syncytial virus. Babies born to mothers with high levels of IgG antibody to RSV were protected against infection with this virus during the first months of life when the risk of severe disease was greatest (24). Similarly, transplacentally acquired antibody protects infants from infection with influenza A virus. A direct correlation was found between age at the time of infection and level of antibody measured in cord serum (25).

MECHANISMS OF PROTECTION BY ANTIBODY

Although some types of antibody neutralize efficiently viruses in vitro, there is no direct evidence that antibody neutralization is a major protective mechanism in vivo. Furthermore, recent work has shown that non-neutralizing monoclonal antibodies passively transferred to mice can prevent lethal Sindbis virus encephalitis (26). This suggests that host protection may be mediated not only by antibodies which neutralize the infectivity of extracellular virus particles but also by those lacking this capacity some of which may react preferentially with virus-infected cells. In the Coxsackie B-3 virus experimental infection of mice, passive transfer experiments have suggested that antibody and host cells collaborate to provide effective resistance against the spread of the virus (27). Antibody dependent cell mediated cytotoxicity, performed by non T, Fc receptor bearing lymphocytes, can efficiently destroy in vitro cells infected with herpes simplex (28), mumps (29), vaccinia (30) or influenza (31) virus. Lysis of infected cells in the presence of specific antibody and complement can also be seen in vitro, and it has been shown that herpes simplex virus-infected cells can be destroyed early in the infectious cycle before the initial production of progeny virus particles (32). It should be stressed, however, that none of these mechanisms has been conclusively demonstrated to be operative in vivo.

MECHANISMS OF ESCAPE FROM PROTECTION BY ANTIBODY

In vitro, viruses can partially escape neutralization by antibody. A study of the kinetics of the formation of the stable combination between virus and antibody indicates that not all the virus particles in the reaction mixture are inactivated at the same rate by neutralizing antibody. This protection results from the presence in the antiserum of non avid, non neutralizing antibody that will combine reversibly with the virus surface, as shown with influenza virus (33). Even viral antigens exposed on the membrane of infected cells can escape recognition by antibody. Thus antibodies to measles virus can modulate and remove measles virus antigens from the surface of infected cells in vitro. This "antigenic modulation" is accompanied by a parallel reduction in the ability of immune lymphocytes to lyse the cells (34). Whether a similar type of mechanism is at work in vivo to protect cells chronically infected with measles virus in patients with subacute sclerosing panencephalitis is a matter of speculation.

Some viruses escape neutralization by changing critical antigenic sites on their external surface. This is clearly the case with influenza viruses, a phenomenon known as antigenic drift. In the mouse, it has been shown that antibodies to strain-specific determinants are highly protective, whereas antibody to crossreactive determinants are not (35). If this is true in man, which is very likely, it could explain why new variants cause epidemics despite the solid immunity induced in a given population by the previous epidemics, associated with a strain closely related, but with a slightly different haemagglutinin than that of the new variant, as discussed previously (36).

DELETERIOUS ROLE OF ANTIBODY RESPONSES

In some experimental models, it has been shown that production of specific antiviral antibody can damage the host. For example, early death from rabies virus infection in immuno-suppressed mice appears to be mediated by rabies-specific antibody or immune B lymphocytes rather than by immune T cells (37). How exactly these immunopathological phenomena are mediated by antibody is not known. In some circumstances, antibody can enhance virus infectivity. Thus non-neutralizing antisera to heterologous serotypes of dengue virus, or highly diluted homologous antisera, promoted dengue infection of mononuclear phagocytes obtained from individuals who had no prior experience with dengue (38). Similarly, antibody-mediated infection of macrophages and macrophage-like cell lines with 17 D-Yellow fever virus has been observed (39). This IgG-mediated phenomenon may facilitate replication and dissemination of the virus. Moreover, non-neutralized, antibody-coated virions may act as immune complexes to trigger monokine secretion. Some of these mediators produced by macrophages, such as prostaglandins, complement, lysosomal enzymes, superoxide anion, plasminogen activator or tumor-necrosing factor may in turn produce pathological reactions. That viruses can circulate for long period of times under the form of immune complexes is now established. For example, circulating immune complexes containing rubella-specific immunoglobulins can be detected in congenital rubella infection many years after birth, and for months after immunization (40). The presence of specific complexes appears to correlate with the late-emerging clinical problems involving several organ systems in congenital rubella.

CELL COOPERATION IN ANTIBODY RESPONSES

Advances in understanding of human immune responses depend, for obvious reasons, on the use of in vitro technique. Whereas in animals it is possible to show the thymus-dependency of a viral antigen by using surgically thymectomized mice, irradiation and reconstitution with bone-marrow cells, as has been done with purified influenza haemagglutinin (41), no clinical situation permits such in vivo demonstration in humans. Fortunately, new in vitro methods are now available that make it possible to induce antiviral antibody production in human leucocytes, as shown with influenza (42) and varicella zoster (43) virus. The in vitro response to influenza antigens has been specially well documented, and shown to be thymus-dependent and HLA-restricted. Studies of the kinetics of specific in vitro antibody production following influenza immunization clearly indicate that memory cells are involved in secondary responses (44). There are good reasons to believe that, like in the mouse (45), these in vitro antibody responses are macrophage dependent. The ability to maintain longterm cultures of interleukin 2-dependent, human helper T lymphocytes has permitted the fine analysis of the mechanisms of T and B cell cooperation in antibody responses to influenza antigens. Such longterm T cell cultures provide specific help for the production of anti-haemagglutinin antibody through soluble HLA-restricted mediators (46). Single clones of these helper T cells can also be used (47). These new methods will permit a better understanding of the intimate mechanisms through which T cells, B cells and macrophages cooperate in antiviral antibody production.

CONCLUSION

Clearly our knowledge of the antibody response to viruses has made considerable progress since modern immunological techniques have been used. The developments of such techniques is rapidly growing, so that further important progress is expected in this field. Indeed much remains to be learned about the mechanisms by which antibody protects or damages the host. The complex interactions between humoral and cellular antiviral responses need to be better understood, and much work is still necessary to appreciate the respective role of the various components of the immune response to viruses. In this respect, each type of virus infection is a model in its own right, since the critical factors of host defence clearly differ according to the virus considered. These notions are important when considering the need for better assays of immune responses. For example, when a new antiviral vaccine is planned, it is essential to know which assay is the more relevant to protection, and which components of immunity have to be predominantly stimulated. In viral infections where antibody responses appear to be important in prevention or recovery, the ability of vaccines to raise long-lived T and B memory cells for the production of antibody with the relevant specificity, class and location in the body should be a major area of future research.

REFERENCES

1. Watson, J.D. Transplantation, 31,313,1981.
2. Virelizier, J.L., Allison, A.C., and Schild, G.C. J. Exp. Med. 140, 1571, 1974.
3. Allison, A.C. Transplant Rev. 19,3,1974.
4. Zweerink, H.J., and Neff, B.J. Infect Immun 31, 436, 1981.
5. Virelizier, J.L. Allison, A.C., Oxford, J., and Schild, G.C. Nature, 266, 52, 1977.
6. Yewdell, J.W., Franck, E., and Gerhard, W. J. Immunol. 126, 1981.
7. Shaw, M.W., Lamon, E.W., and Compans, R.W. Infect. Immun. 34, 1065, 1981.
8. Svehag, S.E., and Mandel, B. J. Exp. Med. 119, 1, 1964.
9. Webster, R.G. Immunology 14, 39, 1968.
10. Lehrich, J.R., Kasel, J.A., and Rossen, R.D. J. Immunol. 97, 654, 1966.
11. Daugharty, H., Davis, M.L., and Kaye, H.S. J. Immunol. 109, 849, 1972.
12. Al-Nakib, W., Best, J.M., and Banatuala, J.E. Lancet 1, 182, 1975.
13. Liu, Y.N., Bona, C.A., and Schulman, J.L. J. Exp. Med. 154, 1525, 1981.
14. Waldman, R.H., Jungensen, P.F., Olsen, G.M., Ganguly, R., and Johnson, J.E. J.Immunol. 111, 38, 1973.
15. Ukkonen, P., Granstrom, M.L., Rasanen, J., Salonen, E.M., and Penttinon, K. J. Med. Virol. 8, 257, 1981.
16. McCullum, R.W. and Zuckerman, A.J. J.Med.Virol. 8, 1, 1981.
17. Niederman, J.C., McCollum, R.W., Henle, G., Henle, W. J. Am. Med. Assoc. 203, 205, 1968.
18. Virelizier, J.L., Lenoir, G., and Griscelli, C. Lancet 2, 231, 1978.
19. Wyatt, H.V. J.Infect.Dis. 128, 802, 1973.
20. Davis, L.E., Bodian, D., Price, D., Butler, J., and Vickers, J. N.Engl.J. Med. 197, 241, 1977.
21. Wilfert, C.M., et al. N. Engl. J. Med. 196, 1485, 1977.
22. Webster, A.D.B., et al. Arch.Dis. Child, 53, 33, 1978.
23. Virelizier, J.L., Griscelli, C. Arch.Fr.Pediatr. 34, 921, 1977.
24. Ogilvie, M.M., Vathenen, S., Radford, M., Codd, J., and Key, S. J.Med.Virol. 7, 263, 1981.
25. Puck, J.M., Glezen, W.P., Frank, A.L., and Six, H.R. J. Infect. Dis. 142, 844, 1980.
26. Schmaljohn, A.L., Johnson, E.D., Dalrymple, J.M., and Cole, G.A. Nature 297, 70, 1982.

27. Rager-Zisman, B., and Allison, A.C. J. Gen. Virol. 19, 329, 1973.
28. Shore, S.L., Black, C.M., Melewicz, F.M., Wood, P.A., and Nahmias, T., J. Immunol. 116, 194, 1976.
29. Harfast, B., Anderson, T., and Perlmann, P. J.Immunol. 114, 1820, 1975.
30. Perrin, L.H., Zinkernagel, R.M., and Oldstone, M.B.A. J. Exp. Med. 146, 949, 1977.
31. Greenberg, S.B., Criswell, B.S., Six, H.R., and Couch, R.B. J.Immunol. 119, 2100, 1977.
32. Cromeans, T.L., and Shore, S.L. Infect. Immun. 31, 1054, 1981.
33. Lafferty, K.J. Virology 21, 61, 1963.
34. Oldstone, M.B.A., and Tishon, A.Clin. Immunol. Immunopathol. 9, 55, 1978.
35. Virelizier, J.L. J.Immunol. 115, 434, 1975.
36. Virelizier, J.L., Allison, A.C., and Schild, G.C. Brit. Med. Bulletin, 35, 65, 1979.
37. Prabhakar, B.S., and Nathanson,N. Nature 290, 590, 1981.
38. Halstead,S.B., and O'Rouske,E.J. J.Exp.Med. 146, 201, 1977.
39. Schlesinger,J.J., and Bandriss,M.W. J.Med.Virol. 8, 101, 1981.
40. Coyle,D.K., Wolinsky,J.S., Buimovici-Klein,E., Moucha,R., and Cooper,L.Z. Infect. Immun. 36, 498, 1982.
41. Virelizier,J.L., Postlethwaite,R., Schild,G.C., and Allison,A.C. J.Exp.Med. 140, 1559, 1974.
42. Callard,R.E. Nature 282, 734, 1979.
43. Souhami,R.L., Babbage,J., and Callard,R.E. Clin. Exp. Immunol. 46, 98, 1982.
44. Mitchell,D.M., Fitzharris,P., Knight,R.A., and Schild,G.C. Clin.Exp.Immunol. 48, 491, 1982.
45. McLaren,C., and Pope,B. J.Immunol. 125, 2679, 1980.
46. Fischer,A., Beverley,P.C.L., and Feldman, M. Nature 294, 166, 1981.
47. Lamb,J.R., Eckels,D.D., Lake,P., Johnson,A.H., Hartzman,R.J., and Woody,J.N. J.Immunol. 128, 233, 1982.

CHAPTER 5

LOCAL IMMUNE RESPONSE TO VIRAL ANTIGENS

Pearay L. Ogra*
Robert C. Welliver
Marie Riepenhoff-Talty

Department of Pediatrics and Microbiology
School of Medicine
State University of New York at Buffalo
Buffalo, New York

INTRODUCTION

It is well known that the primary portals of entry for most human viral infections are limited to the mucous membranes of the respiratory, intestinal and genital tracts. The few agents which are acquired through non-mucosal routes include hepatitis B, and certain arthropod born viruses. After their initial replication in the mucosal surface, many viruses invade the blood stream and produce disease in systemic target tissues. However, a number of other respiratory and enteric viruses produce disease localized at the site of initial mucosal replication, with little or no evidence of systemic involvement. In addition, some evidence is available to indicate that the appearance of antibody or cell-mediated immune responses in the systemic tissues and the absence of sufficient mucosal immunity following certain natural infections or immunization procedures may be potentially hazardous. Thus, the development of effective antiviral immunoprophylaxis must take into account the mechanisms and nature of immune reactivity in systemic and secretory sites and the pathogenesis of specific viral diseases.

DEVELOPMENT OF THE COMMON MUCOSAL IMMUNE SYSTEM

The immunologic reactivity observed in different external

ISBN 0-12-239980-3

mucosal surfaces is generally referred to as the common mucosal immune system. The system appears to function somewhat independently of the immunologic functions in the systemic sites and peripheral blood. It includes the gut-associated lymphoid tissue (GALT), the bronchus associated lymphoid tissue (BALT), and the immunocompetent elements in the genital mucosa, salivary glands, respiratory tract, pharynx, and mammary glands (1). A striking feature of the mucosal immune system is the presence of large quantities of secretory IgA. Other elements of immunity observed in the bloodstream, such as 7S IgA (serum type), IgG, IgM, T lymphocytes, and components of cell-mediated immunity, are also present in various amounts in different mucosal surfaces and their exosecretions (2).

The bronchial lymphoepithelium, Peyer's patches, and other organized lymphoid follicles present in BALT and GALT are replete with antigen-reactive B-cell precursors, particularly those for IgA (3). Several recent investigations have demonstrated that exposure to antigens in the enteric and respiratory tracts is an essential prerequisite for the initial activation of these cells (1) (3). On the basis of the available information, it is generally believed that, following exposure to antigens, the IgA precursor cells undergo proliferation and differentiation into immunoblasts. The antigen-sensitized immunoblasts migrate to the regional lymph nodes and enter the bloodstream via the thoracic duct. During their traffic through the circulation, these cells appear to seed the mucosal surfaces of the genital tract; the ocular, salivary, and pharyngeal tissues; the mammary glands; the subepithelial regions of the upper and lower respiratory mucosa; and the lamina propria of the intestinal epithelium. At these sites, the cells initiate active synthesis of secretory IgA antibody specific for the sensitizing antigens experienced initially in the respiratory tract or enteric lumen (4).

The importance of local mucosal antigenic stimulation in the respiratory and intestinal tracts has been demonstrated by the observation that the titer of specific IgA antibody to poliovirus is highest in intestinal sites that have direct contact with the poliovirus antigen after segmental colonic immunization of subjects with double-barreled colostomies (5). In other studies, intranasal immunization with inactivated poliovaccine induced a specific nasopharyngeal IgA antibody response, often in the absence of any detectable response in the serum (5). The lack of mucosal antibody-producing plasma cells in germfree animals and in human neonates are other examples of the role of local antigenic exposure in the development of mucosal immunity, since such situations are often associated with a significantly reduced mass of microbial and dietary antigens in the respiratory and enteric membranes.

The concept of the common mucosal immune system derived from BALT or GALT is supported by several independent lines of investigation. Studies by Cebra, et al. (6) have shown that cells from rabbit Peyer's patches, when injected into irradiated allogeneic recipients, selectively distribute within the lamina propria and produce primarily IgA antibody, while cells obtained from peripheral nodes of donors appear to home in the peripheral nodes of the recipients and produce predominantly IgG antibody. Similar observations have been made by Rudzik, et al. (7) and by Bienenstock et al. (8), who noted the homing of bronchial lymphocytes to BALT of the recipient animals. Goldblum, et al. (9) found that intestinal immunization of women with a nonpathogenic strain of Escherichia coli resulted in the development of specific secretory IgA antibody activity in the colostrum and milk, although such antibody activity was not observed after parental inoculation of the killed organism. Subsequent studies have provided clear evidence of transfer of IgA precursor cells from the mesenteric lymph nodes to the mammary glands in mice after induction of lactation (1) (3). These observations suggest a selective transfer of antigen-sensitized cells from GALT and possibly BALT to mammary glands. Recent studies have also indicated a selective homing of the cells from the mesenteric lymph nodes and GALT to the subepithelial regions of the female genital tract, particularly the cervix (2).

CELL VIRUS INTERACTIONS IN THE MUCOSAL IMMUNE SYSTEM

The intestinal and respiratory mucosa are endowed with a very sophisticated cellular network. This includes the epithelium, intraepithelial lymphocytes (IEL), lamina propria lymphocytes (LPL), plasma cells and mucosal mast cells, and the subepithelial lymphoid follicles such as the intestinal Peyer's patches. Recently, considerable information has become available regarding their functional characteristics and the nature of interaction with environmental antigens, including certain microbial and viral agents.

TABLE 1. Potential Sites of Cell-Virus Interactions in Mucosal Tissues

1. Epithelium
2. Intraepithelial lymphocytes (IEL).
3. Lamina propria lymphocytes (LPL).
4. Plasma cells
5. Mucosal mast cells.
6. Organized lymphoid follicles - Peyer's patches.
7. Regional lymph nodes.
8. Liver

EPITHELIUM

The mucosal epithelium appears to be heterogenous in terms of the morphology and function of various cellular components (10) (11). An important prerequisite of the pathogenesis of many human viral infections is the replication on the mucosal epithelium or penetration via the mucosal tissues into the systemic circulation (1). Although the mechanisms underlying the viral attachment, replication and/or penetration in the mucosal surfaces are not well defined, several recent observations have provided interesting clues to the nature of mucosal cell-virus interaction. Studies from Wolf,, et al., (12) have suggested that reovirus spares intestinal epithelial cells during their replicative events, with the exception of M cells, (a unique population of epithelial cells with short microvilli), which overlie the luminal surface of the Peyer's patches (10). The M cells are important in sampling of luminal antigens and in their transport across the epithelium. Reovirus appears to adhere selectively to M cells and based on the internalization of the viruses into the cellular cytoplasm, it has been suggested that M cells are the sites where reoviruses penetrate the intestinal epithelium (12).

On the other hand, rotaviruses appear to infect villous enterocytes with the production of pathologic lesions in the intestinal mucosa (13) (14). Although rotaviruses have been recovered from the fecal specimens of subjects of all age groups, clinical disease appears to be uncommon in the immediate newborn period and in older subjects. The nature of rotavirus-mucosal cell interaction has been recently examined in suckling and adult mice employing orally induced infection with mouse rotavirus (MRV) (15). After such infection, MRV antigen could be demonstrated in up to 30% of enterocytes in suckling mice and little or no viral antigen could be observed in the enterocytes of adult mice (over 26 days of age) infected similarly.

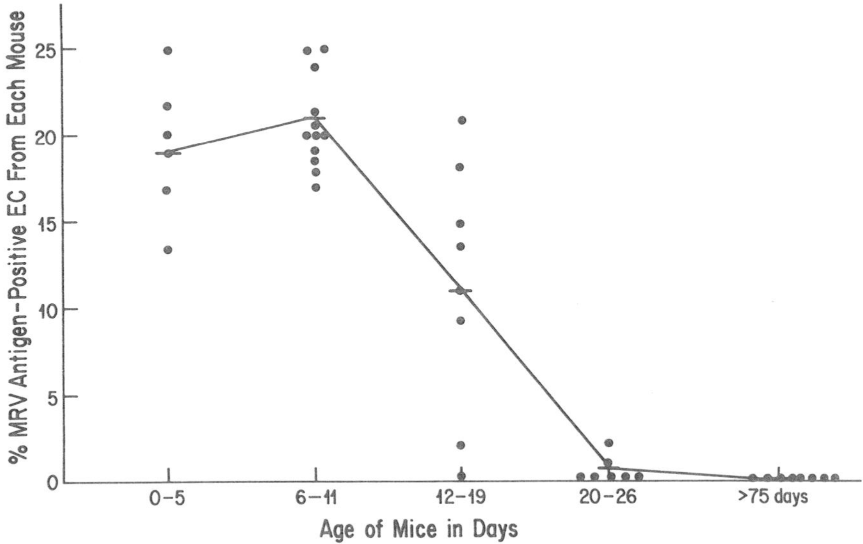

FIGURE 1. Frequency of the enterocytes infected with mouse rotavirus (MRV) after orally induced infection of mice, relative to the age of the animal at the time of infection.

During subsequent studies, isolated dispersed villous enterocytes from uninfected adult or suckling mice were incubated with purified MRV-coated red blood cells. Specific binding of MRV coated RBC to enterocytes as evidenced by formation of rosettes was most pronounced in enterocytes obtained from suckling mice under 10-11 days of age, while only low levels of MRV binding was demonstrable in enterocytes from mice older than 75 days of age. These observations strongly suggest that the degree of virus replication and potential for pathogenicity may be determined by the availability of virus specific receptors on enterocytes.

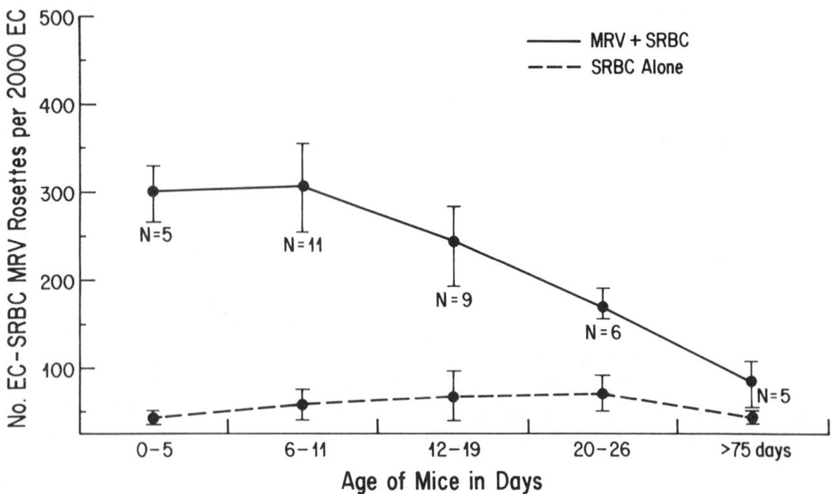

FIGURE 2. Binding of mouse rotavirus (MRV) to uninfected mouse enterocytes as evidenced by rosetting of enterocytes with MRV-coated sheep red blood cells (SRBC), in relationship to the age of the animal at the time of collection of enterocytes.

In addition to virus-specific binding mechanisms, mucosal epithelium is rich in a population of lymphoid cells called intraepithelial lymphocytes (IEL) scattered throughout the epithelium (11) (16) (17). Although their origin is unknown, they appear to be immunologically active and possess a wide spectrum of biologic reactivity. Available information regarding their immunologic properties are summarized in Table 2.

TABLE 2. Characteristics of Mucosal Associated Lymphocytes

Property	Lymphocyte Population Intra-epithelial (IEL)	Lamina propria (LPL)
Cellular Markers		
Mean ± SEM		
T-cells	32±2.0	52±1.3
B-cells	34±2.5	22±1.1
Null cells	34±2.5	26±1.1
IgE Receptors (No. per cell)	>10,000	-
Cytotoxicity in vitro		
ADCC	0	0(+)
SCMC	0	+
MICC	+	+
Natural Killer Cell Activity		
Interferon enhanced	+	-
Antimicrobial Activity		
Antibacterial	+	-
Antiviral	-	-

+ suggestive evidence, 0 - absent
- no available data
(Modified from Chiba, et al., 1981, Tagliabue, 1982, Bienenstock, 1982).

The mucosal lamina propria is replete with plasma cells especially of IgA isotype. In addition, it contains lymphocytes scattered throughout the stroma. The lamina propria lymphocytes (LPL) have not been extensively characterized to date, but seem to differ from IEL as shown in Table 2. No antiviral or antibacterial properties have been attributed to the LPL.

PEYER'S PATCHES

As mentioned previously, a major function of the Peyer's patch (PP) immunocompetent precursor cells is to provide IgA antibody producing cells to the intestinal lamina propria and to other peripheral mucosal surfaces. Recent studies have demonstrated that approximately 40% of PP lymphocytes bear T cell markers. Class specific T suppressor and helper cells have also been observed in Peyer's patches. However, the relative proportion of T suppressor cells appears to predominate (18) (19). The immunologic reactivity of the Peyer's patches differs from other systemic lymphoid tissues (Table 3) and exhibit several limitations in immune responsiveness in in-situ settings (2) as summarized in Table 4.

TABLE 3. Characteristics of Peyer's Patch lymphoid Tissue

Large Lymphocytes
Up to 40% bear T-cell markers, predominance of T suppressors.
Carrier-helper effect in antibody formation.
Cytotoxicity to alloantigen.
Response to alloantigens in MLR, PHA, Con A.
Up to 60% cells L-chain positive, 85% bear surface IgA.
Guy-Grand (1974), McWilliams (1974), Atwater (1978)

TABLE 4. Deficits in Peyer's Patch Immune Reactivity are Characterized by its Inability to:

1. Induce ADCC
2. Mediate optimum GVH
3. Produce antibody to antigen after PO or systemic immunization
4. Present and process antigen by macrophages

Challacombe (1979), Mattingly (1978), Asherson (1977)

ANTIVIRAL ASPECTS OF MUCOSAL IMMUNITY

Role in Protection. The 11S IgA antibody, in association with the secretory component, represents a unique developmental adaptation of immunoglobulins for effective function and optimal survival in the mucosal secretions. Other polymeric immunoglobulins - notably IgM, which is frequently associated with the secretory component - may function similarly, especially in patients with IgA deficiency (20). The monomeric immunoglobulins (IgG, IgD, and IgE), which are present in external secretions in variable amounts, may also function in mucosal defense. Their role in mucosal immunity appears to be secondary and may be apparent especially during states of mucosal inflammation, when their concentrations in the secretions may reach protective levels as a result of increased exudation from the serum antibody pool or following local synthesis in the mucosal tissues (1).

The role of secretory IgA in antibacterial immunity appears to be more complex and less well understood than its role in antiviral immunity. However, several recent investigations have shown that secretory IgA decreases the adhesion of bacteria to the mucous membrane, thereby limiting bacterial colonization and enhancing elimination of the bacteria (23) (24). Based on information obtained with Streptococcus mutans, Vibrio cholerae, and enterotoxin of E. coli, it is now believed that secretory IgA blocks the binding sites on the bacterial cell wall and prevents the attachment of the bacteria or bacterial toxins to the specific receptors on mucosal cell membranes. The secretory antibody has also been shown to effect specific immunity against the uptake of micromolecular and other dietary protein antigens from the intestinal lumen. The elegant studies of Walker and Isselbacher (23) have clearly demonstrated that intestinal antibody interferes with the uptake of nonviable dietary antigens introduced directly into the intestinal lumen in a manner similar to that of viable bacteria. The development of specific antigen-antibody complexes in the glycocalyx appears to prevent the migration of the antigens to the cellular membrane surface (25). This transport arrest may limit the pinocytosis of the antigen by the enterocytes. In other experimental situations, secretory IgA antibody has been observed to interfere with the uptake of serum albumin in the respiratory epithelium. Other studies have shown that secretory IgA, via the formation of immune complexes, increases the degradation of antigens and stimulates the production of mucin by the goblet cells (25). These mechanisms may nonspecifically enhance the elimination of viruses also from the intestinal lumen.

ROLE IN PATHOGENESIS

While it is abundantly clear that secretory IgA antibody is important in determining the course of mucosal infection and uptake of dietary macromolecule, there is appreciable evidence to suggest that protection against illness following viral infection may not be influenced to a great extent by the nature and magnitude of secretory IgA response. For example, studies carried out with respiratory syncytial virus (26) have demonstrated a predictable serum and secretory antibody response following naturally acquired primary or reinfection (Figure 3). However, no significant difference existed for the levels of RSV specific secretory antibody in the nasopharynx between patients with mild illness (upper respiratory infection) and those with more severe disease (bronchiolitis) (26).

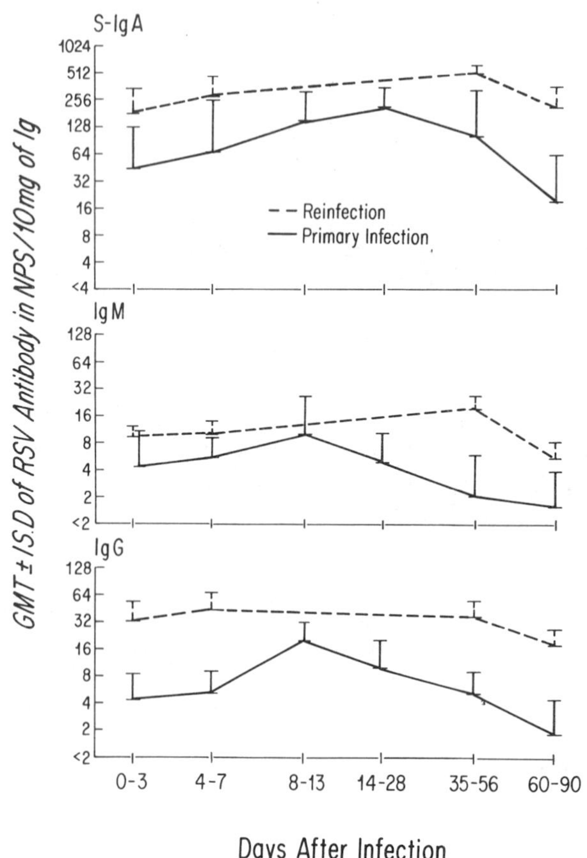

FIGURE 3. Development of antibody response to respiratory syncytial virus (RSV) in nasopharyngeal secretions after primary (-) or reinfection (---) with RSV.

There is no evidence to suggest that secretory IgA antibody has any detrimental role in the pathogenesis or severity of mucosal viral infections, and little information is available about the functional role of other immunoglobulins in the mucosal secretions. During the past few years, several investigators (27-32) have suggested the presence of microbial specific antibody activity in IgE isotype in the serum and in certain select situations in the mucosal secretions (Table 5).

TABLE 5. Antimicrobial Specificity of IgE in Serum or External Secretions

Agent	Presence of IgE Antibody Serum	Presence of IgE Antibody Secretions	Association with Disease	Author
Diptheria toxoid	+	-	-	Nagel (1978)
Tetanus toxoid	+	-	±	Nagel (1978)
Staph. aureus	+	-	±	Schapter(1979)
P. aeruginosa	+	-	-	Shen (1981)
M. pneumoniae	±	-	-	Tipirneni(1980)
Influenza A Vaccine	±	-	-	Michaels(1979
Resp.Syn.Virus	+	+	+	Welliver (1981)
Parainfluenza	-	+	+	Welliver (1982)

+Strong evidence, ± suggestive evidence, - not available.

Recently, studies were carried out by Welliver, et al. (33) (34) in infants and young children with various forms of respiratory illness after infection with respiratory syncytial virus to examine the relation of immune response to the severity of disease. Initial investigations have suggested that most patients with RSV infection exhibit binding of IgE isotype of exfoliated nasopharyngeal epithelium during acute phase of the infection regardless of the severity of the disease. However the continued presence of cell bound IgE was more commonly observed in patients with RSV induced bronchiolitis or asthma than in patients with mild upper respiratory tract infection. Subsequent studies have shown the presence of RSV specific IgE in the nasopharyngeal secretions in most patients with RSV induced reactive airway disease or bronchiolitis. Little IgE antibody to RSV was observed in the secretions of subjects with mild clinical illness without bronchospasm. Furthermore, histamine was detected in some RSV infected patients with all forms of illness. However, it was present significantly more often in and in higher concentration in patients with wheezing. Peak titer of RSV-IgE and concentrations of histamine in nasopharyngeal secretions correlated significantly with the degree of hypoxia. In addition to the alterations in IgE and histamine responses, other studies from Scott, et al., (35) and Welliver, et al. (36) have provided evidence for hyperresponsive pattern of

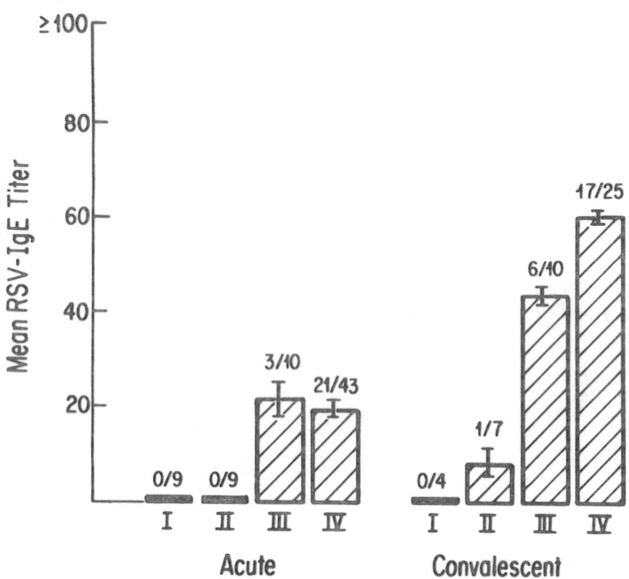

FIGURE 4. Development of IgE response to respiratory syncytial virus (RSV) in the nasopharyngeal secretions. The RSV IgE response is analyzed according to illness group. Group 1 had upper-respiratory-tract disease only, Group II pneumonia without wheezing, Group III pneumonia with wheezing and Group IV bronchiolitis without pneumonia. The acute phase represents the first seven days after the onset of illness, and the convalescent phase the 14th through the 90th day after the onset of illness.

in vitro correlates of RSV specific cell mediated immunity in patients with severe RSV disease. The magnitude of cell mediated immune response in these patients was also correlated with the degree of hypoxia observed during RSV infection (36).

Considerable evidence is available concerning lymphocyte responsiveness and enhanced release of histamine from basophils. Incubation of lymphocytes with viral antigens has been shown to result in release of soluble factor(s) which enhance antigen-induced histamine release from appropriate mediator cells subsequently stimulated with anti-IgE antibody or ragweed antigen E. It has also been suggested that overproduction of IgE in persons with atopy may be due to an imbalance of immunoregulatory T lymphocytes (37-39). Based on these observations, it has been proposed that alterations in T lymphocyte regulatory subsets existing before or at the time of infection with such mucosal viral infections as RSV, and perhaps to other allergens may result in vigorous cellular immune response. Increased elaboration of certain lymphocyte products as a result of such hyperresponsiveness may trigger increased production of specific IgE and thus enhance the release of histamine and possibly other soluble mediators of mucosal damage (34).

REGULATORY ROLE OF MUCOSAL LYMPHOID TISSUE

The classical experiments carried out almost 40 years ago (40) first demonstrated that the oral feeding of a simple chemical such as picryl chloride resulted in hyporesponsiveness to contact hypersensitivity to systemic challenge with the antigen (Chase-Sulzberger phenomenon). More recently, a number of other investigators (41-46) have provided strong evidence for the development of systemic hyporesponsiveness to a variety of antigens administered initially by the oral route (oral tolerance). Available data on the effects of oral vs. systemic priming and challenge on the outcome of systemic or mucosal responses to the challenge exposure are summarized in Table 6. It appears that primary exposure via the oral route with a wide variety of non-replicating antigens or soluble proteins can result in long lasting systemic tolerance. Paradoxically, however, such tolerance is clearly associated with the development of active immune response at the mucosal sites. Systemic tolerance to soluble antigens, haptens and hapten-syngeneic-cell complexes has also been demonstrated after initial exposure by the intravenous route or after continued oral immunization.

Little or no evidence is available regarding the development of systemic tolerance to viral and other replicating agents following mucosal or systemic exposure. Limited field studies carried out by Hanson, et al. (43) in lactating women in Pakistan after immunization with live attenuated poliovaccine have raised the question of mucosal hyporesponsiveness to viral antigens. Oral administration of live poliovaccine in subjects seropositive for polioantibody (presumably as a result of prior natural infection) resulted in a surprisingly significant decrease in preexisting poliovirus specific IgA antibody level in the colostrum and milk, while the level of serum IgG and IgM antibody activity remained unchanged. The possibility of mucosal hyporesponsiveness has also been suggested after systemic priming with cholera antigens (toxoid or LPS) as shown in Table 6. It remains to be determined with certainty whether this observation truly represents mucosal tolerance to infectious agents.

TABLE 6. Effects of the Routes of Priming on the Outcome of Subsequent Re-exposure Challenge

Route of Exposure			Outcome of Challenge		
Priming	Challenge	Antigens	Systemic	Mucosal	Author and Year
Oral	Systemic	Picryl chloride	T	-	Chase (1946)
		SRBC	T	-	Andre (1975)
		OVA	T	(B)?	Challacombe (1980)
		Strep mutans	T	(B)?	Challacombe (1980)
		V.cholerae (LPS)	B	B	Svennerholm (1980)
		AntigenE (ragweed)	T	B	Tomasi (1980)
Systemic	Oral	Poliovirus	B	B	Ogra (1970)
		V.cholera (toxoid)	B	(T)?	Pierce (1980)
			NE	NE	
			T(?)	NE	
Oral	Oral	Polio	B	B	Ogra (1970)
			NE	(T)?	Hanson (1979)
		OVA	T	NE	Tomasi (1980)
		BSA*	T	-	Peri (1981)
Systemic	Systemic	Poliovirus	B	NE	Ogra (1960)
		V. cholerae (LPS)	B	(T)?	Svennerholm (1980)
				NE	
		Haptens	T	-	Claman (1976)
		Hap-syg. cell complex	T	NE	

T=tolerance as evidenced by Ab or DH hyporesponsiveness. B=booster effect, (?) possible effect, NE=no effect, - not available. *Oral priming of lactating dams.

The mechanisms underlying the development of systemic or possible mucosal tolerance remain to be clearly defined, although several possible explanations have been offered

(42). These include removal of immunogenic aggregates by the liver, and presence of antigen-antibody complexes as immunosuppressive factors. However, based on the information summarized above, and the fact that mucosal lymphoid follicles are rich in regulatory (helper and suppressor) T and B activity, it is highly likely that an important primary function of the GALT and possibly the BALT is to limit the development of systemic immune responses without any compromise of the mucosal IgA antibody response. It is reasonably certain that the mucosal immune system is a dynamic immunologic vehicle which operates in a state of equilibrium between the host's internal milieu e.g. hormones, nutrition, age, etc), and the external antigenic environment (e.g. replicating vs. non-replicating, load and patterns of reexposure). Recently Tomasi (42) has proposed that mucosal lymphoid tissues may preferentially produce T suppressor cells for serum IgM, IgG, IgE isotype as well as for delayed hypersensitivity, and T helper cells for the secretory IgA response to soluble proteins. Such regulatory influences may extend to replicating agents under certain circumstances. However, the manner in which different types of regulatory cells are induced in the mucosa may be determined by the inherent nature of the antigen and the predetermined characteristics of its handling by the host. Alterations in mucosal immunoregulatory mechanisms may underlie the mucosal hyporesponsiveness for IgA observed after reexposure to live poliovaccine or for mucosal hyperresponsiveness for IgE demonstrated in patients with RSV induced bronchiolitis.

REFERENCES

1. Ogra, P.L., Fishaut, M. and Gallagher, M.R.: Viral vaccination via the mucosal route. Rev. Infect. Dis. 2:352, 1980.
2. Bienenstock, J. and Befus, A.D.: Mucosal immunology. Immunology 41:249, 1980.
3. Lamm, M.E.: Cellular aspects of immunoglobulin A. Adv. Immunol. 22:223, 1976.
4. Ogra, P.L., Dayton, D.H. Immunology of breast milk. Raven Press, New York, 1979.
5. Ogra, P.L. and Karzon, D.T.: Formation and function of poliovirus antibody in different tissues. Prog. Med. Virol. 13:156, 1971.
6. Cebra, J.J., Crandall, C.A., Gearhart, P.J., Robertson, S.M., Tseng, J., Watson, P.M.: Cellular events concerned with the initiation, expression and control of the

mucosal immune response. In Ogra, P.L. and Dayton, D.H. (ed). Immunology of breast milk. Raven Press, New York, 1979, pp. 1-18.

7. Rudzik, R., Clancy, R.L., Perey, D.Y.E., Day, R.P., Bienenstock, J.: Repopulation with IgA containing cells of bronchial and intestinal lamina popria after transfer of homologous Peyer's patch and bronchial lymphocytes. J. Immunol. 114:1599, 1975.
8. Bienenstock, J., Johnston, N., Perey, D.Y.E.: Bronchial lymphoid tissue I. Morphologic characteristics. Lab. Invest. 28:686, 1973.
9. Goldblum, R.M., Ahlstedt, S., Carlsson, B., Hanson, L.A., Jodal, U., Lidin-Janson, G., Sohl-Akerlund, A.: Antibody forming cells in human colostrum after oral immunization. Nature 257:797, 1975.
10. Owen, R.L. and Jones, A.L.: Epithelial cell specialization within human Peyer's patches: an ultrastructural study of intestinal lymphoid follicles. Gastroenterology 66:189, 1974.
11. Bos, I.R. and Burkhardt, A.: Interepithelial cells of the oral mucosa: Light and electron microscopic observations in germfree, specific pathogen-free and conventionalized mice. J. Oral Pathol. 9:65, 1980.
12. Wolf, J.L., Rubin, D.H., Finberg, R., Kauffman, R.S., Sharpe, A.H., Trier, J.S. and Fields, B.N.: Intestinal M cells: A pathway for entry of reovirus into the host. Science 212:471, 1981.
13. Davidson, G.P., Gall, D.G., Petric, M., Butler, D.G., Hamilton, J.R.: Human rotavirus enteritis induced in conventional piglets. J. Clin. Invest. 60:1402, 1977.
14. Kapikian, A.Z., Kim, H.W., Wyatt, R.G., Rodriguez, W.J., Ross, S., Cline, W.L., Parrott, R.H., Chanock, R.M.: Reovirus-like agent in stools: Association with infantile diarrhoea and development of serologic tests. Science 185:1049, 1974.
15. Riepenhoff-Talty, M., Lee, P-C., Carmody, P.J., Barrett, H.J. and Ogra, P.L.: Age-dependent rotavirus-enterocyte interactions. Proc. Soc. Exp. Biol. Med. (in press).
16. Chiba, M., Bartnik, W., ReMine, S.G., Thayer, W.R., and Shorter, R.G.: Human colonic intraepithelial and lamina proprial lymphocytes: cytotoxicity in vitro and the potential effects of the isolation method on their functional properties. Gut 22:177, 1981.
17. Arnaud-Battendies, F., Bundy, B.M., O'Neill, M., Bienenstock, J., Nelson, D.J.: Cytotoxic activities of gut mucosal lymphoid cells in guinea pigs. J. Immunol. 121:1059, 1978.

18. Guy-Grand, D., Griscelli, C., Vassali, P.: The gut-associated lymphoid system: nature and properties of the large dividing cells. Eur. J. Immunol. 4:435, 1974.
19. McWilliams, M., Lamm, M.E., Philips-Quagliata, J.M.: Surface and intracellular markers of mouse mesenteric and peripheral lymph node and Peyer's patch cells. J. Immunol. 113:1326, 1974.
20. Ogra, P.L.: Ontogeny of the local immune system. Pediatrics 64 (suppl) 765, 1979.
21. Ogra, P.L., Morag, A.: Immunologic and virologic aspects of secretory immune system in human respiratory tract. Dev. Biol. Stand. 28:129, 1975.
22. Ogra, P.L., Morag, A., Tiku, M.L.: Humoral immune response to viral infections. In Notkins, A. L. (ed). Viral Immunology and Immunopathology. Academic Press, New York, 1975, p. 57.
23. Walker, W.A., Isselbacher, K.J.: Intestinal antibodies. N. Engl. J. Med. 297:767, 1977.
24. Williams, R.C., Gibbons, R.J.: Inhibition of bacterial adherence by secretory immunoglobulin A: a mechanism of antigen disposal. Science 177:697, 1972.
25. Walker, W.A., Abel, S.N., Wu, M., Bloch, K.J.: Intestinal uptake of macromolecules. V. Comparison of the in vitro uptake by rat small intestine of antigen-antibody complexes prepared in antibody or antigen excess. J. Immunol. 117:1028, 1976.
26. Kaul, T.N., Welliver, R.C., Wong, D.T., Udwadia, R.A., Riddlesberger, K., Ogra, P.L.: Secretory antibody response to respiratory syncytial virus infection. Amer. J. Dis Child. 135:1013, 1981.
27. McIntosh, K., Ellis, E.F., Hoffman, L.S., et al.: The association of viral and bacterial respiratory infections with exacerbations of wheezing in young asthmatic children. J. Pediat. 82:589, 1973.
28. Nagel, J.E., White, C., Lin, M.S. and Fireman, P.: IgE synthesis in man. II. Comparison of tetanus and diphtheria IgE antibody in allergic and non-allergic children. J. Allerg, Clin. Immunol. 63:308, 1978.
29. Schapfer, K., Baerlocher, K., Price, P., et al.: Staphylococcal IgE antibodies, hyperimmunoglobulienemia E and Staphylococcus aureus infections. New Engl. J. Med. 300:835, 1979.
30. Michaels, A.A., Stevens, M. B. and Adkinson, N.F., Jr.: Detection of influenza vaccine specific IgE. J. Allerg. Clin. Immunol. 63:169, (abstract), 1979.
31. Tipirneni, P., Moore, B.S., Hyde, J.S. and Schauf, V.: IgE antibodies to mycoplasma pneumoniae in asthma and other atopic diseases. Ann. Allergy 45:1, 1980.

32. Shen, J., Brackett, R., Fischer, T., Holder, A., Kellogg, F., Michael, J.G.: Specific Pseudomonas immunoglobulin E antibodies in sera of patients with cystic fibrosis. Infect. Immun. 32:967, 1981.
33. Welliver, R.C., Kaul, T.N. and Ogra, P.L.: The appearance of cell-bound IgE in respiratory-tract epithelium after respiratory-syncytial-virus infection. New Engl. J. Med. 303:1198, 1980.
34. Welliver, R.C., Wong, D.T., Sun, M., Middleton, E., Jr., Vaughan, R.S. and Ogra, P.L.: The development of respiratory syncytial virus specific IgE and the release of histamine in nasopharyngeal secretions after infection. New Engl. J. Med. 305:841, 1981.
35. Scott, R., Kaul, A., Scott, M., Chiba, Y., and Ogra, P.L.: Development in vitro correlates of cell mediated immunity to respiratory syncytial virus infection in humans. J. Infect. Dis. 137:810, 1978.
36. Welliver, R.C., Kaul, A., Ogra, P.L.: Cell mediated immune response to respiratory syncytial virus infection: relationship to the development of reactive airway disease. J. Pediat. 94:370, 1979.
37. Ward, P.A., Dvorak, H.F., Cohen, S., Yoshida, T., Data, R., Selvaggio, S.S.: Chemotaxis of basophils by lymphocyte-dependent and lymphocyte-independent mechanisms. J. Immunol. 114:1523, 1975.
38. Bamzai, A.K., Kretschmer, R.R.: Enhancement of antigen-induced leukocyte histamine release by a mononuclear cell-derived factor. J. Allergy Clin. Immunol. 62:137, 1978.
39. Ida, S., Hooks, J.J., Siraganian, R.P., Notkins, A.L.: Enhancement of IgE-mediated histamine release from human basophils by viruses: role of interferon. J. Exp. Med. 145:892, 1977.
40. Chase, M.W.: Inhibition of experimental drug allergy by prior feeding of the sensitizing agent. Proc. Soc. Exp. Biol. 61:257, 1946.
41. Challacombe, S.J. and Tomasi, T.B., Jr.: Systemic tolerance and secretory immunity after oral immunization. J. Exp. Med. 152:1459, 1980.
42. Tomasi, T.B., Jr.: Oral tolerance. Transplantation 29:353, 1980.
43. Hanson, L.A., Carlsson, B., Cruz, J.R., et al.: Immune response in the mammary gland. In Ogra, P.L., Dayton, D.H. (eds.), Immunology of Breast Milk, Raven Press, New York, 1979, p. 145.
44. Svennerholm, A. M., Hanson, L.A., Holmgren, J., et al.: Different secretory immunoglobulin A antibody responses to cholera vaccination in Swedish and Pakistani women. Infect. Immun. 30:427, 1980.

45. Pierce, N.F.: Suppression of the intestinal immune response to cholera toxin by specific serum antibody. Infect. Immun. 30:62, 1980.
46. Andre, C., Heremans, J.F., Vaerman, J.P., et al.: A mechanism for the induction of immunological tolerance by antigen feeding: antigen-antibody complexes. J. Exp. Med. 142:1509, 1975.

CHAPTER 6

THE ROLE OF COMPLEMENT IN THE ELIMINATION OF VIRUS INFECTION

J.G.P. Sissons

Departments of Medicine and Virology
Royal Postgraduate Medical School
London, England

This volume is primarily concerned with the most effective methods of immunization against viruses. Obviously immunization cannot directly affect the intrinsic efficiency of the complement system - however knowledge of the relative contribution made by complement towards eliminating virus infection might influence decisions about what sort of immune response it is desirable to induce by immunization.

The mechanisms by which the 20 or so proteins of the human complement system interact are now understood in reasonable detail, and the major areas of current interest in complement research are moving towards the molecular genetics and biochemistry of the complement proteins, cellular complement receptors and the role of the system in the induction of the immune response. A schematic outline of the two pathways of complement activation is given in figure 1 and further details are available in recent reviews (1,2).

As is well known, the classical pathway of complement activation is activated when the C1q subunit of the C1 macromolecule binds to IgG or IgM which is either aggregated or complexed with antigen. The activation of C1r and C1s then ensues: C1s sequentially cleaves C4 and C2 with resultant assembly of C4b2b - the classical pathway C3 cleaving enzyme. The activity of C4b2b is restrained by the lability of C2b and to a lesser extent by specific regulatory proteins which inactivate C4 - these are the C4 binding protein and Factor I (Factor I was formerly known as the C3b/C4b inactivator). A schematic outline of the two pathways of complement activation is given in figure 1 and further details are available in recent reviews (1,2).

ISBN 0-12-239980-3

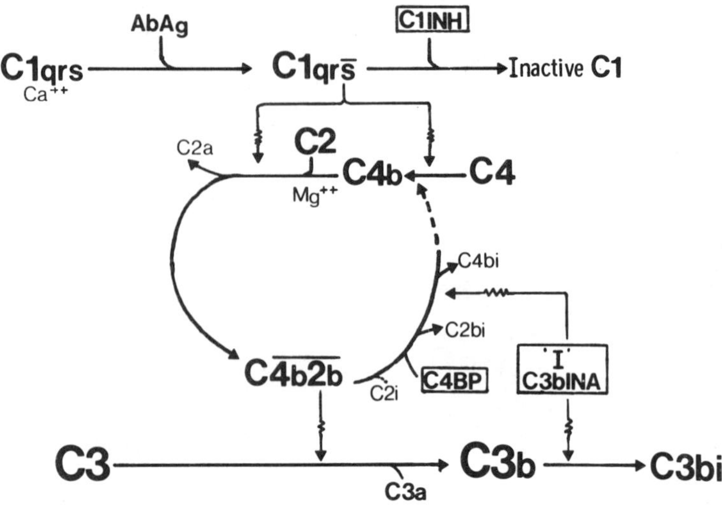

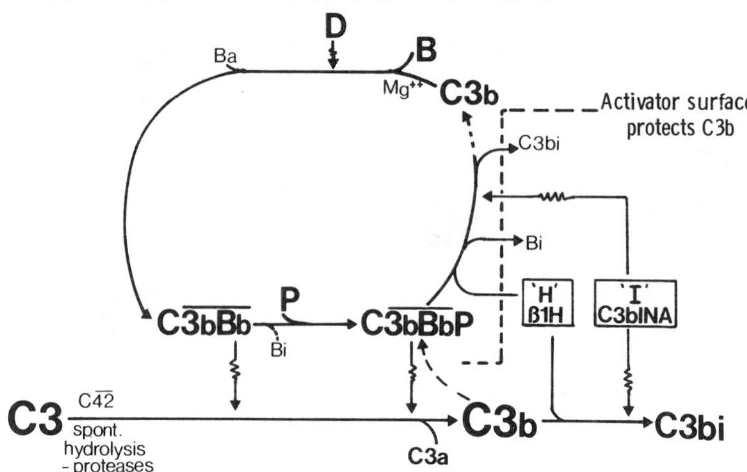

FIGURE 1. Classical Pathway of Complement Activation. Alternative/Amplification Pathway of Complement Activation.

The mechanisms involved in the initiation of the alternative or amplification pathway of complement activation have been clarified by work in the past decade. It appears that C3 undergoes slow spontaneous hydrolysis in plasma with resultant formation of C3b, its major biologically active fragment. This C3b is normally rapidly inactivated in the fluid phase or on the surface of nonactivating particles, by

Factor H and Factor I (formerly designated ß1H and C3b inactivator respectively). However, one property shared by particulate activators of the alternative pathway (e.g. zymoszan, certain gram negative bacteria, erythrocytes of certain species) is that C3b deposited on their surface from the fluid phase is relatively protected from Factor H. This protected C3b can then bind Factor B, which is cleaved by Factor D (a low m.w. serine protease in plasma) to give C3bBb, the C3 cleaving enzyme of the alternative pathway. Its active site is on the 8b fragment and decays rapidly, but the half life of the enzyme is prolonged by properdin (P) which binds to C3b in the bimolecular complex and retards this intrinsic decay. An important point about the alternative pathway is that C3b however generated (whether by the classical pathway, spontaneous hydrolysis, or cleavage of C3 by other proteolytic enzymes) can serve to initiate the amplification of C3 cleavage by the pathway - which is thus a powerful biological positive feedback loop. This emphasizes the importance of the regulatory proteins Factors H and I, as in their absence trivial amounts of C3b may result in unrestrained activation of the pathway. Factor H acts by competitively dissociating Factor B from the C3bB complex and Factor I then cleaves the alpha chain of the C3b molecule, causing its irreversible inactivation.

Following cleavage of C3 further C3b molecules may be incorporated into either C3bBb or C4b2b, giving $C3b_{(n)}Bb$ or C4b2b3b, and C5 cleaving activity is then acquired. Following C5 cleavage, sequential nonenzymatic binding of C6-9 to C5b results in assembly of C5b-9 to form the membrane attack complex (MAC) which inserts into the lipid bilayer of cell membranes producing the familiar complement membrane lesion. Indeed the MAC in isolated form resembles an individual membrane lesion in its ultrastructure.

Experimental work on the role of complement in eliminating virus infection has concentrated on (1) the ability of complement to neutralize virus in the fluid phase, either with antibody or independent of it. (2) the ability of complement to lyse virus infected cells in vitro and (3) the effects of complement depletion or genetic deficiency on handling of virus infections in vivo. From this work evidence has emerged that complement dependent mechanisms can certainly operate to destroy virus and virus infected cells in vitro - however in this author's opinion there is as yet insufficient evidence to justify the assignment to complement of an absolutely necessary role in the clearance of virus infections in humans.

COMPLEMENT DEPENDENT LYSIS AND NEUTRALISATION OF FREE VIRUS

Complement can enhance the antibody dependent fluid phase neutralisation of virus - this observation has been made for a number of different viruses and the loss of viral infectivity may result from aggregation of viral particles, prevention of virus adsorbing to cellular receptors, and (in vivo) opsonizing virus for phagocytosis by cells with C3b receptors. If the virus is enveloped, then it may actually be lysed by antibody and complement and this has been directly demonstrated by electron microscopy for several viruses.

Some viruses can activate complement independently of antibody. Interest in this phenomenon first arose over 30 years ago, when it was shown that influenza, mumps and NDV were neutralised by normal non-immune serum, and later studies with NDV following on the early description of the alternative pathway suggested its involvement in this phenomenon (3,4). Other more recent work has confirmed that NDV can be inactivated by the alternative pathway (5). Studies with Sindbis virus have shown that it can activate both classical and alternative pathways in non-immune serum - this work also suggested that the cell in which the virus was grown influenced the extent to which the virus activated the alternative pathway. It was postulated that this correlated with the extent of sialylation of the viral glycoproteins as determined by the host cell, an analogy being made with other alternative pathway activators where removal of sialic acid residues results in a decreased ability of Factor H to bind to C3b deposited on the particle's surface, and pathway activation (6). It has been clearly shown that murine retro-viruses can activate the classical pathway in human serum by directly binding Clq, independent of antibody (7). They do not activate the classical pathway in murine (or guinea pig) serum - it was suggested this might be a factor explaining the failure to isolate retro-viruses in humans, but this was before the recent description of the human T leukaemia virus. Indeed it is unclear how pertinent any of these observations on antibody independent effects of complement on viruses are to what happens in vivo. The role of complement in humoral immunity to viruses has been thoroughly reviewed elsewhere and full details should be sought there (8,9).

LYSIS OF VIRUS INFECTED CELLS BY COMPLEMENT

Immunologists' interest in the elimination of virus infection tends to focus on the lysis of virus infected cells and particularly on the role of virus specific T cells. However, what is the evidence that complement plays any role in lysing virus infected cells?

There is abundant evidence that virus infected cells can by lysed by antibody and complement in vitro. Much work has been done using heterologous serum as a source of complement, this makes analysis of the mechanism of complement activation in the system more difficult particularly because such serum may contain natural antibody to the cell surface and hence the observations are of less potential relevance to the human situation. However, human serum will lyse cells infected with a variety of different viruses (influenza, measles, herpes viruses) if specific anti-viral antibody and a functional complement system are present. Most of the work discussed hereafter in this section is that of Oldstone and colleagues (10,11,12). They found that integrity of the alternative pathway of complement activation was necessary for human serum to lyse virus infected cells - cells (of epithelial, neuronal and lymphoblastoid origin) infected with the above viruses lyse in the presence of antibody and C2 deficient or C4 depleted serum but not in factor B depleted serum (10). After these observations appeared to establish the generality of the phenomenon we undertook a mechanistic analysis of this dependence on the alternative pathway for lysis using measles virus infected Hela cells as a representative model. Obviously a principal question was why lysis was dependent on antibody and the alternative pathway, when antibody is known to activate complement by binding C1q in the classical pathway of complement activation.

It was clearly confirmed that lysis of virus infected cells could be mediated by the alternative pathway alone by using the purified cytolytic alternative pathway - a system composed solely of the 6 purified proteins of the alternative pathway and the 5 proteins of the MAC (B,D,P,C3,I,H, and C5-9) all at physiological concentration and capable of mediating the functions of the pathway in serum (13). Antibody coated measles infected cells were lysed with a dose response curve similar to that given by C4 depleted serum. Large amounts of IgG antibody ($5x10^6$ molecules bound per cell) were required to produce lysis but the F(ab)2 fragment was as effective as the whole IgG molecule. However, antibody was not actually required for activation of the alternative pathway to occur on the surface of measles virus infected cells. ^{125}I C3b was specifically taken up from the purified alternative pathway of complement activation (B,D,C3,P,I and H) on to infected cells in the absence of antibody, but no lysis occurred (14). Thus the virus infected cell could activate the alternative pathway independent of antibody, but why was antibody required for lysis? Examination of the kinetics of ^{125}I C3 uptake in the absence and presence of antibody showed that C3 uptake was considerably accelerated in the presence of IgG antibody bound to the surface of virus infected cell. Presumably the accelerated C3 uptake increases the number of lytic sites on the cell membrane, and this overwhelms the membrane repair mechanisms of the cell, facilitating its eventual lysis (15). Subsequently it has been shown that surface bound IgG can increase the uptake of C3 on to other known activators of the alternative pathway (rabbit erythrocytes, zymosan), although the molecular basis for this effect is uncertain.

There is work to suggest that cells infected with other viruses (herpes, certain murine retro-viruses) may also activate the alternative pathway independent of antibody. Various lymphoblastoid cell lines also activate the alternative pathway and the ability to do this correlates with their transformation by EB virus (15, reviewed in 11). However the precise membrane structures responsible for the alternative pathway activation in all these various systems, whether the actual viral glycoproteins or other virus specified or virus induced structures, remain to be identified. Nevertheless the process of cell surfaces altered by virus activating the alternative pathway is in accord with the general emerging concept of the alternative pathway as a system of non-specific host defence, which can discriminate between normal host surfaces and those which have been modified by microbial infection or in other ways, or completely foreign structures.

Although relatively large amounts of surface bound IgG antibody are required for lysis of virus infected cells in the above systems it should be emphasized that lysis of virus infected cells by this alternative pathway and antibody dependent mechanism does occur in whole human serum from immune individuals. Furthermore although the classical pathway of complement activation cannot mediate lysis by itself, it is nevertheless activated on the cell surface; however, presumably without the amplification effect of the alternative pathway insufficient lytic sites are created.

ROLE OF COMPLEMENT IN CLEARANCE OF VIRUS INFECTION IN VIVO

It is important to distinguish between the evidence that

complement mediates the immunopathology of virus infections, and that complement plays a necessary role in their elimination. Experimental evidence favouring a role for complement in recovery from virus infection comes from work in which C3 depleted (by cobra venom factor treatment) or C5 deficient mice developed more severe influenza pneumonia with higher mortality, than did control mice (16). CVF treated mice inoculated with Sindbis virus developed more prolonged viremia and higher titres of virus in the brain than controls with intact complement systems, although actual mortality from the infection was not significantly different between the two groups in this particular study (17).

An analysis of the role of complement in the resolution of viral infections in man is made possible by the existence of subjects with genetic dificiencies of complement components. Isolated deficiency of every component of the classical pathway (C1q through C9) has now been described - affected individuals are generally homozygous for a null gene (reviewed in 18). There does appear to be a higher incidence of disease in deficient subjects that is not simply a result of patients with disease being more likely to have their complement measured; nevertheless some deficiencies, particularly C2 deficiency, are compatible with apparently normal health in a proportion of affected subjects (nearly 50% for C2).

The clinical syndromes associated with complement deficiency fall broadly into 3 groups. Patients deficient in components of the classical pathway of complement activation C1q, C1r, C1s C4 or C2 have an increased incidence of "immune complex" diseases, particularly systemic lupus erythematosus and glomerulonephritis; the reasons for this are unknown but the classical pathway of complement activation can solubilize immune complexes in vitro, preventing formation of immune precipitates and it is possible that absence of this function in vivo may impair the clearance of immune complexes. Subjects deficient in C3, or with factor I or H deficiency which results in secondary depletion of C3 consequent upon unrestrained activation of the amplification loop, are prone to repeated bacterial infections rather like agammaglobulinaemic subjects. Finally some patients with deficiencies of components of the membrane attack complex C5-9, and some of the factor I deficient patients, come to notice because of recurrent or disseminated Neisserial infections. One family with properdin deficiency has recently been reported, also presenting with Neisserial infections. Thus far no convincing evidence of a necessary role for complement in eliminating virus infections in humans is provided by these genetic complement deficiencies, unless one speculates that immune complex disease in subjects with C1, C4, and C2 efficiency could result from persistent infection with (so far unidentified!) viruses.

The evidence that complement can be involved in the immunopathology of virus infections is substantial, although not the principal subject of this review. In human (and animal) virus infections it is in situations where immune complexes of antibody and viral antigens circulate and deposit in tissues that evidence of complement activation and tissue deposition also occurs - hepatitis B is a prime example, but systemic complement activation has been demonstrated in primary EBV infection and measles. The complement activation accompanying Dengue shock syndrome is probably important in producing some of the clinical effects, and again results in part from circulating immune complexes.

These are the facts (or some of them at least) - the extent to which they influence the desire to induce antibody by immunisation, in order to engage the complement system, is left to the reader.

REFERENCES

1. Muller-Eberhard HJ, Schreiber RD (1980). The alternative pathway of complement activation. Adv. Immunol. 29:285-310.
2. Lachman PJ, Peters DK. Complement in Clinical Aspects of Immunology. (Blackwell Scientific) 1982.
3. Ginsberg HS, Horsfall FL (1949). A labile component of normal serum combines with various viruses. Neutralization of infectivity and inhibition of hemagglutination by the component. J. Exp. Med. 90:475-495.
4. Wedgewood RJ, Ginsberg HS, Pillemer L (1956). The properdin system and immunity. VI. The inactivation of Newcastle disease virus by the properdin system. J. Exp. Med. 104:707-725.
5. Welsh RM (1977) Host cell modification of lymphocytic choriomengitis virus and Newcastle disease virus altering viral inactivation by human complement. J. Immunol. 118:348-354.
6. Hirsch RL, Winkelstein JA, Griffin DE (1980). The role of complement in viral infections. III. Activation of the classical and alternative complement pathways by Sindbis virus. J. Immunol. 124:2507-2510.
7. Bartholomew RM, Esser AF, Muller-Eberhard HJ (1978). Lysis of oncornaviruses by human serum, isolation of the viral complement (C1) receptor and identification as P15E. J. Exp. Med. 147:844-853.

8. Cooper NR, Welsh RM (1979). Antibody and complement-dependent viral neutralization. Springer Semin Immunopathol 2:285-310.
9. Hirsch RL (1982). The complement system - its importance in the host response to viral infection. Microbiol. Rev. 46:71.
10. Perrin LH, Joseph BS, Cooper NR, Oldstone MBA (1976). Mechanism of injury of virus infected cells by antiviral antibody and complement: participation of IgG, F)ab)$_2$ and the alternative complement pathway. J. Exp. Med. 143:1027-1038.
11. Sissons JGP, Oldstone MBA (1980). The antibody mediated destruction of virus infected cells. Adv. Immunol. 29:209-260.
12. Sissons JGP, Oldstone MBA (1980). Killing of virus-infected cells: the role of antiviral antibody and complement in limiting virus infection. J. Infec. Dis. 142:442-448.
13. Sissons JGP, Schreiber RD, Perrin LH, Cooper NR, Oldstone MBA, Muller-Eberhard HJ (1979). Lysis of measles virus infected cells by the purified cytolytic alternative complement pathway and antibody. J. Exp. Med. 150:445-454.
14. Sissons JGP, Oldstone MBA, Schreiber RD (1980). Antibody independent activation of the alternative complement pathway by measles virus infected cells. Proc. Natl. Acad. Sci. USA 77:559-562.
15. McConnell I, Klein G, Lint TF, Lachman PJ (1980). Activation of the alternative complement pathway by human B cell lymphoma lines is associated with Epstein-Barr virus transformation of the cells. Eur. J. Immunol. 8:453-458.
16. Hicks JT, Ennis FA, Kim E, Verbonitz M (1978). The importance of anintact complement pathway in recovery from a primary viral infection. Influenza in decomplemented and in C5-deficient mice. J. Immunol. 121:1437-1445.
17. Hirsch RL, Griffin DE, Winkelstein JA (1980). The role of complement in viral infections. II. The clearance of Sindbis virus from the bloodstream and central nervous system of mice depleted of complement. J. Infect. Dis. 141:212-217.
18. Lachmann PJ, Rosen FS (1979). Genetic defects of complement in man. Springer Semin. Immunopathol. 1:339-353.

CHAPTER 7

THE IMMUNE BASIS FOR HYPERSENSITIVITY TO VIRAL VACCINES

David T. Karzon

Department of Pediatrics
School of Medicine
Vanderbilt University
Nashville, Tennessee

Hypersensitivity, or as it will be used here, paradoxical response to immunization, has been a problem in the course of development of several vaccines in the past 20 years. In these situations, rather than prevention, immunization has resulted in an exaggerated or exalted response when the agent is next encountered. In each instance the phenomenon was unexpected. The impact upon subsequent thinking and research directions has been significant. First, because pathogenetic mechanism(s) of these untoward responses remain uncertain, there has been renewed vigor in the pursuit of an understanding of the elements of the immune process, especially as related to immunopathology. Second, and in a more pragmatic sense, there has been a shift in interest away from inactivated vaccines to the development of live attenuated strains or purified viral subunit vaccines, at least for viruses of certain groups.

This report will address two inactivated virus vaccines in some detail, measles virus (MV) and respiratory syncytial virus (RSV) (1). Two non-viral vaccines trachoma and Mycoplasma pneumoniae, demonstrate certain analogous features. A similar phenomenon was noted to occur with several low potency, inactivated viral and rickettsial vaccines, although no data were given (2). It is not at all clear that mechanisms are similar in all instances. In fact, it would be expected that the details of the clinical expression of the altered response would vary with the biology of the agent and the pathogenesis of disease expression.

Circumstances of the paradoxical reactions following inactivated measles and RSV vaccines will be described and mechanisms which have been suggested by various investigators will be recounted. Mechanisms which have been suggested to

ISBN 0-12-239980-3

date are not fully satisfying and in this light an effort will be made to reconstruct events which have occurred in man in the language of current mouse immunology.

INACTIVATED MEASLES VACCINE (KV-M)

In the early 1960's, inactivated (or killed) measles virus vaccine (KV-M) was introduced. MV was grown in monkey kidney, chick fibroblast or dog kidney cell culture, concentrated, inactivated with formalin and alum adjuvant added. The vaccines elicited an antibody response and immediate protection in more than 90% of seronegative individuals following 2-3 monthly doses of KV-M with or without a dose of live attenuated measles vaccine (LV-M) within 1-2 months(3-9).

The level of circulating antibody was near that seen in natural infection as measured in CF, HAI or neutralizing antibody systems. Little measles specific sIgA was produced (10). Natural challenge with wild measles virus up to 2 years after immunization demonstrated complete protection or mild illness and a brisk antibody response. The vaccine was licensed and used quite widely in the U.S. It then came as a surprise when reports of adverse reactions appeared four to five years after immunization with KV-M. These reactions took two forms, one associated with natural measles virus reinfection, the second associated with local reactions following subcutaneous injection of LV-M.

PARADOXICAL REACTIONS FOLLOWING NATURAL INFECTION IN CHILDREN PREVIOUSLY VACCINATED WITH KV-M

Beginning in the mid-1960's a syndrome has been recognized which appears two or more years after immunization with KV-M, variously termed atypical, exaggerated or enhanced measles reaction (11,15). The reaction is marked by high fever, tachypnea, myalgia and prostration and often requires hospitalization. Other symptoms include cough, dyspnea, pleuritic chest pain, coryza, abdominal pain, nausea and vomiting. A striking exanthem is present characterized by maculopapular rash with urticaria, purpura, petechial and vesicular lesions. The rash begins and is heaviest on the extremities, especially the legs, and tends to spare the head, neck and trunk unlike natural measles. Edema of the hands and feet is often conspicuous. Pneumonia is frequent, occasionally severe and is characterized by bilateral lymphadenopathy, pleural effusion and unique circumscribed infiltrates or nodular densities which may persist for more than two years (15,16). The constellation of pulmonary findings, especially nodules is unusual and does not occur in natural measles. Eosinophilia has been reported.

REACTIONS FOLLOWING LV-M IN CHILDREN PREVIOUSLY VACCINATED WITH KV-M

Parenteral administration of LV-M given at a later date and not part of the initial monthly series has resulted in moderate to severe local and occasional systemic reactions (17-20). The latter include fever, morbilliform rash and malaise.1 Local reactions consist of erythema, induration, swelling and vesicle formation. The reactions are delayed, with onset 2-6 days after inocluation and persist for 3-7 days, which is unlike the early (6-24 hours) reactions following many vaccine products. These reactions do not occur in an unprimed child.

Thus it appears that immunization with multiple doses of KV-M established an altered immune state in which reintroduction of wild or attenuated measles virus results in an unusual pathological response. The interval between inactivated vaccine and live virus appears to be critical. In general, the local or systemic response occurs several years after initial sensitization and this altered immune state may be lifelong. The longest interval is recorded at 14 years (21).

In a study of the long-term effects of KV-M on the altered immune state, 75 adolescents were revaccinated with LV-M at an interval of 11 to 14 years (20). Ten individuals (13%) had moderate to severe local reactions. The pre-reimmunization determinants of reactions are of interest: 1) low or undetectable circulating antibody 2) a short interval between KV-M and LV-M in the primary series, two months or less and 3) a high level of measles specific sensitized peripheral blood lymphocytes. The latter 3-4 times higher than in individuals with a history of natural measles infection and appeared to be the single most important predictor of reactions. The complement levels were normal in individuals with reactions when measured three weeks after revaccination and in fact were high in five individuals with paradoxical measles during the exanthem stage. An important finding is the apparent "suppression" of lymphocyte stimulation response in individuals given LV-M $\geq$ 3 months after the KV-M series. It has been suggested that serum antibody suppresses lymphocyte activation (22).

POSSIBLE MECHANISMS OF KV-M PARADOXICAL RESPONSE

Several explanations have been offered concerning the mechanism of the paradoxical responses observed.

1. Delayed Type Hypersensitivity (DTH). Children immunized with KV-M demonstrate a positive skin test when tested with measles virus antigen intradermally (23). This is in contrast to the negative skin test in individuals who have had natural measles infection or were immunized with LV-M only. Positive skin tests are obtained using living or inactivated measles antigen and measles virus prepared in cells of homologous or heterologous species. Dermal DTH persists for many years and is frequently present in individuals who have little or no circulating antibody. To confuse this picture positive skin tests have been described in recipients of KV-M using inactivated poliovirus prepared in monkey kidney cells or mumps vaccine prepared in chick embryo fibroblasts (23-26). The latter phenomenon has been ascribed to host tissue sensitization, although the cross antigens are not defined. The presence of alum adjuvant may be significant in the production of DTH. The conjugation of adjuvants with immunogens has been shown to be capable of altering determinants which selectively enhance DTH versus antibody production (27).

Examination of the pulmonary lesion histologically and by immunofluorescence would be instructive, although there has been no opportunity for this.

2. Arthus Phenomenon. The local indurated lesion following immunization with LV-M in a previously KV-M recipient was biopsied and studied by light microscopy and immunofluorescence. An inflammatory infiltrate of lymphocytes, monocytes and neutrophils was observed surrounding blood vessels. IgG,C3 and measles antigen were deposited in blood vessels, findings consistent with an Arthus phenomenon (28). It should be noted that other studies have not been able to demonstrate reduction of circulating C.

The following series of events was hypothesized (28). (a) KV-M produces circulating antibody but not sIgA (10). (b) Wild virus in this circumstance can replicate on mucosal surfaces and spread systemically resulting in a rapid secondary response. Injury is initiated by virus-antibody immune complex localized in the skin and respiratory tract or at the local site of LV-M adminstration.

3. Absence of Fusion (F) Protein in KV-M. Two glycoprotein antigens are associated with MV membrane, fusion (f) protein and hemagglutinin (HA). The F protein is also an hemolysin (HL). Formalin treatment destroys the functional and antigenic integrity of the fusion/hemolysin protein. The F protein is also absent in the Tween-ether preparation of purified HA vaccine which was used in Europe (29,30,31). These preparations result in high titers of hemagglutinin inhibiting (HAI) antibody but are deficient in hemolysin inhibiting (HLI) antibody. Antibody engendered by natural infection or LV-M which does contain HLI is 50-100x more efficient in providing the same level of protection for a given HAI or neutralization content.

In situations other than in recipients of KV-M even a trace amount of measles antibody in the circulation, passively administered as human immune globulin, via blood transfusion or transplacentally is protective or acts as a modifier. The pathogenesis of natural measles infection invovles as obligatory viremia and any measurable amount of antibody which is the result of natural measles infection should be protective. Thus it would appear that measles antibody deficient in anti-F protein is qualitatively different and less efficient in preventing and/or terminating infection. This has been shown in monkeys (32) and in children. A further observation is of interest. Children who received purified HA vaccine, followed by LV-M failed to develop HLI antibody in most instances and even where natural infection followed HA vaccine, there was a poor HLI response (30). It is suggested that the presence of antibody against one of the two surface structural proteins, HA, but not the F protein may set up conditions for an Arthus reaction.

INACTIVATED RSV VACCINE (KV-RS)

A formalin inactivated, concentrated, alum precipitated RSV vaccine grown in monkey kidney cells was studied in four separate field trials. Children five months to ten years of age received two to three doses at monthly intervals. Most seronegative children seroconverted. Vaccinees were challenged in a natural outbreak of RSV one to nine months later. Children immunized with trivalent parainfluenza virus vaccine with or without alum served as controls in some of the trials (34,35,36,37,38).

No protection was evident and the rate of infection in KV-RS vaccinees was not different from the control group. However, the clinical manifestations were paradoxically altered in two ways. (1) The disease expression was more severe and (2) Reinfection disease occurred in children who were somewhat older than the usual peak incidence. For example, in one study (34) 80% of reinfected KV-RS vaccinees required hospitalization and two infants died. Virus was recovered from lung tissue which showed typical bronchiolitis. This may be compared to children receiving an identically prepared parainfluenza vaccine where 5% of RSV infection required hospitalization and there were no deaths. The age effect was unusual in that serious lower respiratory tract disease was frequent in vaccinees who were over six months of age with severe bronchiolitis and pneumonia typically associated with younger infants.

MECHANISMS OF KV-RS PARADOXICAL RESPONSE

Various mechanisms for the KV-RS paradoxical effect have been suggested.

(1) Delayed type hypersensitivity (DTH). Following RSV infection, lymphocyte transformation response to RSV antigen can be demonstrated quite regularly in peripheral blood T cells (39,40,41). The response is evident during actue infection, attains peak levels at two months and falls by five or six months. It thus appears to be transient at least in primary infection. The response is more frequent and vigorous under six months of age and also in patients with severe clinical bronchiolitis or later recurrence of asthma (40,41). There is some overlapping of patients in these age and diagnostic categories. There is a relative "impairment" of antibody response in younger infants in the same group who respond vigorously by lymphocyte transformation (42). RSV specific lymphocyte transformation was studied 2-14 months after immunization with KV-RS or parainfluenza vaccine in one of the original field trials (43). KV-RS immunized children had a more vigorous response than children who had undergone natural infection and equalled that seen in control adults who presumably had experienced multiple infections. It is suggested that while lymphocyte sensitization is not determinative of protection against RSV disease it may contribute to the paradoxical response. It was speculated that transplacentally conferred antigen-specific lymphocyte sensitization may contribute to the pathogenesis of primary infection in young infants. The possibility of maternal transfer of lymphocyte sensitization to several antigens has been described (44,45).

Studies of dermal DTH were not performed in KV-RS vaccinees. Immunization of guinea pigs with KV-RS vaccines prepared in several cell types were sensitized to RSV and also heterologous host cell components. The addition of alum or DPT intensified the dermal test reactions (46). The data parallel the findings in children immunized with KV-M.

2. Arthus Phenomenon. A single explanation was sought for the pathogenesis of natural disease, typically bronchiolitis appearing at 2-6 months of age, in the presence of transplacental antibody, and the events associated with KV-RS. On this basis it has been postulated that the disease results from interaction of serum antibody and RSV antigen in the respiratory tract mucosa of an individual who lacks sIgA. This can occur in the first six months of life in the presence of circulating maternal IgG or following KV induced parenteral antibody. The final pathway may involve an Arthus reaction (47,48).

Prospective studies, on the other hand, have suggested a relative protection of high levels of maternal antibody especially against pneumonia and do not clearly incriminate passive antibody in a pathogenetic role (49,50). The mucosal antibody response has proven difficult to measure by the neutralization test. By immunofluorescent technique specific RSV antibody has been shown to be transient. sIgA antibody appears in secretions within three days of primary RSV infection and IgM and IgG appear within two weeks. All classes disappear by 10-12 weeks. Reinfection results in a booster effect. IgA titers are lower and appear later in infants less than six months of age (51,52).

Gardner (53) examined the lungs of two cases of bronchiolitis and one case of pneumonia who died of RSV. Low concentrations of infectious virus, viral antigen and human globulin were found in bronchiolitis while in pneumonia there was a high titer of virus and antigen but absence of human globulin. He suggests the findings in bronchiolitis to be compatible with an Arthus phenomenon while in pneumonia lesions to be due to direct viral damage. Complement was apparently not sought in this study but was not detected in pathological material in a later report (47). Also, complement levels in serum are not altered in the course of the disease (54).

3. Anaphylaxis. An immediate (type 1) allergic reaction was an alternative mechanism proposed by Gardner. A prior sensitizing infection was presumed but no evidence has since buttressed this line of reasoning.

While serum IgE is not elevated during RSV bronchiolitis, interest has centered on the possibility of IgE in the respiratory tract as a pathogenetic mechanism. IgE was found bound to exfoliated nasopharyngeal cells regularly in the acute phase of RSV infection but was more common and persistent in bronchiolitis or asthma than in mild URI or pneumonia (55). The availability of IgE in the respiratory tract is compatible with a type I allergic reaction, manifest in the wheezing which characterizes severe bronchiolitis. An acute rise of RSV-IgG4 in serum may also be significant in the genesis of bronchiolitis due to bronchospasm (56).

IMMUNOLOGICAL SETTING FOR THE PARADOXICAL RESPONSE

The circumstances involved in the paradoxical response to KV-RS and KV-M have certain common features. These will be reviewed, attempting to identify cogent characteristics of the vaccine and the induced disease process.

TABLE 1. Common Features of Inactivate Measles and RSV Vaccines

1. Formalin inactivated
2. Concentrated, multiple doses
3. Alum adjuvant
4. Membraned virus
5. Fusion protein

Both RS and M virus vaccines were formalin inactivated, highly concentrated and contained alum adjuvant (Table 1). Each was administered in multiple doses. The measles virus F-protein is functionally inactivated and rendered non-antigenic by the formalin treatment. While an RSV specific fusion protein has not been demonstrated, it may be assumed to be represented on the membrane and function in cell fusion. Presumably it is inactivated by formalin as well.

Following KV-M or KV-RS, exposure to infectious virus allows successful reinfection and replication (Table 2). Reinfection in measles must await the fall of circulating antibody to low levels. RSV as a restricted surface infection can successfully replicate during the following annual epidemic, not dampened by circulating antibody.

TABLE 2. Setting for Paradoxical Response*

1. Altered antigen presented to immunologically virgin host.
2. Permissive reinfection.
3. Induction of altered immune state.
    a. inadequate sIgA antibody.
    b. short 1/2 life serum antibody.
    c. qualitatively deficient serum antibody.
    d. increased CMI activity in peripheral blood lymphocytes.
    e. persistent dermal delayed type hypersensitivity.

*A second doctrine of "original antigenic sin"

Reinfection takes place in an altered immune setting. KV does not stimulate mucosal antibody. The serum antibody falls rapidly and at least in the case of measles, is qualitatively handicapped. Despite poor humoral antibody protection, an altered cell mediated immune state is shown by a high lymphocyte transformation response and an aberrantly positive skin test to homologous virus.

It is highly likely that induction of the altered immune state by KV has occurred in immunologically virgin infants and children. Thus the initial presentation of viral antigen to the host is in a physicochemically changed state. This inappropriate perturbation of the immune system may be long lasting and influence all subsequent secondary immune responses.

STUDIES IN THE MOUSE

Given the setting for successful reinfection after KV, an explanation for the exalted pathology is required. Several observations gained from study of viral infection in the mouse model may be contributory to our thinking. Preliminary studies in man reveal significant parallels.

The method of presenting antigen to the immune system clearly has significant implications for the nature of the immune response. The events leading to immune recovery from viral infection and/or the generation of immune pathology constitute a finely balanced network of antigen-cell and cell-cell interactions. In particular, we may draw some generalities concerning the manner in which infectious virus interacts with the immune system compared to inactivated virus. Infectious virus induces a favorable balance of cytotoxic T cells compared to T cells mediating DTH (Td cells). Inactivated virus can induce an exalted DTH response. Both physical forms of virus produce serum antibody. Sendai virus, a natural mouse paramyxovirus pathogen and influenza, an orthomyxovirus readily adaptable to the mouse have been studied extensively. These studies have been reviewed recently (57-65).

Effector T cells are governed by dual specificity for foreign antigen plus a defined region of the major histocompatibility complex. Thus in the mouse there are two subsets of T cells, one H-2 K,D region restricted and the second H-2 IA region restricted. The form of presentation of the virus antigen appears to determine the T cell subset which is stimulated (Table 3) (57).

TABLE 3.

Virus Induction	Subset	H2 Sharing Requirement	Lyt Phenotype	Functional Activity Tc	Td	Th	Ts
LV	1	K,D	1-2+3+	+	+	-	-
LV,KV	2	IA	1+2-3-	-	+	+	-
LV,KV	3	ND	1+2-3-	-	-	-	+

LV=infectious virus (live vaccine)
KV=inactivated virus (killed vaccine)
Tc=cytotoxic T cell, cell mediated lysis (CML)
Td=delayed type hypersensitivity (DTH)
Th=helper T cell
Ts=suppressor T cell
ND=not fully determined

*Ada, et al., Imm. Rev. 58, 5, 1981.

Phenotypic Lyt 23+ cells recognize antigen in association with the K,D restriction site while Lyt 1+ cells recognize antigen in association with the IA site. Fusion of viral membrane with insertion of viral coded glycoproteins into target cell membrane determines a response which is largely K,D region restricted. When viral membrane antigens cannot be incorporated into T cell membrane, processing by macrophage is required, specifying IA region restriction. This is clearly seen with Sendai virus which bears a specific membrane fusion (F) protein. Infectious Sendai virus (F+) activates K,D region restricted Lyt 23+ cells, non-infectious (F-) virus activates IA region restricted Lyt 1+ cells. Virus partially inactivated with UV light fuses cells and abortive infection occurs, behaving as fully infectious virus (66). Influenza virus, although without a specific fusion protein appears to have a functional analogue to the paramyxovirus F protein.

This requires the functional integrity of the N-terminal end of cleaved HA2 glycoprotein (67,68,69).

There is a strong possibility that the K,D restricted subset, i.e., Tc and Td cells are a single population and similarly the IA restricted subset Td and Th are a single population. These subset pairs at least behave entirely in parallel. Infectious influenza virus generates not only K,D but also IA restricted effector T cells possibly because of the presence of a high population of spontaneously inactivated virus present even during infection or it is possible that infectious virus is capable of primary induction of both T cell subsets.

Thus the balance of functional effector T cells is different in infectious versus inactivated virus vaccines. Of specific relevance, KV can activate the IA-restricted Td system differentially and in the absence of a Tc response.

Passive transfer of syngeneic Tc effector lymphocytes results in a reduction of infectious virus in the lung and protects mice against lethal influenza infection. Furthermore, cytotoxic T cells active against an influenza A strain will lyse target cells infected with any homologous or heterologous subtype of A strain. This compares to antibody induced by LV or KV which is HA specific with limited homologous subtype crossing only. The presence of Tc activity induced by infectious virus thus carries the further theoretical advantage of crossprotection with influenza drift or shift strains, beyond that seen with inactivated vaccine (64,70-74). Passive transfer of IA-restricted Td effector cells does not protect and in fact enhances lethality of influenza infection.

TABLE 4. Effects of Virus Infectivity on Suppressor Cells

Virus	Suppression of H-2 Restricted T-Cells
LV → Ts =	IA (Td + Th)
KV → Ts =	K,D (Tc + Td)

Two subsets of Ts cells can be induced, although the H-2 restriction site is not fully defined (Table 4). Infectious influenza or Sendai virus induces Ts which inhibit induction of I-region restricted effector T cells. Inactivated influenza or F- Sendai virus induces Ts which inhibit generation of K,D restricted T cells. The total effect of immunization with inactivated influenza or F- Sendai virus is to reduce cytotoxic T cells and relatively enhance DTH (75).

This differential effect upon distinct T effector cells can be determinative in the balance between immune pathology or recovery.

HYPOTHESIS

The following hypothesis may be constructed. Immunization with KV-M or KV-RS in man produces circulating antibody but in addition induces a high level of DTH response. It is known that KV-M used clinically was F- and the same may be assumed with KV-RS. In addition, there is adequate evidence that adjuvant can enhance the DTH response. Wild virus challenge by the respiratory route (or locally with LV-M), immediately in the case of RSV, and after a period of time necessary for loss of humoral protection in measles, permits viral replication.

In this setting, immune response to viral replication brings into play a set of uniquely sensitized memory cells. This includes a relative excess of the Td function of the DR restricted effector T cell (equivalent to IA in the mouse) and a limitation of the Tc function of the HLA-A-B restricted T cell (equivalent to K,D in the mouse). The reaction to DTH is a mononuclear inflammatory response and has been shown to contribute to the pneumonic process in the mouse (76). It is conceivable that the unusual pneumonitis and the severe cutaneous response to KV-M has a similar pathogenesis. The rash in a typical case of measles may be caused by the appearance of a CMI response which occurs in the early recovery phase of illness along with the disappearance of giant cells and infectious virus. Burnet has termed the measles rash "a diffuse delayed hypersensitivity reaction" (77). This is borne out by observations in patients with deficiency or depression of CMI. Patients with impaired CMI due to thymic aplasia (78) or neoplastic or reticulo-endothelial disease (79) developed fatal giant cell pneumonia due to measles without manifestation of rash at any time.

The following observations are consonant with the hypothesis.

(1) The paradoxical response has involved membraned viruses (and possibly other agents) where cell entry mechanisms normally involve fusion. Poliovirus, for example, which has been used successfully as infectious or inactivated virus vaccine, has a different entry mechanism.

(2) Formalin inactivation of virus destroys the functional integrity of F protein of measles virus and presumably of RSV.

(3) The serum immune response following KV-M is less effective, in that it is deficient in anti-hemolysin/fusion antibody. It also has a shorter half-life. In addition, sIgA is deficient after parenteral administration of KV. These antibody handicaps permit virus reinfection and replication.

(4) Inoculation of LV-M in a previous recipient of KV-M produces a local reaction compatible with DTH, i.e., erythema, induration, vesiculation.

(5) KV-M uniquely induces persisting DTH as measured by a positive skin test to measles virus antigen. This is absent following natural infection or immunization with LV-M. Similar dermal DTH has been induced by KV-RS in the guinea pig.

(6) Based upon well defined murine systems, KV immunization could prepare the immune system to react with a strong DTH and diminished cytotoxic T cell response when restimulated with antigen.

Certain observations do not readily fit or cannot be explained on the basis of current understanding.

(1) Not all membraned fusion-inducing viruses fit the model. For example, parainfluenza virus prepared in a similar fashion was used as a control in KV-RS field trials. Neither protection nor paradoxical response was noted. Also inactivated influenza vaccine has not been shown to cause paradoxical response in man. However, in recent years the vaccine is free of adjuvant. In the mouse the system has to be fine tuned to demonstrate DTH enhancement. In the "negative human experiments" perhaps conditions of host (e.g., prior antigen contact) or vaccine (antigen dose, adjuvant, route, virus surface characteristics) were not appropriate.

(2) Studies of the histology of the early local lesion caused by LV-M after KV-M sensitization revealed the presence of perivascular mixed inflammatory response and deposition of IgG, C3 and measles antigen (28) suggestive of an Arthus phenomenon. A mixed reaction cannot be ruled out.

(3) A unitarian explanation for RSV pathogenesis in the normal infant in the presence of circulating maternal antibody and the KV-RS paradoxical response is not readily apparent. One could speculate that the presence of antibody (leakage in inflamed mucosa) or altered T cell reactivity in the infant (e.g., vigorous Ts or CMI response) may duplicate conditions favoring a low Tc/Td ratio. The latter is essentially invoking a "physiological immaturity" of the developing CMI system for which there is little direct evidence (80,81,82).

(4) The increase in respiratory tract IgE in natural RSV infection suggests a type I anaphylaxis reaction although there are no studies linking anaphylaxis with the paradoxical response.

We are left with many unresolved questions. Categorizing response as "Arthus," DTH, or type I immediate hypersensitivity may well invoke a simplicity which nature doesn't recognize. It is of importance to understand these iatrogenic experiments in order to better understand the total effect which may be anticipated when an antigen is introduced as immunoprophylaxis in man. We have no good animal models demonstrating paradoxical response. Such are needed for study and also for anticipatory safety testing. Parallel investigation of the CMI response to natural infection and antigenic intervention is needed in man (83,70).

REFERENCES

1. Craighead, J.E. Report of a Workshop: Disease Accentuation After Immunization With Inactivated Microbial Vaccines. J. Inf. Dis. 131:749,1975.
2. Cox, H.R., Greenberg,B.G., Kleinman, H., Meier,P. and Ratner, H., Moderator. The Present Status of Polio Vaccines. Part II. III. Med. J. 160,1960.
3. Winkelstein,W.Jr., Jenss,R., Gresham,G.E., Karzon,D.T. and Mosher,W.E. Inactivated Measles Virus Vaccine. III. A Field Trial in Young School Children. J. Amer. Med. Assn. 179:398,1962.
4. Winkelstein,W.Jr., Karzon,D.T., Rush,D. and Mosher,W.E. A Field Trial of Inactivated Measles Virus Vaccine in Young School Children. Protection During 27 Months of Follow-Up. J. Amer. Med. Assn. 194:106,1965.
5. Carter,C.H., Conway,T.J., Cornfield,D., Iezzoni,D.G., Kempe,C.H., Moscovici,C., Rauh,L.W., Vignec,A.J. and Warrne,J. Serologic Response of Children to Inactivated Measles Vaccine. J. Amer. Med. Assn. 179:108,1962.
6. Feldman,H.A., Novack,A. and Warren,J. Inactivated Measles Virus Vaccine II. Prevention of Natural and Experimental Measles with Vaccine. J. Amer. Med. Assn. 179:391,1962.
7. Fulginiti,V.A. and Kempe,C.H. Measles Exposure Among Vaccine Recipients. Response to Measles Exposure and Antibody Persistence Among Recipients of Measles Vaccines. Amer. J. Dis. Child. 106:450,1963.
8. Guinee,V.F., Casey,J.L., Ruthig, D.W., Henderson,D.A., Wingo,S.T., Cockburn,T.A., Nave,F., Thomas,R.E., et al. A Collaborative Study of Measles Vaccines in Five United States Communities. Amer. J. Pub. Health 53:645,1963.
9. Karelitz,S., Berliner,B.C., Orange,M., Penbkharkkul,S., Ramos,A. and Muenboon,P. Inactivated Measles Virus Vaccine. Subsequent Challenge with Attenuated Live Vrius Vaccine. J. Amer. Med. Assn. 184:673,1963.

10. Bellanti,J.A., Sanga,R.L., Klutinis,B., Brandt,B., and Artenstein,M.S. Antibody Responses in Serum and Nasal Secretions of Children Immunized with Inactivated and Attenuated Measles-Virus Vaccines. New Eng. J. Med. 280:628,1969.
11. Rauh,L.W. and Schmidt,R. Measles Immunization With Killed Virus Vaccine. Amer. J. Dis. Child. 109:232,1965.
12. Nader,P.R., Horwitz,M.S., and Rousseau,J. Atypical Exanthem Following Exposure to Natural Measles: Eleven Cases in Children Previously Inoculated with Killed Vaccine. J. Ped. 72:22, 1968.
13. Fulginiti,V.A., Eller,J.J., Downie,A.W. and Kempe,C.H. Altered Reactivity to Measles Virus. Atypical Measles in Children Previously Immunized with Inactivated Measles Virus Vaccines. J. Amer. Med. Assn. 202:1075, 1967.
14. Norrby,E., Lagercrantz,R. and Gard,S. Measles Vaccination VI. Serological and Clinical Follow-up Analysis 18 Months after a Booster Injection. Acta Paediat. Scand. 55:457, 1966.
15. Young,L.W., Smith,D.I. and Glasgow,L.A. Pneumonia of Atypcal Measles. Residual Nodular Lesions. Amer. J. Roentgen., Rad. Ther., & Nuc. Med. 110:439, 1970.
16. Laptook,A., Wind,E., Nussbaum,M. and Shenker,I.R. Pulmonary Lesions in Atypical Measles. Ped. 62:42, 1978.
17. Scott,T.F.M. and Bonanno,D.E. Reactions to Live Measles Virus Vaccine in Children Previously Inoculated with Killed Virus Vaccine. New Eng. J. Med. 277:248, 1967.
18. Fulginiti,V.A., Arthur,J.H., Pearlman, D.S. and Kempe,C.H. Altered Reactivity to Measles Virus. Local Reactions Following Attenuated Measles Virus Immunization in Children Who Previously Received a Combination of Inactivated and Attenuated Vaccines. Amer. J. Dis. Child. 115:671, 1968.
19. Buser,F. Side Reaction to Measles Vaccination Suggesting the Arthus Phenomenon. New Eng. J. Med. 177:250, 1967.
20. Krause,P.J., Cherry,J.D., Naiditch, M.J., Deseda-Tous, J. and Walbergh, E.J. Revaccination of Previous Recipients of Killed Measles Vaccine: Clinical and Immunologic Studies. J. Ped. 93:565, 1978.
21. Haas,E.J. and Wendt,V.E. Atypical Measles 14 Years After Immunization. J. Amer. Med. Assn. 236:1050, 1976.
22. Lai,P.K., Alpers, M.P., and MacKay-Scollay. Development of Cell-Mediated Immunity to Epstein-Barr Herpesvirus in Infectious Mononucleosis as Shown by Leukocyte Migration Inhibition. Inf. and Immun. 17:28, 1977.
23. Lennon,R.G. and Isacson,P. Delayed Dermal Hypersensitivity Following Killed Measles Vaccine. J. Ped. 71:525, 1967a.

24. Lennon,R.G., Isacson,P., Rosales,T., Elsea,W.R., Karzon,D.T. and Winkelstein,W.,Jr. Skin Tests with Measles and Poliomyelitis Vaccines in Recipients of Inactivated Measles Virus Vaccine. J. Amer. Med. Assn. 100:275,1967b.
25. Harris,R.W., Isacson,P. and Karzon,D.T. Vaccine-Induced Hypersensitivity: Reactions to Live Measles and Mumps Vaccine in Prior Recipients of Inactivated Measles Vaccine. J. Ped. 74:552,1969.
26. Isacson,P. and Stone,A. Allergic Reactions Associated with Viral Vaccines. Prog. Med. Virol. 13:239,1971.
27. Coon,J. and Hunter,R. Properties of Conjugated Protein Immunogens which Selectively Stimulate Delayed-Type Hypersensitivity. J. Immunol. 114:1518, 1975.
28. Bellanti,J.A. Biologic Significance of the Secretory A Immunoglobulins. Ped. 48:715,1971.
29. Norrby,E. and Gollmar,Y. Identification of Measles Virus-Specific Hemolysis-Inhibiting Antibodies Separate from Hemagglutination-Inhibiting Antibodies. Infect. & Immun. 11:231,1975a.
30. Norrby,E., Enders-Ruckle,G. and terMeulen,V. Differences in the Appearance of Antibodies to Structural Components of Measles Virus after Immunization with Inactivated and live Virus. J. Inf. Dis. 132:262,1975b.
31. Tyrrell,D.L.J. and Norrby,E. Structural Polypeptides of Measles Virus. J. Gen. Virol. 39:219,1978.
32. Warren,J., Kammer,H. and Gallian,M.J. Immunization of Monkeys with an Inactivated Measles Antigen and Their Response to a Subsequent Measles Infection. Archiv. ges. Virusforschung ii:748,1962.
33. Karzon,D.T., Rush,D. and Winkelstein,W.,Jr. Immunization with Inactivated Measles Virus Vaccine: Effect of Booster Dose and Response to Natural Challenge. Ped. 36:40, 1965.
34. Kim,H.W., Canchola,J.G., Brandt,C.D., Pyles,G., Chanock,R.M., Jensen,K. and Parrott,R.H. Respiratory Syncytial Virus Disease in Infants Despite Piror Administration of Antigenic Inactivated Vaccine. Amer. J. Epid. 89:422, 1969.
35. Fulginiti,V.A., Eller,J.J., Sieber,O.F., Joyner,J.W., Minamitani,M. and Meiklejohn,G. Respiratory Virus Immunization. I.A Field Trial of Two Inactivated Respiratory Virus Vaccines; An Aqueous Trivalent Parainfluenza Virus Vaccine and an Alum-Precipiated Respiratory Syncytial Virus Vaccine. Amer. J. Epid. 89:435,1969.
36. Kapikian,A.Z., Mitchell,R.H., Chanock,R.M., Shvedoff,R.A. and Stewart,C.E. An Epidemiologic Study of Altered Clinical Reactivity to Respiratory Syncytial (RS) Virus

Infection in Children Previously Vaccinated with an Inactivated RS Virus Vaccine. Amer. J. Epid. 89:405,1969.
37. Chin,J., Magoffin,R.L., Shearer,L.A., Schieble,J.H. and Lennette,E.H. Field Evaluation of a Respiratory Syncytial Virus Vaccine and a Trivalent Parainfluenza Virus Vaccine in a Pediatric Population. Amer. J. Epid. 89:449,1969.
38. McIntosh,J. and Fishaut,J.M. Immunopathologic Mechanisms in Lower Respiratory Tract Disease of Infants due to Respiratory Syncytial Virus. Prog. Med. Virol. 26:94,1980.
39. Scott,R., Kaul,A., Scott,M., Chiba,Y. and Ogra,P.L. Development of in vitro Correlates of Cell-Mediated Immunity to respiratory Syncytial Virus Infection in Humans. J. Inf. Dis. 137:810, 1978.
40. Welliver,R.C., Kaul,A. and Ogra,P.L. Cell-Mediated Immune Response to Respiratory Syncytial Virus Infection: Relationship to the Development of Reactive Airway Disease. J. Ped. 94:370, 1979a.
41. Cranage,M.P. and Gardner,P.S. Systemic Cell-Mediated and Antibody Responses in Infants with Respiratory Syncytial Virus Infection. New Eng. J. Med. 5:161,1980.
42. Welliver,R.C., Kaul,T.N. and Ogra,P.L. The Appearance of Cell-Bound IgE in Respiratory Tract Epithelium after Respiratory-Syncytial-Virus Infection. New Eng. J. Med. 303:1198,1980a.
43. Kim,H.W., Leiken, S.L., Arrobio,J., Brandt,C.D., Chanock,R.M. and Parrott,R.H. Cell-mediated Immunity to Respiratory Syncytial Virus Induced by Inactivated Vaccine or by Infection. Ped. Res. 10:75, 1976.
44. Leikin,S., Whang-Peng,J. and Oppenheim,J.J. In Vitro Transformation of Human Cord Blood Lymphocytes by Antigens. Proc. 5th Leuc. Culture Conf. 389,1970.
45. Field,E.J. and Caspary,E.A. Is Maternal Lymphocyte Sensitisation Passed to the Child? Lancet 337,1971.
46. Forsyth,B.R. Development of Delayed Dermal Hypersensitivity in Guinea Pigs Immunized with Inactivated Respiratory Syncytial Virus Vaccine. Proc. Soc. Exp. Biol. Med. 129:777,1968.
47. Chanock,R.M., Kapikian,A.Z. and Mills,J. Influence of Immunological Factors in Respiratory Syncytial Virus Disease of the Lower Respiratory Tract. Arch. Environ. Health 21:347,1970.
48. Chanock,R.M., Parrott,R.H., Kapkikian,A.Z., Kim,H.W. and Brandt,C.D. Possible Role of Immunological Factors in Pathogenesis of RS Virus Lower Respiratory Tract Disease. Perspect. Virol. 6:125,1968.
49. Glezen,W.P., Paredes,A., and Taber,L.H. Abstract of Pathogenesis of Respiratory Syncytial (RS) Virus Bronchiloitis in Infants. Ped. Res. 11:492,1978.

50. Lamprecht,C.L., Krause,H.E. and Mufson,M.A. Role of a Maternal Antibody in Pneumonia and Bronchiolitis Due to Respiratory Syncytial Virus. J. Inf. Dis. 134:211, 1976.
51. Kaul,T.N., Welliver,R.C. and Ogra,P.L. Abstract of Kinetics of Secretory Antibody Response to Respiratory Syncytial Virus (RSV) Infection in Childhood. Ped. Res. 14:559,1980.
52. McIntosh,K., Masters,H.B., Orr,I., Chao,R.K. and Barkin,R.M. The Immunologic Response to Infection with Respiratory Syncytial Virus in Infants. J. Inf. Dis. 138:24,1978.
53. Gardner,P.S.,McQuillin,J. and Court,S.D.M. Speculation on Pathogenesis in Death from Respiratory Syncytial Virus Infection. Brit. Med. J. 327,1970.
54. Sta. Ana., P.P., Arrobio,J.O., Kim, H.W., Brandt,C.D., Chanock,R.M. and Parrott,R.H. Serum Complement in Acute Bronchiolitis (34821) Proc. Soc. Exp. Biol. & Med. 134:499, 1970.
55. Welliver,R.C., Kaul,T.N., Putnam,T.I., Sun,M., Riddleserger,K. and Ogra,P.L. The Antibody Response to Primary and Secondary Infection with Respiratory Syncytial Virus: Kinetics of Class-Specific Responses. J. Ped. 96:808,1980b.
56. Bui,H.D., Imagawa,D.T., Heiner,D.C., St.Geme,J.W.,Jr. and Wright,P.F. Abstract of a Novel Pathogenetic Concept of Wheezing in Respiratory Syncytial Virus (RSV) Bronchiolitis. Submitted to Clinical Research,October 1981.
57. Ada,G.L., Leung,K-N, and Erti,H. An Analysis of T Cell Generation and Function in Mice Exposed to Influenza A or Sendai Viruses. Immunol. Rev. 58:5,1981.
58. Zinkernagel,R.M. and Rosenthal,K.L. Experiments and Speculation on Antiviral Specificity of T and B Cells. Immunol. Rev. 58:131, 1981.
59. Leung,K.N. and Ada,G.L. Cells Mediating Delayed-Type Hypersensitivity in the Lungs of Mice Infected with an Influenza A Virus. Scand. J. Immunol. 12:393,1980a.
60. Leung,K.N. and Ada,G.L. Two T-Cell Populations Mediate Delayed-Type Hypersensitivity to Murine Influenza Virus Infection. Scand. J. Immunol. 12:481, 1980b.
61. Leung,K.N., MaK,N.K. and Ada,G.L. The Inductive Requirements for the Primary in vitro Generation of Delayed-Type Hypersensitivity Response to Influenza Virus in Mice. Immunol. 44:17,1981.
62. Lin,Y.L. and Askonas, B.A. Crossreactivity for different type A influenza viruses of a cloned T-killer cell line. Nature (Lond). 288:164,1980.

63. Lin,Y.L. and Askonas,B.A. Biological Properties of an Influenza A Virus-Specific Killer T Cell Clone, Inhibition of Virus Replication in vivo and Induction of Delayed-Type Hypersensitivity Reactions. J. Exp. Med. 154:225,1981.
64. Webster,R.G. and Askonas,B.A. Cross-Protection and Cross-Reactive Cytotoxic T cells Induced by Influenza Virus Vaccines in Mice. Eur. J. Immunol. 10:396,1980.
65. Liew,F.Y. Regulation of Delayed-Type Hypersensitivity to Pathogens and Alloantigens. Immunol. Today 3:18,1982.
66. Cascardo,M.R. and Karzon,D.T. Measles Virus Giant Cell Inducing Factor (Fusion Factor) Virol. 26:311,1965.
67. Lazarowitz,S.G. and Choppin,P.W. Enhancement of the Infectivity of Influenza A and B Viruses by Proteolytic Cleavage of the Hemagglutinin Polypeptide. Virology 68:440,1975.
68. Rott,R. The Structural Basis of the Function of Influenza Virus Glycoproteins. Med. Microbiol. Immunol. 164:23,1977.
69. Kurrie,R., Wagner,H., Rollinghoff,M. and Rott,R. Influenza Virus-Specific T Cell-Mediated Cytotoxicity: Integration of the Virus Antigen into the Target Cell Membrane is Essential for Target Cell Formation. Eur. J. Immunol. 9:107,1979.
70. McMichael,A.J., Gotch,F., Cullen,P., Askonas,B. and Webster,R.G. The Human Cytotoxic T Cell Response to Influenza A Vaccination. Clin. Exp. Immunol. 43:276,1981.
71. Armerding,D. and Liehl,E. Induction of Homotypic and Heterotypic T- and B- Cell Immunity with Influenza A Virus in Mice. Cell. Immunol. 60:119,1981.
72. Braciale,T.J. Immunologic Recognition of Influenza Virus-Infected Cells. II. Expression of Influenza A Matrix Protein on the Infected Cell Surface and its Role in Recognition by Cross-Reactive Cytotoxic T Cells. J. Exp. Med. 146:673, 1977.
73. Biddison,W.E., Doherty,P.C. and Webster,R.G. Antibody to Influenza Virus Matrix Protein Detects a Common Antigen on the Surface of Cells Infected with Type A Influenza Viruses. J. Exp. Med. 146:690, 1977.
74. Lamb,J.R., Eckels,D.D., Phelan,M., Lake,P. and Woody,J.N. Antigen-Specific Human T Lymphocyte Clones: Viral Antigen Specificity of Influenza Virus-Immune Clones. J. Immunol. 128:1428,1982.
75. Liew,F.Y. and Russell,S.M. Delayed-Type Hypersensitivity to Influenza Virus. Induction of Antigen-Specific Suppressor T Cells for Delayed-Type Hypersensitivity to Hemagglutinin During Influenza Virus Infection in Mice. J. Exp. Med. 151:799, 1980.

76. Ennis,F.A., Wells,M.A., Butchko,G.M. and Albrecht,P. Evidence that Cytotoxic T Cells are Part of the Host's Response to Influenza Pneumonia. J. Exp. Med. 148:1241,1978.
77. Burnet,F.M. Measles as an Index of Immunological Function. Lancet 2:610,1968.
78. Nahmias,A.J., Griffith,D., Salisbury,C. and Yoshida,K. Thymic Aplasia with Lymphopenia,Plasma Cells, and Normal Immunoglobulins. J. Amer. Med. Assn. 201:729, 1967.
79 Enders, J.F., McCarthy,K., Mitus,A. and Cheatham,W.J. Isolation of Measles Virus at Autopsy in Cases of Giant-Cell Pneumonia Without Rash. New Eng. J. Med. 261:875,1959.
80. Chiba,Y., Fitzpatrick,P., Patel,P., Scott,R. and Ogra,P.L. Age Related Differences in Cellular Immune Response to Vaccine Induced Rubella infection. Microbiol. Immunol. 22:325,1978.
81. Pisciotta,A.V., Westring,D.W., DePrey,C. and Walsh,B. Mitogenic Effect of Phytohaemagglutinin at Different Ages. Nature 215:193,1967.
82. Kay,M.M.B. and Makinodan,T. Immunobiology of Aging: Evaluation of Current Status. Clin. Immunol. & Immunopathol. 6:394,1976.
83. McMichael,A.J. and Askonas,B.A. Influenza Virus-Specific Cytotoxic T Cells in Man; Induction and Properties of the Cytotoxic Cell. Eur.J.Immunol. 8:705,1978.

II

INFLUENZA

CHAPTER 8

STUDIES ON THE PATHOGENICITY OF INFLUENZA VIRUS FOR FERRETS AS A MODEL FOR INFLUENZA IN MAN

H. Smith
C. Sweet
R. Husseini

Department of Microbiology
University of Birmingham
Birmingham, England

Influenza in the ferret was used as the model because the syndrome is similar to that in man, namely a predominantly upper respiratory tract infection with little lung involvement (1). Comparisons of the behaviour in ferrets of the parent strains and virulent and attenuated clones of the recombinant influenza virus A/PR/8-A/England/939/69 (H3N2), particularly clones 7a and 64d, (1-6) produced the following conclusions.

FACTORS AFFECTING INFECTION OF THE UPPER RESPIRATORY TRACT

Virulent and attenuated strains showed similar abilities to infect the nasal mucosa rapidly and heavily during the first day after intranasal inoculation, but thereafter the virulent strains persisted longer at higher levels. During the second and third days, before the main impact of the immune response, the upper respiratory tract infections of all strains were reduced by the influence of inflammatory phagocytes, non-specific humoral inhibitors, interferon and fever; but only in the case of fever could differential effects on virulent and attenuated strains be detected (1,2). The replication of virulent strains in organ cultures of nasal turbinate tissue was inhibited less than that of attenuated strains at the elevated temperatures that occur in ferrets during days 2 and 3 after intranasal inoculation (1,2). Experimental reduction of the fever in infected ferrets produced a higher and more prolonged upper

ISBN 0-12-239980-3

respiratory tract infection, more so for an attenuated strain than for a virulent strain (3). Thus, ability to replicate in the upper respiratory tract at fever temperatures is a major factor in the virulence of influenza virus, at least for the members of the recombinant system examined.

THE ORIGIN OF FEVER

In ferrets influenza fever is due to the liberation of endogenous pyrogen from the phagocytes of the inflammatory response in the upper respiratory tract (1). Insufficient virus escapes from the respiratory tract for fever to result from the respiratory tract for fever to result from systemic interaction with the phagocytes in the spleen, liver and elsewhere (1). Virulent strains produce more fever than attenuated strains and the differential effects may be due to either the presence of less virus or induction of less inflammatory cells in the case of infection with attenuated strains.

THE NATURE OF INFECTION IN THE LOWER RESPIRATORY TRACT

Virulent and attenuated strains showed much greater differences in their abilities to infect the lower than the upper respiratory tract. The reasons for these differences lie in differential abilities of the strains to infect the airways of the lower respiratory tract. Quantitative assessment of virus infectivity, cellular virus antigen by fluorescent antibody, and histological damage in the external bronchi and three zones (hilar, intermediate and outer) of the lung lobes showed that even for virulent strains alveolar infection was almost nonexistent and viral activity was confined to the airways, particularly the bronchi (4,5). The lack of alveolar infection was not due to inability of alveolar cells to support replication of influenza virus but to factors which prevent attack of these susceptible cells and to the extremely small release of virus from them if they are attacked (6).

IMPLICATIONS FOR INFLUENZA IN MAN

The results of this work on ferret influenza suggest the following for influenza in man. First, it is worth investigating whether treatment of fever with antipyretics exacerbates the infection and prolongs shedding of virus which has epidemiological implications. Second, the unpleasant constitutional effects of influenza such as headache, malaise, myalgia, shivering and nausea may, like the fever, be due to liberation of endogenous pyrogen from purely local virus-phagocyte interactions in the upper respiratory tract since such effects have followed administration of human leucocyte pyrogen to volunteers (1). Third, some strains may cause more severe disease than normal by virtue of an ability to attack bronchial tissue in the lower respiratory tract.

REFERENCES

1. Sweet, C., Smith, H. Pathogenicity of influenza virus. Microbiol. Rev. 44:303-330, 1980.
2. Husseini, R.H., Sweet, C., Collie, M.H., Smith, H. The relation of interferon and nonspecific inhibitors to virus levels in nasal washes of ferrets infected with influenza viruses of differing virulence. Br. J. Exp. Pathol. 62: 87-93, 1981.
3. Husseini, R.H., Sweet, C., Collie, M.H., Smith, H. Elevation of nasal viral levels by suppression of fever in ferrets infected with influenza viruses of differing virulence. J. Infect. Dis. 145: 520-524, 1982.
4. Sweet, C., McCartney, J.C., Bird, R.A., Cavanagh, D., Collie, M.H., Husseini, R.H., Smith, H. Differential distribution of virus and histological damage in the lower respiratory tract of ferrets infected with influenza viruses of differing virulence. J. Gen. Virol. 54: 103-114, 1981.
5. Husseini, R.H., Sweet, C., Collie, M.H., Smith, H. Distribution of viral antigen within the lower respiratory tract of ferrets infected with a virulent influenza virus. J. Gen. Virol. submitted.
6. Sweet, C., Bird, R.A., Husseini, R.H., Collie, M.H., Smith, H. Production and release of influenza virus from organ cultures of ferret lower respiratory tract tissues. J. Gen. Virol., submitted.

CHAPTER 9

MURINE CYTOTOXIC T-CELLS IN INFLUENZA

Brigitte A. Askonas

Patricia M. Taylor

National Institute for Medical Research
Mill Hill, London

INTRODUCTION

Recent work has shown that in contrast to the variant specificity of neutralising and protective antibodies, cytotoxic T-cells (T_C) generated by influenza infection in mouse and man in large part do not discriminate between serologically distinct type A influenza viruses (10,27,6,18). This means that T_C induced by infected with say A/USSR virus will recognize and lyse cells infected with any of the type A influenza viruses, but will not see type B influenza infected cells. It therefore becomes important to establish whether such virus crossreactive T-cells generated by infection can be protective against challenge of a host with a heterologous type A virus, particularly since protection by antibodies is restricted to the homologous virus or a very close drift variant. In the previous paper by A. McMichael the problem of influenza specific T_C in man and of their recognition of influenza virus in conjunction with HLA A or B molecules is discussed; once more suggestive evidence for a correlation between level of cytotoxic T-cell memory and absence of virus shedding in a study with volunteers is presented. The mouse model provides the possibility of obtaining more data in regard to the biological function of T_C in vivo by cell transfer studies. Cytotoxic T-cells are mature cells which appear to be rather short-lived, while their precursors or T_C memory cells are longer lived recirculating lymphocytes without the ability to lyse virus infected cells. But stimulation with histocompatible infected cells in vitro, or in vivo challenge with virus generate T_C within very few days (3-4 days) (1);

ISBN 0-12-239980-3

T-helper cells amplify this response, and these are equally crossreactive for different subtypes of A virus (4,20). Cytotoxic T-cells appear in the lungs of infected cells within 3-4 days (1,11). Infection leads to high levels of T_C memory in mice (50-100 fold increase in T_C precursor frequency) (4), and the memory persists over many months (4). Whether this is a reflection of the persistence of some influenza virus or a long lived cell type is not clear.

Since neutralising antibodies induced by infection or vaccination are mainly directed to the variable regions of the haemagglutinin molecule (HA), it becomes important to determine whether T_C memory cells can be protective rather than deleterious against infection with influenza viruses within a type. If so, vaccination methods would need reassessment, since inactivated whole virus vaccines are very poor inducers of long lasting T_C memory cells, and the virus subunit (HANA) vaccine does not appear to induce any virus crossreactive T_C or memory for such cells (24,7). An added difficulty in the development of adequate virus preparations is the ever elusive nature of the cytotoxic T-cell receptor and its recognition of virus and products of the major histocompatibility complex (MHC) (the K and D regions of the mouse H-2 and HLA A or B in man) (26).

In this paper we should like to discuss experiments in a mouse model system that relate to the role and properties of cytotoxic T-cells in influenza by examining T_C clones in vivo and in vitro as well as the question of antigen recognition pattern of T_C. In addition we shall comment briefly on some preliminary attempts to induce better T_C memory with inactivated virus preparations; however antigen presentation with H-2 even on liposomal surfaces so far has not led to a significantly improved generation of T_C memory cells. While secondary stimulation in vitro by means of liposomal preparations is effective, just as secondary stimulation with killed virus (28), priming of mice with liposomal preparations induces far lower T_C memory than infective virus (Hackett, Taylor and Askonas, manuscript in preparation).

RECOGNITION PATTERN OF T-CELLS IN INFLUENZA INFECTION

T-cells see viral antigens in conjunction with MHC products at cell surfaces and their recognition pattern is therefore very different from that of B-cells. T_C are restricted to the K and D regions of H-2 while T-helper (T_H) cells amplifying both antibody responses and T_C generation are I-region restricted; yet both T_H and T_C

can crossreact with all type A influenza viruses (not with type B influenza) in contrast to the variant specific antibodies (e.g. 20,23,10,27,6,8). A subset of both T_H and T_C appear to be A virus variant specific; recently the recognition by a T_C clone of such specificity has been mapped to the virus polymerase gene (5) and another one at Mill Hill to genes coding for virus internal proteins (Townsend and Skehel, to be published). The determinants recognised by A virus crossreactive or specific T_H and T_C thus remain elusive. It has not been possible to effectively block A virus crossreactive T_C with monoclonal or polyclonal antibodies to HA, neuraminidase (NA), nucleoprotein (NP) or Matrix (M-) proteins in several laboratories. Although a synergistic inhibition of cytotoxicity was demonstrable with one out of many monoclonal antibodies to HA and an anti-H-2^k (3), it was clear that this was by steric hindrance rather than binding to the T-cell recognition site, since the anti-HA did not bind to cells infected with different subtypes of A influenza virus, while the T_C lysed cells infected with any type A influenza virus. Recognition of viral components, such as matrix (M-) protein or nucleoprotein (NP) by type A virus crossreactive T_H is still controversial. After immunisation of mice with M-protein, Liew reports T-cell help for antibody formation (21). In our hands, mice primed by infection, on challenge with whole virus show A virus crossreactive T_H for antibody responses, but these T_H show no activity on challenge with M-protein, viral cores, or HANA in vivo, even when presented on liposomal preparations (23). Human T-cell clones with T_H-cell markers have been shown to proliferate with HA, M-protein, HA, NA or NP (16). However, in studies with T_C this has not yet been established. Some influenza specific T_C clones also show alloreactivity and can lyse an allogeneic uninfected cell of a certain haplotype in addition to the syngeneic infected cell (9,2). This raises the possibility that T_C see self-molecules altered by interation with viral components expressed at the cell surface or virus-self interaction molecules (14). On the other hand the restricted alloreactivity is generally lower than the lysis of infected self-targets. It is hoped that mapping of the recognition by T_C clones of viral and self molecules and gene cloning of the T-cell receptor will elucidate target cell recognition in the near future.

WHAT IS THE ROLE OF T_C IN INFLUENZA?

Much work has shown that the appropriate neutralising

antibody present before the host's contact with infective virus is able to protect against infection (22). However, the ability of the virus to change its surface glycoprotein coat, and the fact that the virus antigenic sites for antibody are the variable regions of the haemagglutinin molecule preclude efficient immunisation possibilities against future influenza variants. Under these circumstances it becomes of particular importance to understand the biological function of T_C in vivo. Work in recent years, has indicated that T-cells are important for recovery from influenza infection and control of virus shedding: once more transfer of influenza immune T-cells into congenic mice can reduce lung virus titres as long as a donor and host share K or D regions of H-2 (25). This K or D restriction implicates T_C as the active cell type in inhibiting virus replication. In contrast I region restricted T-cells from influenza A infected mice, although able to induce delayed skin reactions, do not lead to a reduction in lung virus titre (1,25). Since spleen consists of a highly complex mixture of T-cell subpopulations, it is difficult to assign any given activity to a single cell type. We therefore studied the biological activity of mouse clones of T_C specific for type A influenza virus. Such clones can be grown over long time periods in the presence of antigen and T-cell growth factor(s) (TCGF) present in Concanavalin A stimulated rat spleen cell supernatants (17).

The first influenza specific T_C clone selected (17) (derived from H-2^d BALB/c mice) (referred to as L4) grew slowly, adhered to plastic and showed an absolute growth requirement for TCGF but not for antigen. It lysed cells infected with different subtypes of A virus and this was the first evidence that the viral crossreactivity among type A influenza viruses was the property of a single clone rather than of a polyclonal T_C population. Its effect on the course of influenza infection was studied in vivo by transferring L4 cells intravenously into syngeneic hosts 24 hours after infection. The result showed that T_C transfer led to survival of the host after a lethal intranasal infection of lightly irradiated mice. Following a non-lethal intranasal infection of lightly irradiated mice. Following a non-lethal intranasal infection, transfer of T_C clone L4 resulted in reduction of the lung virus titre by 2-3 logs of either homologous or heterologous type A virus (17). Thus cloned T_C are able to limit the spread of virus.

Electron microscopic analysis of clone L4 showed the very close contact with the target and extended psudopods over a broad area of type A virus infected target cells, but no such contact when the target cell was infected with type B influenza (13). A very highly organized Golgi zone and prominent microtubules suggested that this cell can release macromolecules. This indication could be supported by two additional properties of this clones:

(1) Transfer of small numbers of L4 cells into the mouse footpad in the presence of purified type A influenza virus led to a 24 hour skin reaction; this was antigen specific and did not result on challenge with type B influenza virus (17). The histology of the footpads (kindly examined by F.Y. Liew, Wellcome Laboratories) showed macrophage infiltration suggesting the release of macrophage or chemotactic factors (not yet defined) the the Lyt-2 positive cytotoxic T-cell clone with high killing activity. Further support for the activity of Lyt-2 positive cells in inducing DTH comes from transfer experiments by Ada and colleagues (1) which demonstrated that both I region restricted and K or D region restricted immune T-cells were able to transfer delayed skin reactions to influenza.

(2) With A. Morris (Warwick) we also tested for the release of another mediator, that is interferon (IFN). During a 6 hour contact between clone L4 cells (5×10^5/ml) and type A virus infected H-2^d target cells, 100 units of immune (γ)-IFN were released by the L4 cells (19). The release of interferon mapped to the recognition of the appropriate target cells by clone L4. Histocompatible targets infected with type A virus did lead to IFN release by the cloned T_c, while the same was not true after contact with a target cell it does not recognise - for example H-2^b cells infected with A/X31 virus. On the other hand clone L4 showed some alloreactivity and could also lyse uninfected H-2^k cells (2). This recognition was reflected in the release of IFN after contact with infected or uninfected H-2^k BW 5167 target cells (Table 1).

Very recent work with additional clones demonstrated that not all T_c clones have identical properties. Taylor selected further influenza specific T_c clones by following essentially the method of Braciale et al. (8). Cloning and maintenance of the cells was in the presence of antigen (e.g. irradiated, A virus infected spleen cells) plus TCGF (a rat spleen cell supernatant only pulsed with Con A). T_c clone T5/5 (also BALB/c) was highly cytotoxic and lysed histocompatible target cells infected with any type A influenza virus, it grew rapidly with an approximate division time of around 24 hours, did not adhere to plastic and was small in size. This clone was able to release high levels of γ-IFN in the presence of concanavalin A, but released only barely detectable amounts of γ-IFN after contact with its correct target cell overnight (Table 2).

TABLE 1. Antigen Induced Release of γ-Interferon by T_C Clone L4

T_CClone L4	Infected Target Cells	γ-IFN (U/ml)	Target Cell Lysis
+	–	<3	–
–	+	<3	–
+	A/X31-H-2^d	100	++
+	A/X31 BW H-2^{k*}	45	+
+	A/X31 H-2^b	<3	–
+	A/X31 H-2^{dm2}	<3	–
+	B/HK H-2^d	<3	–

Clone L4 derived from BALB/c mice (H-2^d), maintained in TCGF. 5 x 10^5 L4 cells/ml, 6 hour assay. Some of the data and Interferon (IFN) assays, has been described by Morris et al (19).

*BW 5147 cells (H-2^k) are also recognised by clone L4 (2) which is alloreactive for H-2^k only in addition to its specificity to H-2^d plus type A influenza virus. Clone L4 does not lyse influenza infected H-2^{dm2} mutant targets (2).

TABLE 2. Interferon Production by an Antigen Dependent T_C Clone (T/5/5) from BALB/c Mice

Hrs of Incubation	5μg/ml Con A	Target Cells	γ-Interferon U/ml
5	–	A/X31-P815*	0
5	–	A/X31-P815	0
24	–	A/X31-P815	17
24	–	B/HK-P815	0
5	+	–	794
24	+	–	19,950

5 x 10^5 cells/ml of clone T5/5 were incubated in RPMI medium/10 FCS with virus infected target cells or Concanavalin A as indicated. The killer cells (clone T5/5) /target ratio was 5:1 and the clone lysed A virus infected target cells, but not B-virus infected targets.

*P815 cells (H-2^d) were infected with type A influenza virus (A/X31) or type B influenza virus (B/HK).

This raises the question whether it is the antigen induced release of γ-IFN which leads to a protective effect of T_C. Clone T5/5 did not limit the spread of virus after transfer of cells into infected hosts. Further work is required before any conclusions can be reached regarding the role of γ-IFN release, but one might predict that it is the γ-IFN which is essential to prevent the spread of virus after lysis of an infected cell which is assembling virus particles or contains them intracellularly.

TABLE 3. Properties of Two Influenza Specific Cytotoxic T-Cell Clones

	Clone L4°	Clone T5/5*
TCGF dependent	+	+
Antigen dependent	–	+
Plastic adherence	+	–
Size	large, granular	small, clear
Growth rate	slow	rapid'

°Lin and Askonas (17)
*P.M. Taylor, to be published.
'Division time is 20-24 hours.

Table 3 summarises the difference in properties of the two T_C clones studied. There is also need to ascertain that such T-killer cells do not induce pathology. In the following paper Dr. Ennis, will describe further support for the importance of immune T-cells in clearing virus in thymus deprived mice. Although in nude mice the onset of lung inflammation is delayed somewhat, nu/nu hosts die of lung consolidation and are unable to clear the virus from the lung unlike normal mice. A secondary transfer of in vivo stimulated T_C into these infected nude mice leads to less pathology and clearance of virus from the lung in the absence of neutralising antibody (see paper by Dr. Ennis).

KILLED VIRUS PREPARATIONS INDUCE ONLY LOW LEVELS OF T_C MEMORY

Earlier work has shown that influenza infection induces longlasting memory for A virus crossreactive T_C and confers on the host heterotypic immunity (crossprotection against challenge with a heterolous type A virus) in the absence of appropriate neutralising antibodies (24). However, after administration of inactivated virus preparations to mice, only low levels of A virus crossreactive T_C memory cells were detected (7). The only exception was a short lasting crossprotection observed after 2 injections of inactivated virus. HANA vaccine was unable to induce A virus crossreactive T_C (24). T_C, in view of the A virus crossreactivity and their biological properties, may well be responsible for crossprotection, be it complete or only partial, leading to less severe symptoms and infective processes. It is not clear why inactivated viruses in general are so much poorer in inducing cytotoxic T-cells, but this is connected to the T-cell recognition and the insertion of viral components into the cell membrane. In fact inactivated viruses which fuse easily into the cell membrane e.g. Sendai virus, effectively prime for cytotoxic T-cell activity (12). We therefore made some preliminary attempts to improve the presentation of influenza virus components to T-cells by incorporation of viral components into the surface of liposomal vesicles in the presence or absence of appropriate membrane glycoproteins and MHC products. Fig. 1 illustrates such an experiment. The assay for A virus cross-reactive T_C memory was as follows as described previously (24): BALB/c mice were primed intranasally by infective virus or i.m. with a variety of killed virus preparations. After varying time intervals, the spleen cells were suspended and T_C memory was assayed by culturing in vitro with A virus infected target cells (of a different influenza subtype as that used for priming the mice). After 5 days cytotoxicity was assayed on A virus infected P815 (H-5^d) target cells. While intranasal infection leads to very high levels of influenza A virus crossreactive T_C memory cells (more than six months (4)), inactivated virus preparations lead to much lower memory for A virus specific cytotoxicity when tested as early as 3 weeks; with time this memory declines further. Whole virus incorporated into liposomal membranes (23) marginally improved this result (Fig. 1).

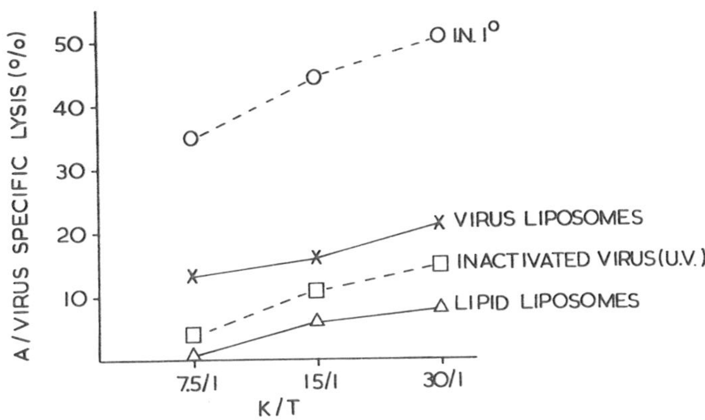

FIGURE 1. Generation of Tc Memory by Various Immunisation Methods.

Priming for influenza specific T_C memory cells by various immunisation methods.

BALB/c mice were primed by different means as indicated below. Assay for T_C memory at different intervals after priming was as follows: Spleen cell suspensions from primed donors were stimulated in vitro with syngeneic A/X31 infected lymphoblasts for 5 days, and Figure 1 illustrates the resulting cytotoxic activity assayed on A/X31 P815 target cells (H-2^d). For details of the method see ref. 27,28. Results expressed in A virus specific lysis of A virus infected targets after subtraction of lysis of uninfected P815 cells.

O——O	1°: I.N. 8 HAU A/JAP/305 (in vitro challenge 6 months later).
X----X	1°: i.m. 5μg A/JAP/Bel liposomes, (in vitro challenge 22 days later)
△----△	1°: i.m. 5 μg lipid liposomes, (no virus) (in vitro challenge 22 days later)
□----□	1°: i.m. 5 μg U.V. irradiated purified A/JAP/Bel, (in vitro challenge 17 days later)

The presence of H-2^d MHC antigen extracted from cellular membranes (not illustrated) had no additional effect. On calculation of the lytic units induced by 10^7 spleen cells, priming with virus liposomes resulted in 30% of T_C memory compared to intranasal infection, and U.V. irradiated virus in about 13% of T_C memory resulting from influenza infection. However, in a series of experiments, comparing inactivated virus preparations and liposomes, the differences in priming led us to conclude that the effect of liposomes was marginal rather than reproducibly significant. The liposomes were prepared essentially as described in reference 15, and lipids and plasma membrane proteins were extracted from H-2^d P815 or spleen cells (23, Hackett, Taylor and Askonas, manuscript in preparation). Our preliminary attempts thus have not improved the results reliably and it is hoped that a better molecular understanding of T-cell recognition will aid in devising more effective immunisation procedures for T-cell priming.

SUMMARY

In conclusion, the properties of mouse immune T-cells and influenza specific cytotoxic T-cell clones in vivo and in vitro suggest that cytotoxic T-cells represent an important arm of immune defense against influenza infection, particularly for recovery from an infection and clearance of virus from infected tissues. In contrast to variant specific antibodies, a major proportion of cytotoxic T-cells and T-helper cells generated by infection does not distinguish between serologically distinct subtypes of type A influenza virus. Thus the recognition pattern of MHC restricted cytotoxic and helper T-cells is different from that of B-cells; however, the determinants recognized by T-cells at the surface of influenza infected histocompatible cells, whether the T-cells are A virus crossreactive, or look more subtype specific, remain to be elucidated.

By examining the properties of cytotoxic T-cell clones, it could be shown that one such clone inhibits virus replication in vivo and releases γ-IFN on contact with an infected target cell it recognises. However, not all T_C clones possess the same properties and further studies are required to assess whether these differences can be attributed to different developmental stages of the T-cell. Whether the virus protective effect relates to antigen induced release of interferon also needs to be evaluated further.

The type A virus crossreactivity of cytotoxic T-cells has important implications in regard to possible crossprotection against different subtypes of influenza virus within a type and yet present vaccination procedures are poor in inducing long-lasting cytotoxic T-cell memory.

REFERENCES

1. Ada, G.L., Leung,K.N. and Ertl,H. (1981). An analysis of effector T-cell generation and function in mice expressed to influenza A or Sendai viruses. Immunol. Rev. 58:5.
2. Askonas,B.A. and Lin,Y.L. (1982). An influenza specific T-killer clone is restricted to H-2L^d and crossreacts with K^k region. Immunogenetics in press.
3. Askonas,B.A. and Webster,R.G. (1980). Monoclonal antibody to haemagglutinin and to H-2 inhibit the crossreactive T-cell population induced by influenza. Eur. J. Immunol., 10,151.
4. Askonas,B.A., Mullbacher,A. and Ashman,R.B. (1982). Cytotoxic T-memory cells in virus infection and the specificity of helper T-cells. Immunol. 45:79.
5. Bennink,J.R., Yewdell,J.W. and Gerhard,W. (1982). A viral polymerase involved in recognition of influenza-virus infected cells by a cytotoxic T-cell clone. Nature 296:75.
6. Braciale,T.J. (1977). Immunologic recognition of influenza virus-infected cells. I. Generation of a virus-strain specific and a virus-reactive subpopulation of cytotoxic T-cells in the response to type A influenza viruses of different subtypes. Cell. Immunol. 33:423.
7. Braciale,T.J. and Yap,K.L. (1978). Role of viral infectivity in the induction of influenza virus specific cytotoxic T-cells. J. Exp.Med. 147:1236.
8. Braciale,T.J., Andrew,M.E. and Braciale,V.L. (1981). Heterogeneity and specificity of cloned lines of influenza-virus specific cytotoxic T lymphocytes. J. Exp. Med. 153:910.
9. Braciale,T.J., Andrew,M.E. and Braciale,V.L. (1981). Simultaneous expression of H-2 restricted and alloreactive recognition by a cloned line of influenza virus-specific cytotoxic T-lymphocyte. J. Exp. Med. 153:1375.
10. Doherty,P.C., Effros,R.B. and Bennink,J. (1977). Heterogeneity of the cytotoxic response of thymus derived lymphocytes after immunisation with influenza virus. Proc. Natl. Acad. Sci. 74:1209.
11. Ennis,F.A., Martin,W.J. and Verbonitz,M.W. (1977). Haemagglutinin-specific cytotoxic T-cell response during influenza infection. J. Exp. Med., 146:893.
12. Gething, M.J., Koszinowski,U. and Waterfield,M. (1978). Fusion of Sendai virus with the target cell membrane is required for T-cell cytotoxicity. Nature 274:689.
13. Hackett,C.J., Sullivan,K. and Lin,Y.L. Ultrastructure of an influenza virus specific cytotoxic T-cell clone and

its interaction with P815 and macrophage targets (1982). Cellular Immunol. 68:276.

14. Hunig,T.R. and Bevan,M.J. (1982). Antigen recognition by cloned cytotoxic T lymphocytes follows rules predicated by the altered-self hypothesis. J. Exp. Med. 155:111.
15. Kagawa,Y. and Racker,E. (1971). Partial restriction of the enzymes catalysing oxidative phosphosylation. Reconstitution of vesicles catalysing ^{32}p ATP exchange. J. Biol. Chem. 246:5477.
16. Lamb,J.R., Eckels,D.D., Phelan,M., Lake,P. and Woody,J.N. (1982). Antigen-specific human T-lymphocyte clones: viral antigen specificity of influenza virus immune clones. J. Immunol. 128:1428.
17. Lin,Y.L. and Askonas,B.A. (1981). Biological properties of an influenza A virus-specific killer T-cell clones. J. Exp. Med. 154:225.
18. McMichael,A.J. and Askonas,B.A. (1978). Influenza virus specific cytotoxic T-cells in man: induction and properties of the cytotoxic cell. Eur. J. Immunol. 8:705.
19. Morris,A.G., Lin,Y.L. and Askonas,B.A. (1982). Immune interferon release when a cloned cytotoxic T-cell line meets its correct influenza-infected target cell. Nature 295:150.
20. Reiss,C.S., Burakoff,S.J. (1981). Specificity of the helper T cell for the cytotoxic T lymphocyte response to influenza viruses. J. Exp. Med. 154:541.
21. Russell,S.M. and Liew,F.Y. (1980). Cell co-operation in antibody responses to influenza virus I. Priming of helper T-cells by internal components of the virion. Eur. J. Immunol. 10, 791.
22. Schulman,J.L. (1975). In: Influenza viruses and influenza (Ed. By Kilbourne,E.D.) P.373. Academic Press, New York and London.
23. Thomas,D.B., Hackett, C.J., Askonas,B.A. (1982). Evidence of two T-helper populations with distinct specificity in the humoral response to influenza A viruses (1982). Immunology, in press.
24. Webster,R.G. and Askonas,B.A. (1980). Crossprotection and crossreactive cytotoxic T-cells induced by influenza virus vaccines. Eur. J. Immunol. 10:396.
25. Yap,K.L., Ada,G.L. and McKenzie,I.F.C. (1978). Transfer of specific cytotoxic T lymphocytes protects mice inoculated with influenza virus. Nature (Lond.), 273:238.
26. Zinkernagel,R. and Doherty,P.C. (1979). MHC-restricted cytotoxic T-cells - studies on the biological role of polymorphic major transplantation antigens determining T cell restriction - specificity function and responsiveness. Adv. Immunol. 27:51.

27. Zweerink,H.J., Courtneidge,S.A., Skehel,J.J., Crumpton,M.J. and Askonas,B.A. (1977). Cytotoxic T-cells kill influenza virus infected cells but do not distinguish between serologically distinct type A viruses. Nature 267:354.
28. Zweerink,H.J., Askonas,B.A., Millican, D., Courtneidge,S.A. and Skehel,J.J. (1977). Cytotoxic T-cells to type A influenza virus: viral haemagglutinin induces A strain specificity while infected cells confer cross-reactive cytotoxicity. Eur. J. Immunol. 7:630.

CHAPTER 10

CYTOTOXIC LYMPHOCYTE RESPONSES TO INFLUENZA VIRUS

Francis A. Ennis*

Martha A. Wells**

*Department of Medicine
University of Massachusetts Medical Center
Worcester, Massachusetts, USA

**Division of Virology
Bureau of Biologics
Food and Drug Administration
Bethesda, Maryland

INTRODUCTION

The mechanisms responsible for the prevention of and recovery from viral infections in humans is the theme of this volume. For many years, pathologists have known that mononuclear cell infiltrates are a characteristic of inflamed tissues during the course of acute virus infections, as opposed to bacterial infections where the predominant cell present is the polymorphonuclear leukocyte. Although polymorphonuclear leukocytes are present in virus infected inflammatory responses, the mononuclear cell infiltrate is considered to be a characteristic of the host response to the virus infection. The role of these cells in response to virus infections remains to be elucidated. The lymphoid cells present in the areas of inflammation presumably are a variety of lymphocytes of both B and T cell lineage. Although some information has been described regarding the percentages of macrophages, and lymphocytes with Ig^+ or θ antigen on the surface of these cells in the course of infection (1) more detailed information has been developed by the use of passive transfer experiments with various populations of lymphocytes being transferred to virus infected hosts.

This progress has been made since the finding of

ISBN 0-12-239980-3

Zinkernagel and Doherty (2) that a specific lymphocyte, the cytotoxic-T lymphocyte, (CTL) recognized and killed virus infected target cells which possessed both the viral and the cells (H-2) antigens in common with the virus antigen used to stimulate the lymphocyte and the self antigen of the killer lymphocyte. These specific killer cells could be identified following virus infection, or immunization, and studies using these markers were performed to evaluate the in vivo function of these cells. In addition, another effector lymphocyte, the natural killer (NK) cell has been described; these cells unlike the cytotoxtic-T lymphocyte can be detected in the circulation of normal nonimmune mice and humans, and NK activity appears to be increased shortly after virus infection begins. In addition, the killing activity is not restricted by self antigens and is not virus specific (3). We will summarize some of the observations which have been made using these markers of in vitro cytotoxicity in conjunction with passive transfer experiments performed in mice infected with influenza, and these cytotoxic lymphocyte responses which have been observed in humans during the course of infection with influenza virus or after immunization with influenza virus vaccines.

ANTIBODY : PREVENTION OF INFLUENZA

Before proceeding to summarize observations from experiments dealing with cell mediated host immune responses to influenza infection, we should briefly review the evidence for the role of antibody in influenza infection. It has been known for many years that the presence of circulating and local antibodies to the hemagglutinin of the challenge influenza virus aided in the prevention of influenza infection. This information was primarily obtained from animal model experiments, and the results suggested that resistance against challenge with influenza viruses could be correlated with the presence of antibody to the surface antigen of the virus used in challenge. Fazekas de St. Groth demonstrated that the transfer of antibodies from immune mice protected recipient mice against intranasal challenge with virus, and the level of protection correlated with the amount of antibody in the local secretions (4). Using recombinant viruses, Schulman demonstrated a decrease in the pulmonary virus titers of mice that had been immunized with a virus which shared the surface antigen of the challenged virus, but had an antigenically distinct hemagglutinin. Immunity to the hemagglutinin was quantitatively greater than that observed in mice with immunity only to the neuraminindase (5). Using hyperimmune rabbit serum prepared against isolated proteins of influenza virus, Virelizer demonstrated that antibody to the hemagglutinin conferred significant protection against challenge if administered before or very soon after virus was administered; however, antibody to the nucloprotein on matrix protein were not protective (6). Similarly, we reported that the passive transfer of antibody from donor mice that had received inactivated influenza vaccine protected recipients against death from challenge, provided that antihemagglutinin antibody was detectable in the circulation of the recipient mice at the time of challenge. This protection by antibody was not observed 12 hours after viral challenge (7). In a series of studies using ferrets, Potter et al (8), also demonstrated resistance against challenge provided the recipient animals had antibody present in the circulation or respiratory secretions at the time of challenge.

The information available in humans on the role of antibody in the prevention of influenza infection is much less detailed. It is however known that there is a general correlation between the susceptibility of groups of individuals to influenza virus infection and the presence of antibody to the hemagglutinin in the serum of the challenged population. Hobson et al (9) demonstrated this in a series of studies in which individuals challenged with a variety of influenze viruses were assessed for illness. Although these studies did not include measurements of local antibody, there was a convincing correlation between the presence and level of serum antibodies to the hemagglutinin and resistance against challenge. More recent information which supports the concept that antibody is very important in protection against influenza challenge comes from volunteer studies in which local antibodies have been measured using sensitive techniques. Clements and Murphy (unpublished observations) found that the presence of IgA antibody in the nasopharayngeal secretions to the hemagglutinin of the challenge virus correlated with resistance to challenge, using an ELISA procedure. Couch et al demonstrated a correlation between local antibody in this case IgG and resistance to challenge (10). Even more convincing evidence for the protection afforded by antibody against natural influenza challenge was reported by Puck et al who followed babies in the first 6 months of life during an epidemic of influenza A infection. There was a significant correlation between the titer of antibody to the hemagglutinin present in the cord blood at the time of birth and protection against influenza (34).

That type of information supports the hypothesis that antibodies are effective in the prevention of disease caused by influenza virus. Presumably the mechanism of protection afforded by antibody is, at least in part, due to neutural-ization of some of the input virus in the respiratory tract. However, the evidence from passive transfer studies in experimental animals would indicate that shortly after infection is underway, administration of antibody would not appear to be helpful to infected recipients.

At present, there is no similar data available concerning the possible role of other host responses in prevention of infection. Although it may be hypothesized that the presence of memory CTL might result in a more aggressive local cell mediated immune response early during the course of influenza virus replication of the respiratory tract, and thus limit infection and reduce clinical disease, data have not been presented to support this possibility. In addition to the possible direct role that CTL may play in resistance against challenge, indirectly they may act to limit infection and reduce disease by the elaboration of gamma interferon which has been recently reported in humans following influenza virus administration, (11) and in mice using a cloned T lymphocyte cell line specific for influenza virus (12). Despite the possibilities that these immune responses may contribute to resistance against influenza challenge, we and others have focused our efforts primarily on analyzing the roles of cytotoxic lymphocyte in recovery from virus infection following initiation of infection, rather than on their potential role in resistance against challenge.

CYTOTOXIC LYMPHOCYTES: RECOVERY FROM INFECTION

Following the observation by Zinkernagel and Doherty that H2 restriction was a characteristic of virally induced cytotoxic-T lymphocytes induced by viruses, several laboratories independently explored the role of these cells in response to influenza virus infection. Yap and Ada (12) demonstrated that H-2 restricted cytotoxic-T lymphocytes developed as a response to influenza virus in mice. Zweerink et al (13) using secondarily in vitro stimulated murine lymphocytes demonstrated a broadly crossreactive subtype memory cytotoxic-T lymphocyte response in mouse spleen cells following influenza infection. We reported (15, 16) the induction of a subtype specific, as well as crossreactive subtype specific cytotoxic-T lymphocyte response during the course of primary infection of mice and also observed the cross subtype reactive T-cell response following secondary in vitro stimulation. Braciale demonstrated that there were subtype specific CTL responses observed following secondary stimulation with purified hemagglutinin and also noted subtype crossreactive response following secondary stimulation in vitro with infectious virus (17).

These experiments naturally lead to studies designed to analyze the role of these virus influenza specific CTL in the course of recovery from infection. Yap et al (18) demonstrated that transfer of secondarily stimulated influenza specific CTL reduced the virus titer in the lungs of mice challenged with influenza A virus, and this reduction was due to a T-cell with Ly 1-2+ characteristics. We reported that during the course of infection of nude mice, influenza virus was never cleared from their lungs (19) and that transfer of spleen cells with H2 restricted, influenza specific CTLs resulted in the clearance of virus in resolution of influenza pneumonia in immunocompetent Balb/c mice, as well as their nude counterparts (20). In addition, we noted that the transfer of immune spleen cells without CTL activity induced very high levels of antibody responses early during the course of infection in recipient mice, this did not result in clearance of infectious virus from the lungs of recipients, nor did it prevent their death from challenge (20). Additional evidence that antibody was not important in the resolution of recovery from influenza pneumonia, was the fact that the recipients of the secondarily stimulated spleen cells which had high H-2 restricted influenza specific cytotoxicity had no detectable antibodies following transfer of these cells, but survived lethal challenge and cleared the virus from their lungs. Subsequently, Lin and Askonas have demonstrated a similar protective effect using a murine influenza specific cloned CTL line. Recipients of this cloned CTL lined had a significant reduction in pulmonary virus titers (21). Thus, several laboratories have convincingly demonstrated that influenza specific cytotoxic-T lymphocytes are important in the recovery of mice after influenza infection is underway.

The mechanism of protection afforded by the transfer of cytotoxic-T lymphocytes to influenza challenged mice remains to be determined. Although we expected that the reduction in clearance of virus from the target organ was secondary to in vivo destruction of cells with virus antigens on their surface prior to complete cycles of infection, it is now clear that these cells release factors which may contribute to clearance of the virus to the target organ. Morris, Lin and Askonas (12) have shown that the influenza specific clone CTL line which aided in recovery influenza infection releases gamma interferon when it recognizes its correct target cell in vitro. We have reported that lymphocytes obtained from humans shortly after immuniation with influenza antigens produce high amounts of gamma interferon in vitro when stimulated by autologous lymphocytes infected with influenza virus (11). These observations imply that the cytotoxic-T lymphocytes upon transfer to animals with influenza pneumonia may accomplish the virus clearance by the release of factors such as gamma interferon in the target organ which might be associated with viral clearance, in addition to destruction of the virus infected cell by the specifically sensitized CTL.

CYTOTOXIC LYMPHOCYTE RESPONSE OF HUMANS TO INFLUENZA VIRUS

Two laboratories independently demonstrated that humans have influenza specific memory cytotoxic-T lymphocytes in their peripheral blood. McMichael et al demonstrated the presence of HLA restricted influenza specific T lymphocytes in the circulation of adults by restimulation in vitro with virus infected autologous lymphocytes (22). Shaw and Biddison demonstrated a similar HLA restricted influenza specific CTL response (23). This research is described in detail in the chapter in this volume by McMichael. We have used their methods to determine whether influenza infection or immunization to induce HLA restricted virus specific CTL responses.

In our initial small study, we failed to detect an increase in influenza specific HLA restricted cytotoxic activity in three volunteers following administration of an H3N2 strain of influenza virus, although the volunteers appeared to be infected. In a second study, we were able to detect low levels of directly measurable cytotoxic-T lymphocyte activity in the circulation of 4 of 5 volunteers following the administration of an H1N1 strain of virus (24). Subsequently, we performed a larger study and measured the cytotoxic-T lymphocyte responses which could be directly detected using freshly obtained peripheral blood lymphocytes, as well as an increase in the level of influenza specific memory CTL activity assayed after in vitro restimulation with autologous infected lymphocytes. That study was performed in volunteer medical students in Sheffield, England, in 1980-81 (25). Briefly, we were able to detect increased levels of influenza specific HLA restricted cytotoxic activity in the majority of the recipients of each of three types of influenza vaccines including a live attenuated H1N1 vaccine, a whole virus inactivated vaccine, and a surface antigen prepared vaccine. The volunteers were young adults with a mean age of 19 years and few had pre-existing antibody to the H1N1 strains used to make these vaccines. The majority of these volunteers were probably undergoing primary infection with a virus of the H1N1 subtype since those viruses have not circulated between 1957 and 1977 when these subjects were born and maturing. However, these subjects undoubtedly have been repeatedly naturally infected with influenza viruses in the H2N2 and H3N2 subtype, and apparently their brisk cytotoxic-T lymphocyte responses were stimulated by the crossreactive antigen(s) responsible for inducing CTL responses to influenza infection. The vast majority of the volunteers developed both serum antibody and influenza specific cytotoxic lymphocyte responses. There were however, several exceptions where only one was infected in the absence of the other. In addition, it was clear that the cytotoxic responses observed were overwhelmingly HLA restricted, that is, there was a highly statistically significant correlation ($P < .001$) between the ability of a volunteer's lymphocyte to lyse a virus infected target cell and the sharing of at least one HLA type A or B in common between the stimulator lymphocyte and the infected target.

In addition to this study which demonstrated that young adults developed brisk increase in their HLA restricted memory CTL responses following immunization with influenza H1N1 antigens, we performed two smaller studies in volunteers who were infected with live H1N1 virus at the common cold research unit in Salisbury, England. The results of those studies (26) indicate that shortly following introduction of influenza virus into the respiratory tract, humans develop augmented natural killer cell activity. This is detected using peripheral blood PBLs obtained early following infection (days 3 and 6) before the CTL responses described above were detected. In addition to the increased natural killer cell activity, the volunteers also had levels of serum interferon present at the same increased early period following virus administration.

Thus, it is clear that influenza infection in adults results in an increase in the nonspecific natural killer cell activity early during the course of influenza infection and subsequently an increase in their influenza specific HLA restricted cytotoxic-T cell responses. The possible role of natural killer cells in the control of influenza or other virus infections remains to be determined. There are however, data from three laboratories which indicate that natural killer cells do not appear to play as obvious a role in clearance of influenza virus infection as the virus specific H-2 restricted CTLs which was summarized above. Leung and Ada (22) have reported that beige mice ($bg^{+}bg^{+}$) mice which have decreased killer cell activity appear to have similar pulmonary virus titers during the course of influenza infection, as their counterparts which have normal natural killer cell activity. Shimomura et al reported a lack of clearance of pulmonary virus (28) despite NK activity in nude and irradiated mice in influenza infected mice. In adoptive transfer experiments we have observed (29) that clearance of pulmonary virus from challenged mice requires the presence of detectable cytotoxic-T lymphocyte activity and that no such correlation existed for natural killer cell activity. Thus, the evidence to date would indicate that cytotoxic-T lymphocytes are needed to clear the virus from the infected animal's lungs and not NK cells. This is also supported by the absence of viral clearance in T-deficient mice who do have higher levels of natural killer cell activity than their immunocompetent counterparts. These data, however, do not rule out the possibility that early during the course of infection before virus H-2 restricted CTLs are detectable, natural killer cells may aid in control of the infection. Such an hypothesis appears likely since we have observed in both nude mice and their Balb/c immunocompetent counterparts a drop in pulmonary virus titers of about 1 $\log_{10}$ early during the course of infection in the absence of any immune intervention.

RECENT RESULTS AND QUESTIONS TO ANSWER

Regarding the role of cytotoxic-T lymphocytes in aiding in recovery of influenza infection in humans, it is important to determine the effect of immunization regimens on these cells. In mice it is clear (30) that inactivated antigens can induce these responses, but appear to be less effective as primary antigens (31). We are attempting to determine in the murine system whether the presence of memory influenza specific CTLs prior to infection is associated with resistance against challenge similar to the reports described above which have demonstrated effects for antibody. Given the evidence that antibodies appear to be effective in aiding the host resist challenge and that cytotoxic-T lymphocytes are effective the host recover from challenge, we did not expect to obtain information to indicate that memory cytotoxic-T lymphocytes would contribute in the resistance against challenge. Preliminary experiments (Wells and Ennis unpublished observations) suggest, however, that the presence of detectable memory influenza specific CTLs even in the absence of antibody, appears to be associated with significant protection of subsequently challenged mice. The reader should refer to McMichael's chapter in this volume in which he reports results which suggest that the presence of memory CTL activity in humans who do not have detectable serum antibodies appear to be associated with a decrease amount of virus shedding of challenge volunteers. Another area of our interest is the relationship between gamma interferon production by the virus specific CTLs and the control of virus infection in the infected host. We have begun experiments in the murine model to address the question of whether gamma interferon in the mechanism of recovery solely rather than virus specific lysis accomplished by the effector or cytotoxic-T lymphocyte. Another research interest in our laboratory involves the antigens responsible for induction of the influenza specific CTL response and the production of gamma interferon. It is clear that cross subtype reactive antigens can induce both CTL and gamma interferon responses. The information on the specificity of the inducible CTL response was summarized above and more recent work by Braciale (32) and Lamb et al (33) have indicated that there are clones of both subtype specific and cross subtype reactive T lymphocytes induced by influenza infection. In addition, T lymphocyte memory responses were induced by purified protein such as matrix and nucleoprotein by Lamb et al (33). There is less information available on the nature of the crossreactive antigen responsible for gamma interferon production, but it would appear that at least some of the crossreactive antigen may be due to shared hemagglutinin determinants (Ennis unpublished observations).

CONCLUSION

The reports in this volume by McMichael et al and Askonas et al along with the data reviewed here provide some specific detailed information which has been developed in the past few years which provide a solid base for discussion about the roles of cytotoxic-T lymphocytes, natural killer cells, and gamma interferon in the response of the host infected with influenza virus. It is clear that these in vitro assays have relevance to control and recovery from infection with influenza. The best evidence to date deals with the H-2 restricted influenza specific CTL and their correlary, the HLA restricted CTL in man. These experiments have used influenza as a model to address questions of generic interest to researchers dealing with immune responses of humans to viruses. It is clear already that these intensive efforts have shed light not only on our understanding of the role of cell mediated immune responses in influenza infection in mice and humans, but also stimulated research into the cell media that immune responses of humans to infection with other viruses. For example herpes simplex virus, measles virus and cytomegalo virus virus which are described in detail in other chapters in this volume. Thus, in the past five years tremendous progress has been made in our understanding and immune responses to viruses and their antigens, and it can safely be predicted that in the next 5 to 10 years this area of research will be extremely productive and result in a vastly improved understanding of how humans respond to infections with viruses.

REFERENCES

1. Wyde,P.R., Peavy,D.L. and Cate,T.R. Morphological and Cytochemical Characterization of Cells Infiltrating Mouse Lung after Influenza Infection. Inf. Immun. 21:140-146, 1978.
2. Zinkernagel,R.M. and Doherty,P.C. MHC-restricted cytotoxic-T cells: Studies on the biological role of polymorphic major transplantation antigens demonstrating T-cell restriction - specificity, formation and responsiveness. Advances Immunol. 27:51, 1979
3. Welsh,R.M., Zinkernagel,R. Heterospecific cytotoxic cell activity induced during the first three days of acute lymphocytic choriomeningitis virus infection in mice. Nature 268, 646-664, 1977.
4. Fazekas de St.Groth,S., Donelly,M. Studies in experimental immunology of influenza IV. Protective value of active immunization. Anst. J. Exp. Biol. Med. Sci. 28. 61, 1950.
5. Schulman,J.L. Effects of Immunity of Transmission of Influenza: Experimental Studies. Prog. Med. Virol. 12, 128-160, 1970.
6. Virelizier,J.L. Host defenses against influenza virus: The role of anti-haemagglutinin antibody. J.Immunol. 115, 434-437, 1975.
7. Ennis,F.A., Wells,M.A., Barry,D.W., Daniel,S., Manischewitz,J. Host defence mechanisms against influenza infection II Protection of mice with vacines against A/Port Chalmers/1/73 and B/Hong Kong/5/72. Postgrad. Med. J., 52, 338-344, 1976.
8. Potter,C.W., Oxford,J.S., Shore,S.L., McLaren,C., Stuart-Harris,C. Immunity to influenza in farrets. I. Response to live and killed virus. Brit. J. Exp. Path. 53, 153-167, 1972.
9. Hobson,D., Curry,R.L., Beare,A.S., Ward-Gardner,A. The role of serum hemagglutination-inhibnitory antibody in protection against challenge infection with A2 and B viruses. J. Hyg. 70, 767-777, 1972.
10. Couch,R.B., Kasel,J.A., Six,H.R., Cate,T.R. The basis for immunity to influenza in man. In Nayak,D.P.,

Fox,C.F. Genetic Variation among Influenza Viruses. ICN-UCLA Symposia on Molecular and Cellular Biology XXI, 535-546, 1981.

11. Ennis,F.A., Meager,A. Immune interferon produced to high levels of antigenic stimulation of human lymphocytes with influenza virus. J. Exp. Med. 1981, 1279-1289.
12. Morris,A.G., Lin,Y.L., Askonas,B.A. Immune interferon release when a cloned cytotoxic T cell line meets its correct influenza infected target cell. Nature, 295, 150-152, 1982.
13. Yap,K.L., Ada,G.L. Cytotoxic T cells specific for influenza virus infected target cells. Immunology 32, 151-159, 1977.
14. Zweerink,H.J., Courtneidge,S.A., Skehel,J.J., Crumpton,M.J., Askonas,B.A. Cytotoxic T cells kill influenza virus infected cells but do not distinguish between serologically distinct influenza A virus. Nature 267, 354-356, 1977.
15. Ennis,F.A., Martin,W.J., Verbonitz,M.W. Haemagglutinin specific cytotoxic T cell responses during influenza infection. J.Exp.Med. 146,843-898, 1977.
16. Ennis,F.A., Wells,M.A., Butchko,G.M., Albrecht,P. Evidence that cytotoxic T cells are part of the host's response to influenza pneumonia. J.Exp. Med. 148, 1241-1249, 1978.
17. Braciale,T.J. Immunologic recognition of influenza infected cells. 1.Generation of virus stain specific and cross-reactive subpopulations of cytotoxic T cells in response to type A influenza virus infection of different subtypes. Cell Immunol. 33, 423-426, 1977.
18. Yap,K.L., Ada,G.L., McKenzie,I.F.C. Transfer of specific cytotoxic T lymphocytes protects mice inoculated with influenza viruscs. Nature 273, 238-239, 1978.
19. Wells,M.A., Albrecht,P., Ennis,F.A. Recovery from a viral respiratory tract infection. I. Influenza pneumonia in normal and T deficient mice. J.Immunol., 126, 1036-1041, 1981.
20. Wells,M.A., Ennis,F.A., Albrecht,P. Recovery from a viral respiratory tract infection II. Passive transfer of immune spleen cells to mice with influenza pneumonia. J. Immunol. 126, 1042-1046, 1981.
21. Wells,M.A., Ennis,F.A., Albrecht,P. Recovery from a viral respiratory tract infection II. Passive transfer of immune spleen cells to mice with influenza pneumonia. J.Immunol. 126, 1042-1046, 1981.
22. McMichael,A.J., Ting,A., Zweerink,H.J., Askonas,B.A. HLA restriction of cell mediated lysis of influenza virus infected human cells. Nature 270, 524-526, 1977.

23. Shaw,S., Biddison,W.E. HLA-linked genetic control of the specificity of human cytotoxic T cell responses to influenza virus. J.Exp.Med. 149, 565-575, 1979.
24. Daisy,J.A., Tolpin,M.D., Quinnan,G.V., Rook,A.H., Murphy,B.R., Mittal,K., Clements,M.L., Mullinix,M.G., Kiley,S.C., Ennis,F.A. Cytotoxic cellular immune responses during Influenza A infection in human volunteers. In: Bishop,D.M.L., Compams,R.W. (eds.). The replication of negative strand virus, 443-448, Elsevier/North-Holland, 1981.
25. Ennis,F.A., Rook,A.H., Yi-Hua,Q., Schild,G.C., Riley,D., Pratt,R., Potter,C.W. HLA restricted virus specific cytotoxic T lymphocyte responses to live and inactivated influenza viruses to live and inactivated influenza viruses. Lancet 887-891, 1981.
26. Ennis,F.A., Meager,A., Beane,A.S., Yi-Hua,Q., Riley,D., Schwarz,G., Schild,G.C., Rook,A.H. Interferon induction and increased natural-killer cell activity in influenza infections in man. Lancet 891-893, 1981.
27. Leung,K.N. and Ada,G.L. Induction of natural killer cells during murine influenza virus infection. Immunobiol. 160, 352-366, 1981.
28. Shimomura,E., Zuyutai, and Ishida,N. Characterization of cells infiltrating the lungs of X-irradiated and nude mice after influenza virus infection. Microbiol. Immunol. 26:129-138, 1982.
29. Wells,M.A., Daniel,S., Djeu,J.Y., Kiley,S.C. and Ennis,F.A. Recovery from a Viral Respiratory Tract Infection: IV. Specificity of Protection by Cytotoxic T Lymphocytes. J.Immunol., in press.
30. Ennis,F.A., Martin,W.J., Verbonitz,M.W. Cytotoxic T lymphocytes induced in mice by inactivated influenza vaccine. Nature 266, 418-419, 1977.
31. Reiss,C.S., Schulman,J.L. Cellular immune responses of mice to influenza virus vaccines. J.Immunol. 125, 2181-2188, 1980.
32. Braciale,T.J., Andrew,M.E., Braciale,V.L. Heterogeneity and specificity of cloned lines of influenza virus specific cytotoxic T lymphocytes. J. Exp. Med. 153:910-923, 1981.
33. Lamb,J.R., Eckels,D.D., Lake,P., Johnson,A.H., Hartzman,R.J., Woody,J.M. Antigen-specificity and MHC restriction of influenza-virus immune clones. J.Immun. 128:233-238, 1982.
34. Puck,J.M., Glezen,W.P., Frank,A.L., Six,H.R. Protection of infants from infection with influenza A virus by transplacentally acquired antibody. J.Inf.Dis., 142:844-849, 1980.

CHAPTER 11

DELAYED TYPE HYPERSENSITIVITY TO INFLUENZA VIRUS

F.Y. Liew

Department of Experimental Immunobiology
The Wellcome Research Laboratories
Beckenham, Kent, England

Beveridge and Burnet in 1944 (1) made the original observation that in many people the intradermal injection of influenza virus was followed by a skin lesion which clinically resembled a tuberculin reaction. Habershon et al (2) confirmed this finding using purified influenza virus and showed that the histology of the lesion was compatible with a delayed-type hypersensitivity (DTH). Furthermore, Cole and Molyneux (3) observed in man a strong correlation between DTH and in vitro lymphocyte proliferation to purified influenza antigens. DTH to purified influenza virus was also reported in mice injected with purified matrix protein in Freund's complete adjuvant (4). More recently, DTH to influenza virus was systematically studied in the mouse model by us (5-7) and by Leung and Ada (8-10). In this report, attempts will be made to review the DTH reactivity to influenza virus in the experimental model. The regulation of DTH and the biological significance of this cell-mediated immunity in terms of pathogenesis and host defence will also be discussed.

CHARACTERISATION OF DTH TO INFLUENZA VIRUS

Mice infected with an aerosol of influenza virus or immunised with purified UV-inactivated whole virus or viral subunits develop a transient DTH which peaks 5-7 days after immunisation. The level of DTH is greatly enhanced and sustained when mice are injected intraperitoneally 2 days prior to immunisation with 100-200 mg/Kg of cyclophosphamide (5). The DTH reactivity is maximal at 24 h after elicitation, has the classical tuberculin-type histology and is transferable by immune Ly 1+2- T cells but not by immune serum (8).

ISBN 0-12-239980-3

DTH induced by deoxycholate treated subviral particles or the matrix protein of the influenza virus is type specific, i.e. DTH induced by the particles or matrix protein of type A virus cross-reacts with all type A viruses but not with any type B influenza virus. On the other hand, DTH induced by the purified monomeric form of haemagglutinin (monomer HA), derived from bromelain treatment of the virion, shows subtype specificity. Thus DTH induced by the monomer HA of X31 virus (H_3) does not cross-react with PR8 virus (H_0). However, DTH induced by monomer HA of one subtype cross-reacts significantly with all the drift variants of the same subtype. Therefore it appears that the effector T cells of DTH do not discriminate between the antigenic variants of influenza virus which are distinguishable by serology. DTH induced by infectious A virus administered as aerosol (5) or subcutaneously (8) cross reacts with all the A viruses. This is as expected since the internal components of the virus which are common among all the subtypes are capable of inducing DTH. What is unexpected is that DTH induced by subcutaneously injected purified UV-inactivated virus shows extensive crossreactivity, reacting even with egg grown Sendai virus. This non-specific reaction appears to be due to host-derived materials (egg) since the DTH elicited with virus grown in a different host cell (Vero cell) is type specific.

These host derived materials form an integral part of the lipid bilayer of the virus, rather than contaminants resulting from ineffective purification of the virus. When the virus is treated with deoxycholate, the non-specific DTH-inducing material is recovered with the polymeric form of the haemagglutinin and neuraminidase but not with the spikeless particles, although similar purification steps (sucrose gradient centrifugation) are used to recover both the materials. Such host derived materials causing non-specific delayed hypersensitivity appear to be a common feature of all commercially prepared influenza vaccines and may be partly responsible for the undesirable pyrogenicity of these products (C.M. Brand and F.Y. Liew, submitted). So far, attempts to reduce this non-specific reactivity by chemical means without diminishing the immunogenicity of the virus have not been successful, although absorption and elution of the virus with chicken red blood cells somewhat reduces this host derived reactivity (unpublished data). The reasons for this are at present unclear.

The influence of the major histocompatibility gene products on the manifestation of DTH to viral antigens has been extensively studied (Table 1). The cells mediating DTH to infectious lymphocytic choriomeningitis virus are restricted only to the K and D subregions of the H-2 (11), whilst the cells mediating DTH to reovirus (12), and infectious sendai virus are K, D and 1-A region restricted (8). DTH induced by infectious sendai virus are K, D and 1-A region restricted (8). DTH-induced by infectious herpes simplex virus (HSV-1), injected virus, DTH response to inactivated virus is 1-A restricted, whereas DTH induced by influenza virus is restricted by K, D and 1-A subregions. Thus the genetic requirement for the expression and probably the induction of DTH to viral antigens is highly dependent upon the replicating nature of the virus which in turn is conditioned by the route and form (infectious or inactivated) of the viral antigen presentation by the antigen presenting cells.

TABLE 1. Genetic restriction of DTH to viral antigens in mice

Virus	H-2 restriction	Reference
LCM (infectious)	K,D,	Zinkernagel,1976 (11)
Reovirus(infectious)	K,D,I-A	Weiner et al,1980(12)
Sendai virus:		
infectious	K,D,I-A	Leung et al,1980 (8)
inactivated	I-A	
Influenza virus:		
infectious	K,D,I-A	Leung et al,1980 (8)
inactivated	I-A	Liew,1980(unpublished)
HSV (infectious)	I-A	Nash et al,1981 (13)

T-HELPER CELLS FOR DTH TO INFLUENZA VIRUS

After various preliminary attempts, it was found that mice primed with matrix protein of influenza virus produced significantly higher levels of DTH to viral haemagglutinin upon boosting with the whole virus, as compared with unprimed mice (7). This helper effect is adoptively transferable by Lyt-1+2- T cells primed with matrix protein using the protocol in Fig. 1. The T-helper cells are antigen specific since priming with matrix protein from type A virus only potentiates the DTH response to type A but not type B virus. The helper cells also appear to act in the classical "carrier-hapten" associative recognition manner as the effect is only evident when the boosting antigen consists of both matrix protein and haemagglutinin presented in physical association (Fig.2).

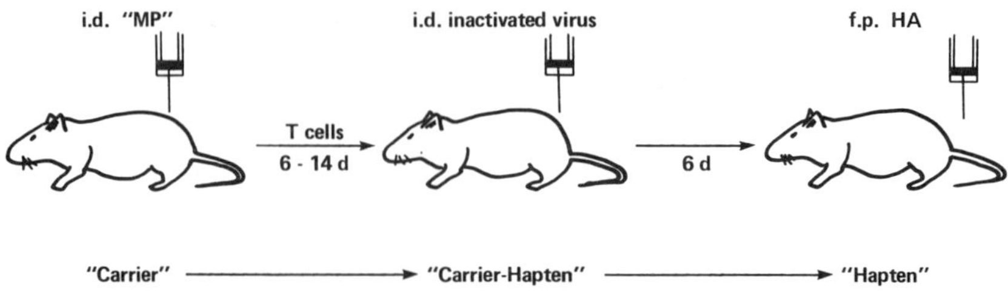

FIGURE 1. Protocol for the demonstration of T-helper cells for DTH to influenza virus. Normal CBA mice 10-12 weeks old were primed intradermally (i.d.) with 10μg of matrix protein (MP). Various times after priming splenic Ig- cells were harvested and transferred i.v. at 10^8/recipient into normal syngeneic mice which were infected i.d. immediately with 10μg of purified UV-inactivated virus. 6 days later these mice together with controls were injected in the footpad with 1μg of monomeric haemagglutinin (HA). DTH was expressed as 24 h footpad thickness increase. The analogy with the classic carrier-hapten system is indicated, where MP=carrier, HA= hapten and the intact virus = carrier-hapten. The priming effect is not likely to be due to the small amount of haemagglutinin present in the matrix protein preparation, since priming with the whole virus which contains both matrix protein and haemagglutinin did not lead to enhancement of DTH to haemagglutinin. Indeed, priming by haemagglutinin suppresses the subsequent DTH response to haemagglutinin when challenged with the whole virus. More recently, T-helper cells for the generation of antigen-specific DTH to influenza virus have also been demonstrated in vitro (10) and to herpes simplex virus in vivo (A.A. Nash, and P. Wildy in this volume). Thus, the features of T-T help in DTH to viral antigens apparently parallel those of T-B help in antibody synthesis.

SUPPRESSOR T CELLS FOR DTH TO INFLUENZA VIRUS

Mice infected with influenza virus by aerosol develop a transient DTH response which peaks around 5-7 days, thereafter it is barely detectable. Such reactivity can be greatly enhanced and sustained if the mice are pretreated with 100-200 mg/Kg cyclophosphamide 2 days prior to infection. Since cyclophosphamide has been shown in vivo (14) and in vitro (15) to enhance DTH by eliminating suppressor T cell

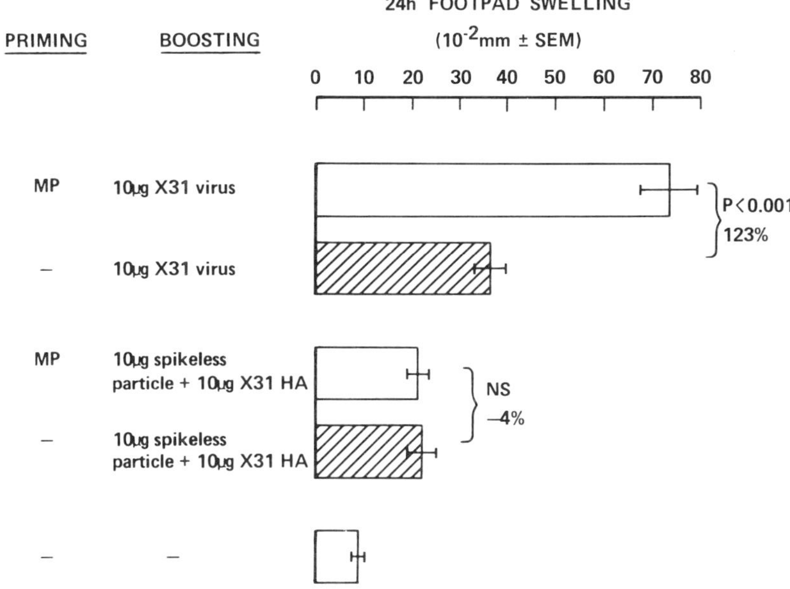

FIGURE 2. The helper effect is expressed only when boosted with intact whole virus particles. Mice were either primed i.d. with 10µg of MP (A/Jap/Bel) or left unprimed and boosted i.d. 6 days later with the antigens indicated. DTH was elicited with 1 µg of 31 monomeric HA 6 days after boosting. n = 5. All groups were significantly different from negative controls (at least $p < 0.05$).

precursors (though this may not be the only mechanism involved, see ref. 16), it is possible that suppressor T (T_S) cells are involved during influenza virus infection. Indeed, antigen-specific T_S cells for DTH, analogous to those induced by erythrocyte antigens (17) and contact sensitizing antigens (18) are readily generated during influenza virus infection (6). Using a protocol similar to that shown in Fig. 1 (except that the priming is by aerosol of infectious virus) it has been shown that the T_S cells are Lyt-1+2- and Ia- (Table 2) and therefore unlikely to be cytotoxic T (T_C) cells.

They first appear 2 weeks after infection and can be detected in the spleen for at least 40 days thereafter. The T_S cells are specific for a subtype of haemagglutinin and do not affect DTH to other antigenic epitopes of the virus. T-helper cells for antibody response to haemagglutinin are induced concomitantly with the T_S cells for DTH. However it is unlikely that these helper cells are responsible for the suppression of DTH, since passive transfer of immune serum does not affect the induction nor the expression of DTH to hemagglutinin (6). A T_S cell system similar to this has also been demonstrated in mice injected i.v. with UV-inactivated reovirus (19). In infection of mice with

TABLE 2. Effect of treatment of suppressor T cells with antiserum and complement*

Donor spleen cells (10^8) treated with	DTH** ($x10^{-2}$mm)	Suppression	p+
Untreated	51.0± 5.6	58.6	<0.005
Anti-Thy-1.2+C'	97.9± 5.9	1.5	NS
Anti-Lyt-1.1+C'	80.9±13.2	22.2	NS
Anti-Lyt-2.1+C'	28.2± 4.7	86.4	<0.001
Anti-Ia^k+C'	37.0± 2.3	75.6	<0.002
Normal serum +C'	40.2± 7.6	71.7	<0.005
Normal cells	99.1± 4.6	0	-
Negative controls	17.0± 4.6	-	-

*Spleen cells from mice infected 2 weeks before with an aerosol of Rec X-31 virus were treated with monoclonal serum and complement as indicated. The treated cells were transferred i.v. into syngeneic recipients which were immunised immediately after cell transfer with 10μg of purified UV-inactivated X31 virus. 6 days later DTH was elicited in the footpad with 10μg of the X31 virus.

**DTH is expressed as the difference in footpad thickness increase 24 h after antigen injection.

+All p values compared with the group transferred with normal cells, n=5, NS=not significant.

herpes simplex virus, it was also found that i.v. doses of living avirulent mutant strains or UV-inactivated virulent viruses can produce a state of tolerance that is specific for DTH and is readily transferable by splenic T cells (20).

It has been proposed that suppressor and helper T cells differ in their functional specificity repertoires (21) such that certain determinants on a macromolecule are "helper epitopes" whilst others may by "suppressor epitopes." If this is so, one could postulate that the matrix protein which preferentially induces T-helper cells for DTH and for antibody synthesis (22) against the haemagglutinin is a "helper epitope", whereas the haemagglutinin, or part of it which is capable of inducing specific suppressor T cells for DTH, is a "suppressor epitope" in the immune response to influenza virus. In this system, it is important to note the difference between the suppression of DTH during infection and the apparent lack of suppression by immunisation with inactivated virus. Inactivated viruses when injected into the host may passively attach to the host's antigen-presenting cells via their haemagglutinin, thus providing equal presentation probability to both the "suppressor epitope" (haemagglutinin) and the "helper epitope" (matrix protein). The net effect will be a nullification of each other's effect. In contrast, replicating viruses mainly express viral subunits such as haemagglutinin on the surface of host cells (23). Thus there may be presentation advantage for the "suppressor epitope" during infection leading to the predominant activation of suppressor T cells by haemagglutinin. The precise mechanism of the preferential induction of suppression or enhancement of the immune response to macromolecules with multi-determinants is, of course, at present unknown and is currently a subject of intense investigation. It may well be that the "helper epitopes" have stronger affinity for the products of the I-A/E subregion gene (the so called helper gene). The "suppressor epitopes", on the other hand, may associate more readily with the determinants encoded by the I-J subregion gene (the so called suppressor gene). The interaction of exogenous antigens with the major histocompatibility complex (MHC) gene products leading to activation or suppression of T cell activity remains a tantalising question.

GENERAL CONSIDERATIONS

Since the first description of DTH by Zinsser (24) in 1921 based on the tuberculin-type skin reaction which developed in sensitized guinea pigs, considerable insight into the detailed mechanism of this cell mediated phenomenon has been achieved. Today, DTH is defined as an immunologically specific inflammatory reaction maximal at 24-48 h and with a characteristic histologic appearance of infiltration with mononuclear cells. The reaction is transferable by T lymphocytes whose induction and manifestation are restricted by products of the MHC (25). A subset of antigen specific precursor T cells, upon stimulation by antigens presented in the context of MHC determinants on antigen presenting cells, differentiate and become sensitized T cells, which are destined to mediate a DTH response (Fig. 3).

This subset of T cells, T_D cells, bears the Lyt-1+2-Ia- phenotype. There are reports that some Lyt-1-2+,Ia- can also mediate local DTH when passively transferred together with antigen in the footpads of mice (10,26). However, the

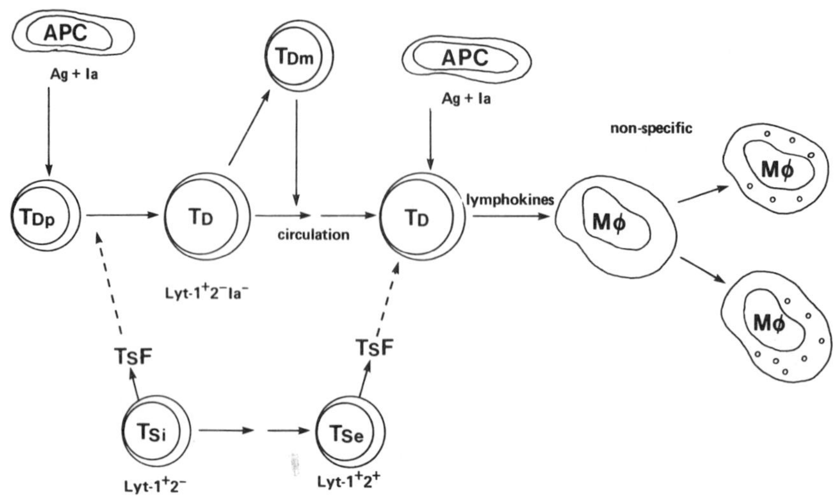

FIGURE 3. Schematic representation of DTH induction, manifestation and regulation. APC=antigen presenting cells of undefined cell type, Ag=antigen, Ia=I region associated antigen, TDP=precursor of T cell mediating DTH (T_D), TDM=memory T_D, Mo=macrophage, TSi=Suppressor T cells for induction of T_D, TSe=suppressor T cells for the expression of T_D, TSF=suppressor T cell factor. Interrupted arrows represent inhibition.

relationship between these and the recirculating Lyt-1 bearing T_D cells is at present unclear. Some of the T_D cells may differentiate separately to become memory cells for DTH. These specifically sensitized T_D cells form a longlived recirculating pool which may play an important role in immunological surveillance. The mature T_D cells react with specific antigen, again presented in the context of MHC determinants on antigen-presenting cells, by proliferation and release of soluble mediators (lymphokines) which attract and activate a nonspecific population of macrophages. The nonspecific bone-marrow derived macrophages, upon activation by lymphokines, continue to proliferate and infiltrate at the site of reaction and become predominant in the lesion. Thus the final effector phase of DTH involves the nonspecific engulfment and destruction of pathogens by these activated macrophages which are the ultimate effector cells.

By arming the host macrophages nonspecifically, the DTH response may produce severe host tissue damage, particularly if infections occur in vital organs. Thus, from the evolutionary standpoint, it is critical that DTH reactivity be kept in optimum balance. It is therefore not surprising that

DTH response has turned out to be tightly regulated by suppressor T cells in most situations. At least two distinct types of T_S cells for DTH have been demonstrated: those suppressing the induction of DTH (T_Si) and those interfering with the expression of DTH (T_Se). The effector of both these T_Si and T_Se is at present unclear. They may be of the same cell lineage at various stages of antigen driven differentiation, or alternatively, they may represent members of a cascade whose activation is interdependent on each other. The existence of T_S cells capable of suppressing both the affector and the effector phases of DTH no doubt contributes towards the effectiveness of regulation of this potentially harmful immune response.

In the case of influenza virus, although T-helper cells for DTH could be induced in vivo by matrix protein, in natural infection by aerosol, suppressor T cells appear predominant soon after virus uptake and remain active long after clearance of the virus in readiness, perhaps, against later reinfection. This persistent presence of specific suppressor T cells could be of a significant evolutionary advantage, since there is no evidence that DTH is an important arm of immunity against influenza virus infection. On the contrary, in influenza pneumonia in mice, T_D cells clearly contribute to the pathology (lung consolidation) resulting in an increased early mortality (9).

TABLE 3. Effect of T_S Cells for DTH on the Mortality Induced by T_D Cells in A/PR8 Infected Mice

Infection (d0 aerosol)	Cells transferred (d1,i.v.)	Mortality
A/PR8	-	3/10
A/PR8	T_D + T_N	9/10
A/PR8	TD + TS	2/10

Groups of 10 CBA mice were infected by an aerosol (LD50) of A/PR8 virus and 24 h later transferred i.v. with various cell combinations as indicated. The cells were prepared as follows: splenic Ig- cells (T_D) from CBA mice primed (i.p.) 3 weeks earlier with 10μg of purified UV-inactivated PR8 virus were cultured for 5 days with syngeneic spleen cells infected with PR8 virus in the presence of an equal number of Ig- cells from normal spleen (T_N) or from spleens of mice infected two weeks earlier with an aerosol of PR8 virus (T_S). At the end of culture, viable cells were harvested and transferred at 6 x 10^7/recipient. Mortality was recorded up to 28 days after infection.

Since DTH is deleterious to the host and antigen specific suppressor T cells for DTH can be readily generated, it may be expected that interaction of T_S and T_D would result in the cancellation of this detrimental effect of T_D in infected mice.

Results shown in Table 3 demonstrate that this, may be the case. When CBA mice were infected with LD_{50} dose of A/PR8 virus, 3/10 died by day 28. When these mice were transferred with 3 x 10^7 T_D cells one day after infection, only 1/10 survived. However, if the T_D cells were incubated with spleen cells containing T_S cells and then transferred to infected mice 8/10 of the recipients survived. The T_S cells have been characterised extensively (6) and appear to be Lyt-1+2- (F.Y.Liew and S.M. Russell, in preparation).

These results suggest, as far as I am aware, for the first time the beneficial effect of specific suppressor T cells towards the host against a potentially lethal viral infection. They also complement the metazoal parasite model where I-J+ T_S cells adoptively reduce the granuloma formation (which is related to DTH response) in mice chronically infected with Schistosoma mansoni (27). However, it should be emphasized that DTH response should be extremely beneficial to the hosts in systems where the primary targets of the infectious organisms are macrophages. The generation of T_S cells for DTH in these instances would therefore be detrimental to the survival of the hosts. Indeed, in Leishmania tropica infection in mice, fatality to the protozoon is the result of the generation of antigen-specific T_S cells for DTH have clearly established the in vivo relevance of suppressor T cells beyond the mere experimental effect of an in vitro phenomenon.

REFERENCES

1. Beveridge, W.I.B. and Burnet, F.M. (1944). A cutaneous reaction to the influenza viruses. Med. J. Aust. 1, 85.
2. Habershon, R.B., Molyneux, M.E., Slavin, G., Loewi,G. and Tyrrell,D.A.J. (1973). Skin tests with influenza virus. J. Hyg. (Camb.), 71, 755.
3. Cole,P.J. and Molyneux,M.E. (1975). Lymphocyte reactivity to influenza virus in man. Immunology, 29, 749.
4. Webster,R.G. and Hinshaw, V.S. (1977). Matrix protein from influenza A virus and its role in cross-protection in mice. Inf. and Immunity, 17, 561.
5. Liew,F.Y., Russell,S.M. and Brand, C.M. (1979). Induction and characterisation of delayed-type

hypersensitivity to influenza virus in mice. Eur. J. Immunol., 9, 783.

6. Liew,F.Y. and Russell,S.M. (1980). Delayed-type hypersensitivity to influenza virus. Induction of antigen-specific suppressor T cells for delayed-type hypersensitivity to haemagglutinin during influenza virus infection in mice. J. Exp. Med., 151, 799.
7. Liew,F.Y. (1981). Recognition of the hapten carrier system in infectious diseases. In Immunological recognition and effector mechanism in infectious diseases. Eds. G. Torrigiani and R. Bell, Schwabe and Co. A.G. Basel. Chapter 1, pp. 1-12.
8. Leung,K.N., Ada, G.L. and McKenzie,I.F.C. (1980). Specificity, Ly phenotype, and H-2 compatibility requirements of effector cells in delayed-type hypersensitivity response to murine influenza virus infection. J. Exp. Med. 151, 815.
9. Leung,K.N. and Ada, G.L. (1980). Cell mediating delayed-type hypersensitivity in the lungs of mice infected with an influenza A virus. Scand. J. Immunol. 12, 393.
10. Leung,K.N. and Ada, G.L. (1981). Effect of helper T cells on the primary in vitro production of delayed-type hypersensitivity to infleunza virus. J. Exp. Med., 153, 1029.
11. Zinkernagel,R.M. (1976). H-2 restriction of virus-specific T-cell-mediated effector functions in vivo. II. Adoptive transfer of delayed-type hypersensitivity to murine lymphocytic choriomeningitis virus is restricted by the K and D region of H-2. J.Exp.Med., 144, 776.
12. Weiner,H.L., Greene, M.I. and Fields,B.N. (1980). Delayed hypersensitivity in mice infected with reovirus. I. Identification of host and viral gene products responsible for the immune response. J. Immunol., 125, 278.
13. Nash, A.A., Phelan,J. and Wildy,P. (1981). Cell-mediated immunity in herpes simplex virus-infected mice: H-2 mapping of the delayed-type hypersensitivity response and the anti-viral T cell responses. J. Immunol., 126, 1260.
14. Gill,H.K. and Liew,F.Y. (1978). Regulation of delayed-type hypersensitivity. III. Effect of cyclophosphamide on the suppressor cells for delayed-type hypersensitivity to sheep erythrocytes in mice. Eur. J. Immunol., 8, 172.
15. Shand, F.L. and Liew,F.Y. (1980). Differential sensitivity to cyclophosphamide of helper T cells for humoral responses and suppressor T cells for delayed-type hypersensitivity. Eur.J.Immunol. 10, 480.

16. Milon,G. and Marchal,G. (1978). Increased infiltration by monocytes in delayed type hypersensitivity site following cyclophosphamide treatment. Immunology, 35, 989.
17. Ramshaw,I.A., Bretscher,P.A. and Parish,C.R. (1976). Regulation of the immune response. I. Suppression of delayed-type hypersensitivity by T cells from mice expressing humoral immunity. Eur. J. Immunol., 6, 674.
18. Asherson,G.L. and Zembala,M. (1974). Suppression of contact sensitivity by T cells in the mouse. I. Demonstration that suppressor cells act on the effector stage of contact sensitivity; and their induction following in vitro exposure to antigen. Proc. R. Soc. London (Biol.), 187, 329.
19. Greene,M.I. and Weiner,H.L. (1980). Delayed hypersensitivity in mice infected with reovirus. II. Induction of tolerance and suppressor T cells to viral specific gene products. J. Immunol. 125, 283.
20. Nash,A.A., Phelan,J., Gell,P.G.H. and Wildy,P. (1981). Tolerance and immunity in mice infected with herpes simplex virus: studies on the mechanism of tolerance to delayed-type hypersensitivity. Immunology, 43, 363.
21. Sercarz,E.E., Yowell,R.L., Turkin,D., Miller,A., Araneo,B.A. and Adorini,L. (1978). Different functional specificity repertoires for suppressor and helper T cells. Transpl. Rev., 39, 108.
22. Russell,S.M. and Liew,F.Y. (1979). T cells primed by influenza virion internal components can cooperate in the antibody response to haemagglutinin. Nature, 280, 147.
23. Hackett,C.J., Askonas,B.A., Webster,R.G. and VanWyke,K. (1980). Quantitation of influenza virus antigens on infected target cells and their recognition by crossreactive cytotoxic T cells. J.Exp.Med., 151,1014.
24. Zinsser,H. (1921). Studies on tuberculin reaction and on specific hypersensitiveness in bacterial infection. J. Exp. Med., 34, 495.
25. Miller,J.F.A.P., Vadas,M.A., Whitelaw,A. and Gamble,J. (1976). Role of major histocompatibility complex gene products in delayed-type hypersensitivity. Proc. Natl. Acad.Sci. USA, 73,2486.
26. Lin,Y.L. and Askonas,B.A. (1981). Biological properties of an influenza A virus-specific killer T cell clone. Inhibition of virus replication in vivo and induction of delayed-type hypersensitivity reaction. J.Exp.Med., 154, 225.
27. Green,W.F. and Colley,D.G. (1981). Modulation of Schistosoma mansoni egg-induced granuloma formation: I-J restriction of T cell-mediated suppression in a chronic parasitic infection. Proc. Natl. Acad. Sci. USA 78, 1152.

28. Howard,J.G., Hale,C. and Liew,F.Y. (1981). Immunological regulation of experimental cutaneous leishmaniasis. IV. Prophylactic effect of sublethal irradiation as a result of abrogation of suppressor T cell generation in mice genetically susceptible to Leishmania tropica. J. Exp. Med., 153,557.
29. Liew,F.Y., Hale,C. and Howard,J.G. (1982). Immunologic regulation of experimental cutaneous leishmaniasis. V. Characterisation of effector and specific suppressor T cells. J. Immunol., 128, 1917.

III

HERPES SIMPLEX VIRUS

CHAPTER 12

IMMUNITY IN RELATION TO THE PATHOGENESIS OF HERPES SIMPLEX VIRUS

A. A. Nash
P. Wildy

Department of Pathology
University of Cambridge
Tennis Court Road
Cambridge, U.K.

In this review we consider separately the three important areas of herpes simplex virus pathogenesis, namely the primary, the latent and the recurrent phases of infection. As the information on herpes pathogenesis in man is still rudimentary, we will concentrate mainly on some relevant animal models of the human disease. In particular emphasis will be placed on the role of the immune response during viral pathogenesis. In doing this it is important to acknowledge that the study of experimental infection is very much second best for two reasons. First, herpes simplex virus is not a natural parasite of laboratory animals and variation between species is to be expected (1). Secondly, the means of infection are necessarily contrived so that the outcome may result greatly from variable factors such as age of host, dose of virus, or route of infection and some of these factors will be considered and made use of here.

THE PHASE OF PRIMARY INFECTION

Variable Factors

Route. Various routes of infection have been used experimentally but only those which seem relevant to natural human infections will be considered here.

It is clear from several studies that the LD_{50} doses of herpes virus types 1 and 2, injected i.v. or i.p. into susceptible mice are smaller than the LD_{50} of mice injected

ISBN 0-12-239980-3

s.c. Presumably this is because in these cases the virus gains access to the CNS more readily. Indeed, following on i.v. injection, virus can be isolated from the adrenal gland after 1 or 2 days and from the spinal cord after 3-5 days (1,2). It is therefore likely that access to the CNS following i.v. injection is via the adrenal gland or coeliac plexus. Infective virus is seldom found in other tissues e.g. spleen, lung, heart, blood, whatever the route of entry. In a detailed study of Balb/c and A/J mice injected intravaginally Walz et al. (3) observed virus antigen in vaginal, uterine and cervical epithelial cells, as well as cervical and uterine glandular epithelium, myometrium and local autonomic ganglion cells. Progression to the CNS is often swift with infective virus detected after 4 to 5 days (2,4). The other route commonly used, intradermal or subcutaneous infections is considered in more detail below.

Genetic Attributes of Virus

Avirulent variants of herpes virus have of course been used to advantage in the study of herpetic infection. For example thymidine kinase negative mutants are recognized to be relatively avirulent (5,6) and induce latency less readily than wild-type virus (7). Further facts which produce quite unexpected pathological effects have been described (8). But here we wish to consider only unmodified (i.e. virulent) naturally occurring viruses.

A few striking differences are to be found between type 1 and type 2 herpes simplex virus, for instance with type 2, but not type 1, virus injected i.p. or i.v., a focal necrotic hepatitis is frequently observed after 4 days in some mouse strains (2,9). In a recent comparative study between various recent isolates and laboratory strains of types 1 and 2 virus, injected intravaginally, type 1 virus replicated to higher titres in the vaginal mucosa, but type 2 isolates produced a higher mortality and greater frequency of latent infections in the lumbosacral ganglia of surviving animals (10). Interestingly, type 2 virus injected intranasally produced a higher mortality, but type 1 produced a higher incidence of latency in the trigeminal ganglia. It appears to be a general finding that type 2 isolates are more neurovirulent than type 1 isolates; yet in man almost all cases of encephalitis are caused by strains of type 1 virus (11).

In a study using type 1 herpes strains producing predominantly stromal or epithelial infections, Centifanto-Fitzgerald et al (12) found that the disease pattern in ocular herpetic infections was genetically determined by the virus. Using recombinants of the two strains they mapped the genes determining the ocular disease pattern to 0.70 to 0.83 units of the type 1 genome.

Age of Animal

It has been recognized for years that the behavious of herpes virus in animals was considerably modified by their age. While i.c. injections of neonatal or adult mice gave similar LD_{50} values, there were great differences in the LD_{50} on peripheral inoculation (13,14). Not surprisingly therefore death rates in neonatal herpes with types 1 and 2 are similar (15).

A Standard Animal Model

Of the various models studying the cutaneous herpes type 1 infection (a natural infection route of man) perhaps the best characterized is the mouse ear model, originally described by Hill, Field & Blyth (16). In this model moderate doses ($10^4$to 10^5 p.f.u.) of a standard recent isolate are inoculated intradermally or subcutaneously into the ear flap of a standard mouse (5-6 weeks old). Though some liberties have had to be taken in adapting this model for immunological experiments it has been of the greatest possible use.

Soon after infection, almost exclusively of epithelial cells, the local multiplication of virus begins and can readily be followed for at least 7 days. Inflammation can be recorded in single mice by the measurement of ear thickness and histological confirmation is simple in a mouse's ear. The fate of the original inoculum is readily assessed using isotope labelled virus and the progression of infected virus to lymph node, sensory ganglia and other tissues can readily be followed. The productively infected cells in the dorsal root ganglia have been identified as neurons (Field, personal communication).

Genetic Attributes of Animals

The severity of a particular herpes infection is also dependent upon the genetic constitution of the host. This is particularly relevant in mice, where Lopez (17) has shown that C57BL strains are very resistant, Balb/c and CBA of intermediate resistance and AKR and A/J quite susceptible to an i.p. infection with type 1 virus. We have to some extent confirmed these findings in mice injected subcutaneously: C57BL10 mice replicate type 1 virus (strain SC16) less efficiently than AKR or A/J mice and have a lower mortality than them (Nash & Field, unpublished observations).

Infection of athymic nude mice in the ear flap leads to local replication of virus with no abatement after 7 days, but a persistent, spreading lesion which is obviously uncontrolled by the host. The virus seems to spread sequentially to the dorsal root ganglia, spinal cord, brain and adrenal glands. Virus has also been observed in the coeliac plexus, cardiac plexus and also the eye on the ipsilateral side (18). These animals usually die 2 to 3 weeks after infection, a feature which contrasts with the much earlier mortality found in immunocompetent animals.

Clearly the severity and nature of the primary infection will depend largely on the route, the nature of the virus, the dose used and resistance mechanisms of the host.

Natural Resistance Mechanisms

We believe that resistance mechanisms operate at a very early stage after infection; most probably involving natural killer cells (19), interferon (20), and macrophages. (Such mechanisms are clearly important in athymic nude mice which are quite resistant to i.p. infection, in contrast to their susceptibility to s.c. infection of the ear). The macrophage appears to play a central role in the recovery from herpes infections. In type 2 i.p. infections, resistance is sex-linked and dependent upon the integrity of macrophage function (9). As already discussed infection of young animals with herpes leads to a high mortality, compared to adult animals. Resistance to i.p. infections develops rapidly during the first few weeks of life and corresponds to the maturation of the macrophage system (14). Furthermore, treatment of mice with silica particles or antimacrophage serum produced a rapid mortality beginning 5 days after infectiuon and resulting in high titres of virus in the liver and virus-induced hepatic necrosis (21). Clearly impairment of macrophage function will also lead to a failure to induce specific immune responses, another important response involved in the early elimination of virus.

Immune Response During the Primary Infection: Cell Mediated Immunity

The finding that athymic (nu/nu) mice are susceptible to intradermal herpes infections implies that T cell mediated responses are essential for antiviral immunity. Such observations are consistent with the severity of primary and recurrent diseases encountered in patients with predominantly T cell immunodeficiencies (22). Although it has been known for some time that the adoptive transfer of immune spleen cells can protect the recipient against a lethal herpes infection (23,24) the nature of the cell types involved have only recently been investigated (25). T cell subpopulations involved in anti-hperes immunity has been extensively investigated in the mouse ear model (26,27,28). Four to five days after an ear inoculation of herpes virus type 1 (strain SC16) the lymph nodes draining the infected pinna contain cytotoxic T cells, T cells mediating delayed hypersensitivity (DH) and T cells involved in protective immunity. The DH-T cells are Lyt $1^{+}2^{-}$ and restricted by the IA subregion of the H-2 complex. Protective T cells are also Lyt $1^{+}2^{-}$ but are restricted by the H-2K (D) and IA regions. Antiviral immunity in this system is determined by adoptive transfer of immune lymph node cells to infected syngeneic recipients, the DH response is measured after 48 hrs and the infective herpes titres after 4 days. A strong correlation between DH and the rapid elimination of infective herpes in the ear has recently been reported by Nash & Ashford (28). The finding that DH correlates with protective immunity in our model shows parallels with allograft rejection in the mouse. Delayed hypersensitivity and allograft rejection both correlate and are mediated by Lyt $1^{+}2^{-}$ and not Lyt $1^{-}2^{+}$ cells (29). As both systems involve a response against altered self or foreign epithelial cells, then the analogy is reasonable one.

Antibody Mediated Responses

In man defects of humoral immune responses (hypogammaglobulinemia) does not seem to interfere with the control of herpes viruses (22). This finding was confirmed experimentally using the mouse-ear model. The B-cell responses of mice were suppressed by the regular administration of anti-IgM antibodies from birth (30). Such animals had depleted B cell dependent areas in spleen and lymph nodes, no detectable serum IgM and reduced IgG levels. Following infection in the ear, no serum neutralizing antibodies or total herpes specific IgG antibodies could be detected, yet the animals recovered from the infection normally. CMI responses were unaffected by such treatment. However, we noted that the incidence of latency in B cell suppressed animals was higher than in controls and there was a more florid primary infection of the dorsal root ganglia and spinal cord. This suggested that specific antibody was effective in restricting the spread of herpes to the nervous system, a finding that was confirmed by the passive transfer of antibody to nude mice. As described above the virus spreads sequentially from the ear pinna to the dorsal root ganglia and spinal cord and in nude mice this is easy to measure. However in nudes given neutralizing polyclonal or monoclonal antibodies 3 days after infection, little or no virus could be recovered from the dorsal root ganglia or spinal cord 11 days later, despite virus titres in the ear flap comparable to controls (18). Non-neutralising monoclonal antibodies against the same glycoprotein were ineffective in restricting virus in the nervous system. Taken together these data suggest an important role for antibody in restricting the spread of virus to the peripheral and control nervous system, possibly by neutralising virus at peripheral nerve endings and synaptic junctions. We note that virus clearance from the pinna was only achieved following the transfer of immune lymphoid cells.

The importance of specific anti-herpes antibody as a protective response in the primary infection phase has been the subject of other reports (31,32). In particular antibody mediated neutralisation was considered important only if present at the time of infection. After 8 hours post infection, protective mechanisms depended on the presence of an intact Fc piece which probably indicates a role for antibody dependent cell cytotoxicity (32). However, it should be noted in many of these systems one is studying passively administered antibody responses against a background of developing cell-mediated immunity. Furthermore, since the endpoint in many of these experiments is mortality, then the protective effects attributed to antibody could be operating in the way described by Kapoor et al (18,30).

THE LATENT PHASE

In both man and in mouse models, as the primary infection is eliminated, a long lived immune response involving memory T-cells and antiherpes antibodies is found. The virus in the meantime has established itself as a latent infection in the ganglion innervating the primary infection site. The ganglionic cell harbouring latent virus is the neuron (33,34). However, other sites have been implicated namely the skin in a guinea pig model (35) and the brain (36,37); the particular cells involved in these cases have not been identified. The state of the virus genome during this particular period is still a subject of speculation (1). Although the new evidence favours a static form of latency, in which the virus exists integrated with host DNA or as episomal DNA, with either no expression, or partial expression of viral genes being observed (38,39). Alternatively, it has been suggested that a dynamic form of latency could exist with reactivated virus cycling to and from the primary infection site establishing new latent foci. In the latently infected host a combination of both forms seem likely.

Is there immune control of latent infections? The finding that virus could only be recovered from latently infected ganglia after a period in culture or co-cultivation with a sensitive monolayer, prompted investigators to consider the possibility that immunologcial factors maintain the latent state, since when the ganglia were removed from the host, virus reactivations readily occur. Stevens & Cook (40) originally proposed that immune mechanisms were important for maintaining latency, since when latently infected ganglia were transplanted into immune or non-immune mice, the extent of virus reactivation was markedly reduced in the immune animals. Furthermore they found the adoptive transfer of anti-herpes IgG was effective in reducing the level of virus reactivation. It is perhaps difficult to imagine antibody per se inhibiting a reactivation event in a neuron, but the studies of Stevens & Cook suggest that once such an event occurs, extracellular spread with the ganglion is inhibited.

Recently the role of antibody in maintaining latency has been questioned (41). In these experiments latency was established in mice given high doses of virus, followed 2 days later by rabbit anti-herpes antibodies. The protecting antibodies were allowed to decay to 'undetectable' levels (i.e. $<1/8$ neutralization titre) and any subsequent rise in neutralizing antibody responses would be of mouse origin and presumably in response to a reactivation event. In mice traumatized so as to induce a reactivation, the neutralization titre was observed to rise. Since in only a small percentage of mice not traumatized was there an increase in neutralization titres noted, clear evidence was provided that antibody was not required for maintaining the latent state. This model does not however consider any role for T cells or their products in maintaining latent infections or indeed a role for non-neutralizing antibodies and ADCC or interferon.

That T cells or their products could conceivably be involved in maintaining latency was suggested by experiments of Kapoor et al (manuscript in preparation). They established latent infections in athymic nude mice by transferring 2×10^7 immune lymph node cells, which were effective in controlling the primary infection. Fourteen days after infection the ganglia were removed and assayed for latent virus by reactivation. In half the latency positive ganglia no neutralising antibody responses were detected, implying latency in the presence of T cells, but in the absence of specific antibody. Interestingly in this model, if the dose of immune cells given 3 days after infection was increased to

7×10^7 cells/nude recipient, then in 90% of the animals no latent virus was reactivated, when the ganglia were assayed 4 weeks later. In only 40% of the animals was specific antibody detected. The suggestion that high doses of immune T cells (including DH-T cells and cytotoxic T cells) can prevent or even 'eliminate' latent infections is intriguing and deserving of further investigation.

THE PHASE OF REACTIVATION, RECURRENCE AND RECRUDESCENCE

It is abundantly clear that periods of stress, pregnancy, trauma, excessive sunlight or organ transplantation can lead to reactivation of herpes which manifests itself as recrudescent lesions or cold sores. The repeated outbreaks suffered by some individuals is restricted to one or few dermatomes (reviewed in 42,1). The mechanism of reactivation of virus is not understood, although it is reasonable to assume it involves a physiological change of the latently infected neuron. Various hypotheses have been advanced, to account for reactivation and recurrence including the ganglion trigger hypothesis and the skin trigger hypothesis (43). Essentially the ganglion trigger hypothesis proposes that following a reactivation event in a ganglion, virus travels back along the peripheral nerves and establishes an infection in the skin. The stimulus for this event comes initially from outside the ganglion, e.g. the skin. In the skin trigger hypothesis, the assumption is made that virus is periodically seeded to the skin and it is only following periods of trauma, prostaglandin release etc. that conditions in the skin favour virus replication and hence recurrent disease. It is however likely that both events are required in recurrence disease.

In animal models recurrence is achieved with varying success. For example in the guinea pig, recurrence is more demonstrable than in the mouse. Here only certain outbred strains have been useful as models for studying recurrent disease (44). The incidence of recurrence is increased if certain traumatizing agents e.g. cellophane tape, chemicals such as xylene or 'dry-ice' are used or by immunosuppression. Clearly the nature of the immunosuppression is important. Openshaw et al (45) have shown that reactivation of virus in the ganglion and recurrences at the primary infection site (i.e. the lip) can be achieved with cyclophosphamide and X-irradiation. The problem here is in deciding whether the depression of immune surveillance results in reactivation and recurrences or whether these agents directly affect the ganglia and local skin environment. Other workers using antithymocyte serum and corticosteroid treatment did not increase the recurrence rate in the ear model (46). On the other hand massive immunosuppression i.e. adult thymectomy, X-irradiation to lethal doses and antithymocyte serum treatment was required to produce reactivation of virus in the local sensory ganglia and in the brain of latently infected mice (47). Similar treatments are often found with immunosuppressed patients undergoing bone-marrow transplantation, where the incidence of herpes-induced encephalitis is high (Kay, personal communication).

This type of evidence clearly suggests that immune mechanisms could be important in controlling recurrent virus episodes, and that such mechanisms are resistant to moderate immunosuppressive regimes.

Immune Control During Recurrent Infections

Recurrences often take place in the face of high levels of circulating neutralizing virus antibodies. Indeed this has often been used as an argument against the role of antibody in controlling herpes infections. Attention was therefore focused on the role of protective T cells. In this respect the observation of Shillitoe et al (48,49) are relevant that patients undergoing recurrences have reduced or absent levels of MIF producing lymphocytes in their circulation. As MIF production correlates well with DH responses in vivo, then this data implies that defects in T cell surveillance mechanism is an important criteria in recurrences. Similar findings have been made for herpes type 2 in the guinea-pig recurrence model (50). The cause of these breakdowns in immune surveillance may be many. One possibility is the observation that B suppressor cells, which appear to regulate the intensity of DH reactions to the virus are observed during the latent period of infection and could represent a possible interruptor of normal immune surveillance (51). Another possibility is the presence of T cell suppressors which are induced following a i.v. injection of infectious herpes (52). This response is long lived and is specific for suppressing the induction of DH responses to the virus. The cells mediating this type of suppression appear to be Lyt $1^{+}2^{-}IJ^{+}$ and Lyt $1^{-}2^{+}IJ^{+}$ cells (Nash & Gell, submitted for publication). Although these suppressor cells recognize only a 'type-specific' determinant they are capable of suppressing DH responses to presumed type-specific and type common determinants. This immunoregulating mechanism is specific for DH responses, since specific antibody responses and cytotoxic T cell responses are not affected (28). The animals with this split

T cell tolerance effect are still capable of eliminating infectious virus challenges, but the effect of these mechanisms in controlling recurrences is unknown, since the particular inbred strains used in these studies i.e. Balb/c and CBA, do not readily produce recurrent disease.

Despite the various possibilities discussed in this section, it is perhaps surprising that with the various advances made in the fields of virology and immunology in recent years that we should still be puzzled by the events leading to herpes recurrences. If immune control is, as we believe, important in determining whether recurrent virus is eliminated subclinically or not, then the cell types involved and their susceptibility to immunosuppression represent important areas for future investigation.

EPILOGUE

In this review we have considered the importance of animal models in understanding some of the fundamental problems surrounding herpes virus pathogenesis. Although there are shortcomings from studying such models, the basic mechanisms underlying latency and recurrences are likely to be similar between species, and consequently such mechanisms are more readily investigated in experimental animals. In particular, the T cell mechanisms important during the control of cutaneous herpes infections may provide important clues as to the immune control of recurrent disease in man. Similarly the recent findings that anti-herpes antibodies are effective in controlling the spread of virus to the peripheral and central nervous system, may serve to rekindle interest in the importance of the humoral response in man.

REFERENCES

1. Wildy, P., Field,H.J. & Nash,A.A. 1982. Classical herpes latency revisited. In Virus Persistence, (ed. Mahy, B.W.J., Minson, A.C. & Darby, G.K.), Cambridge Univ. Press. pp. 133-167.
2. Renis, H.E., Eidson,E.E., Mathews, J. & Gray, J.E. 1976. Pathogenesis of herpes simplex virus types 1 and 2 in mice after various routes of inoculation. Infect. Immun. 14:571-578.
3. Walz, M.A., Price, R.W., Hayashi, K., Katz, B.J. & Notkins, A.L. 1977. Effect of immunization on acute and latent infections of vaginouterine tissue with herpes

simplex virus types 1 and 1. J. Infect. Dis. 135, 744-752.
4. Morahan,P.S., Breinig,M.C. & McGeorge,M.C. 1977. Immune responses to vaginal or systemic infection of Balb/c mice with herpes simplex virus type 2. J. Immunol. 119, 2030-2036.
5. Field,H.J. & Wildy,P. 1978. The pathogenicity of thymidine kinase-deficient mutants of herpes simplex virus in mice. J. Hyg. Cambridge 81, 267-277.
6. Field,H.J. & Darby,G. 1980. Pathogenicity in mice of strains of herpes simplex virus which are resistant to acyclovir in vitro and in vivo. Antimicrobial Agents & Chemotherapy 17, 209-16.
7. Tenser,R.B., Miller,R.L. & Rapp, F. 1979. Trigeminal ganglion infection by thymidine kinase negative-mutants of herpes simplex virus. Science 205, 915-917.
8. Field,H.J., Anderson,J.R. & Wildy,P. 1982. Atypical patterns of neural infection produced in mice by drug resistant strains of herpes simplex virus. J. Gen. Virol. 59, 91-99.
9. Mogensen,S.C. 1980. Genetics of macrophage-controlled natural resistance to hepatitis induced by herpes simplex virus type 2 in mice. In Genetic Control of Natural Resistance to Infection and Malignancy, ed. Skamene, E., Kongshavn, P.A.L. & Landy, M., pp. 291-296. Academic Press, New York.
10. Richards, J.T., Kern, E.R., Overall,J.C. & Glasgow,L.A. 1981. Differences in neurovirulence among isolates of herpes simplex virus types 1 and 2 in mice using four routes of inoculation. J. Infect. Dis. 144, 464-471.
11. Nahmias,A.J. & Roizman,B. 1973. Infection with herpes simplex viruses 1 and 2 (part 3). N. Engl. J. Med. 289, 781-789.
12. Centifanto-Fitzgerald,Y.M., Yamaguchi, T., Kaufman, H.E., Tognon, M. & Roisman, B. (1982). Ocular disease pattern induced by herpes simplex virus is genetically determined by a specific region of viral DNA. J. Exp. Med. 155, 475-489.
13. Johnson,R.T. 1964. The pathogenesis of herpes virus encephalitis. I. Virus pathways to the central nervous system of suckling mice demonstrated by fluorescent antibody staining. J. Exp. Med. 119, 343-356.
14. Hirsch, M.S., Zisman,B. & Allison, A.C. 1970. Macrophage and age-dependent resistance to herpes simplex virus in mice. J. Immunol. 104, 1160-1165.
15. Whitley, R.J., Nahmias,A.J., Visintine,A.M., Fleming,C.L. & Alford,C.A. 1980. The natural history of herpes simplex virus infection of mother and newborn. Pediatrics 66, 489-494.

16. Hill,T.J., Field,H.J. & Blyth, W.A. 1975. Acute and recurrent infection with herpes simplex virus in the mouse: a model for studying latency and recurrent disease. J. Gen. Virol. 28, 341-353.
17. Lopez, C. 1975. Genetics of natural resistance to herpes virus infections in mice. Nature 258, 152-153.
18. Kapoor, A.K., Nash,A.A., Wildy,P., Phelan,J., McLean,C.S. & Field,H.J. 1982a. Pathogenesis of herpes simplex virus in congenitally athymic mice: the relative roles of cell-mediated and humoral immunity. J. Gen. Virol. 60, 225-233.
19. Lopez,C. 1980. Genetic resistance to herpes infections: role of natural killer cells. In Genetic Control of Natural Resistance to Infection and Malignancy, ed. Skamene, E., Kongshavn, P.A.L. & Landy, M. pp.253-265. Academic Press (New York).
20. Kirchner,H., Engler,H., Zawatsky,R. & Schroder, C.H. 1980. Studies of resistance of mice against herpes simplex virus. In Genetic Control of Natural Resistance to Infection and Malignancy (ed. Skamene,E., Kongshavn,P.A.L. & Landy,M. p. 267-276. Academic Press.
21. Zisman,B., Hirsch,M.S. & Allison,A.C. 1970. Selective effects of anti-macrophage serum, silica and anti-lymphocyte serum on pathogenesis of herpes virus infection of young adult mice. J. Immunol. 104, 1155-1159.
22. Merigan, T.C. & Stevens,D.A. 1971. Viral infections in man associated with acquired immunological deficiency states. Fed. Proc. 30, 1858-1864.
23. Oakes,J.E. 1975. Role for cell mediated immunity in the resistance of mice to subcutaneous herpes simplex infection. Infect. Immun. 12, 166-172.
24. Ennis,F.A. 1973. Host defense mechanisms against herpes simplex virus. II. Protection conferred by sensitized spleen cells. J. Infect. Dis. 127, 632-638.
25. Howes,E.L., Taylor, W., Mitchison,N.A. & Simpson,E. 1979. MHC matching shows that at least two T-cell subsets determine resistance to HSV. Nature 277:67-68.
26. Nash,A.A., Field,H.J. & Quartey-Papafio,R. 1980. Cell mediated immunity in herpes simplex virus-infected mice: induction, characterization and antiviral effects of delayed type hypersensitivity. J. Gen. Virol. 48, 351-357.
27. Nash,A.A., Phelan,J., Gell,P.G.H. & Wildy,P. 1981. Tolerance and immunity in mice infected with herpes simplex virus. Studies on the mechanism of tolerance to delayed type hypersensitivity. Immunology 43, 363-369.

28. Nash,A.A. & Ashford,N.P.N. 1982. Split-T cell tolerance in herpes simplex virus-infected mice and its implication for antiviral immunity. Immunology 45, 761-767.
29. Loveland,B.E. & McKenzie,I.F.C. 1982. Delayed-type hypersensitivity and allograft rejection in the mouse: correlation of effector cell phenotype. Immunology 46, 313-320.
30. Kapoor,A.K., Nash,A.A. & Wildy, P. 1982b. Pathogenesis of herpes simplex virus in B-cell suppressed mice: the relative roles of cell-mediated and humoral immunity. J.Gen.Virol. 61, 127-131.
31. Worthington,M., Conliffe, M.A. & Baron,S. 1980. Mechanism of recovery from systemic herpes simplex virus infection. I. Comparative effectiveness of antibody and reconstitution of immune spleen cells on immunosuppressed mice. J. Infect. Dis. 142, 163-173.
32. Oakes,J.E. & Lausch,R.N. 1981. Role of Fc fragments in antibody-mediated recovery from ocular and subcutaneous herpes simplex virus infections. Infect. Immun. 33, 109-114.
33. Cook,M.L., Bastone,V.B. & Stevens,J.G. 1974. Evidence that neurons harbour latent herpes simplex virus. Infect. Immun. 9, 946-951.
34. McLennon,J.L. & Darby,G. 1980. Herpes simplex virus latency: the cellular location of virus in dorsal root ganglia and the fate of the infected cell following virus activation. J. Gen. Virol. 51, 233-243.
35. Scriba,M. & Tatzber,F. 1981. Pathogenesis of herpes simplex virus infection in guinea pigs. Infection & Immunity 34, 655-661.
36. Cabrera,C.V., Wohlenberg,C., Openshaw,H., Rey-Mendez,M., Puga,A. & Notkin,A.L. 1980. Herpes simplexvirus DNA sequences in the CNS of latently infected mice. Nature (Lond.) 288, 288-290.
37. Brown,S.M., Subak-Sharpe,J.H., Warren,K.G., Wroblewska,Z. & Kiprowski,H. 1979. Detection by complementation of defective or uninducible (herpes simplex type 1) virus genomes latent in human ganglia. Proc. Natl. Acad. Sci. USA 76, 2364-2368.
38. Green,M.T., Cartney,R.J. & Dunkel,C. 1981. Detection of an immediate early herpes simplex virus type 1 polypeptide in trigeminal ganglia from latently infected animals. Infection & Immunity 34, 987-992.
39. Galloway,D.A., Fenoglio,C.M. & McDougall,J.K. 1982. Limited transcription of herpes simplex virus genome when latent in human sensory ganglia. J. Virol. 41, 686-691.
40. Stevens,J.G. & Cook,M.L. 1974. Maintenance of latent herpetic infection. An apparent role for anti-viral IgG. J. Immunol. 113, 1685-1693.

41. Sekizawa,T., Openshaw,H., Wohlenberg,C. & Notkins,A.L. 1980. Latency of herpes simplex virus in absence of neutralizing antibody: model of reactivation. Science 210, 1026-1028.
42. Wheeler,C.E.Jr. 1975. Pathogenesis of recurrent herpes simplex infections. J. Invest. Dermatol. 65, 341-346.
43. Hill,T.J. & Blyth,W.A. 1976. An alternative theory of herpes simplex recurrence and a possible role for prostaglandins. Lancet i, 397-399.
44. Harbour,D.A., Hill,T.J. & Blyth,W.A. 1981. Acute and recurrent herpes simplex in several strains of mice. J. Gen. Virol. 55, 31-40.
45. Openshaw,H., Puga,A. & Notkins,A.L. 1979. Latency and reactivation of herpes simplex virus in sensory ganglia of mice. Developments of Immunology 7, 301-306.
46. Blyth,W.A., Harbour,D.A. & Hill,T.J. 1980. Effect of immunosuppression on recurrent herpes simplex in mice. Infect. Immun. 29, 902-907.
47. Kastrukoff,L., Long,C., Doherty,P.C., Wroblewska,Z. & Koprowski,H. 1981. Isolation of virus from brain after immunosuppression of mice with latent herpes simplex. Nature 291, 432-433.
48. Shillitoe,E.J., Wilton,J.M.A. & Lehner,T. 1977. Sequential changes in cell-mediated immune responses to herpes simplex virus after recurrent herpetic infections in humans. Infect. Immun. 18, 130-137.
49. O'Reilly,R.J., Chibbaro,A., Anger,E. & Lopez,C. 1977. Cell mediated responses in patients with recurrent herpes simplex infections. II. Infection associated deficiency of lymphokine production in patients with recurrent herpes labialis or genitalis. J. Immunol. 118, 1095-1102.
50. Donnenberg,A.D., Chaikof,E. & Aurelian,L. 1980. Immunity to herpes simplex virus type 2: cell mediated immunity in latently infected guinea pigs. Infect. Immun. 30, 90-109.
51. Nash,A.A. & Gell,P.G.H. 1980. Cell mediated immunity in herpes simplex virus infected mice: suppression of delayed hypersensitivity by an antigen-specific B lymphocyte. J. Gen. Virol. 48, 359-364.
52. Nash,A.A., Phelan,J. & Wildy,P. 1981. Cell mediated immunity in herpes simplex virus-infected mice: H-2 mapping of the delayed type hypersensitivity response and the antiviral T cell response. J. Immunol. 126, 1260-1262.

CHAPTER 13

CELL-MEDIATED IMMUNE RESPONSE TO HERPESVIRUS INFECTIONS

Carlos Lopez

Sloan-Kettering Institute for Cancer Research
New York, New York

INTRODUCTION

The immune response is capable of interacting with a herpes simplex virus type 1 or 2 (HSV-1 or HSV-2) infection on several different levels (1) (see description of HSV pathogenesis by Nash in this volume). Defense mechanisms could be active to inhibit a primary infection from becoming established at the site of inoculation. These or other systems may localize the infection and keep it from becoming disseminated. The immune response probably helps clear an established infection and protects against a second challenge with HSV-1 or HSV-2. Resistance mechanisms may also inhibit the development of latent virus infections. In addition, defense mechanisms might be required to control reactivated virus and thus limit lesion formation. Lastly, the immune response is probably responsible for at least some of the damage (immunopathology) associated with the virus infection. In this discussion, I will restrict my comments to the mechanisms thought to interact with a primary herpesvirus infections. The systems to be discussed might also control reactivated virus infections (2) either indirectly by limiting the incidence of latent infection or directly at the site of reactivation. Although these are interesting possibilities, little new data is available on these and they will therefore, not be discussed here.

Defense against an invading herpesvirus infection depends on a number of different cell populations and humoral factors acting in concert to limit and clear the infection (3). The mechanisms involved in this defense include both non-specific and specific immune responses. Non-specific responses are induced immediately after the infection begins and require no previous exposure to the foreign agent. Specific, or

ISBN 0-12-239980-3

adaptive immune responses, are usually not detected until three to five days after the infection begins. The non-specific (or natural resistance) mechanisms usually thought to be important in herpesvirus infections include macrophages, interferon, and natural killer cells. Evidence will be discussed of a possible role for these mechanisms in resistance to HSV-1 and HSV-2 infections. The adaptive immune responses induced against herpesvirus infections include antibody and T-cell mediated delayed hypersensitivity and cytotoxic responses. Since most data suggests that neutralizing antibody is protective against HSV-1 only when given before or at the same time as the virus infection, antibody is thought to be protective against a second exposure to HSV-1 or HSV-2 but is not an important role for cell-mediated immune responses in the clearing of an established subcutaneous herpesvirus infection. Although this subject will be covered more fully in the chapter by Nash et al (in this volume), this mechanism will also be discussed here in order to consider the role it might play in resistance to a primary infection.

METHODS OF STUDY OF RESISTANCE MECHANISMS

Although HSV-1 and HSV-2 are usually self limiting infections which clear up in one to three weeks in normal, healthy individuals, infections in immunosuppressed patients can be unusually severe (1,4). The latter are usually more widespread, take far longer to heal, and can even be lifethreatening. Since the immunosuppressive treatments appeared to diminish cell-mediated immunity but often not antibody responses, the former was defined as necessary for resistance. However, these treatments suppressed many different cell types and studies failed to define specifically the deficiencies resulting in increased susceptibility. These results led to a number of mouse studies attempting to use relatively selective immunosuppression to define mechanisms of resistance. Although more selective than the multi-drug regimens used in many of the patient groups, these studies still had similar drawbacks. This has been well documented recently by Schlabach et al (5), who showed that an antithymocyte antisera suppressed macrophage functions during the first few days after treatment. If mice were inoculated with HSV-1 during this early period, the mice appeared to be very susceptible to HSV-1 but if inoculated after macrophage function returned to normal and when T-cells were still suppressed, then treated mice were no more susceptible.

Although the anti-thymocyte sera was thought to be selective, its other (unexpected) function was in fact, responsible for increased susceptibility.

In recent years, genetic models of resistance to HSV-1 and HSV-2 have been described (6,7). There have been several advantages to working with these models. First, cell transfer and bone marrow reconstitution experiments have been possible. Second, when mechanisms are found which might be responsible for resistance, studies can be carried out to determine whether these functions segregate with genetic resistance. There are, however, possible artifacts of these models which must be considered. For example, HSV-1 and HSV-2 are not indigenous to the mouse and, since herpes viruses appear to have evolved with their hosts, it is possible that resistance mechanisms in the mouse might be different than those in man. Thus observations made in the study of the mouse must be carried over to the study of man to determine whether they play a role in human resistance as well. The preliminary data developed to date suggests that these models have not lead us astray.

NATURAL RESISTANCE MECHANISMS

In the normal adult host there are a number of primary barriers to infection (see ref. 7 for further detail). This section will review the data which indicates that macro phages, natural killer cells, and interferon are important resistance mechanisms against herpesvirus infections.

A. Macrophages

Newborn mice have been shown to be much more sensitive to an intraperitoneal (IP) infection with HSV-1 than were adult mice (8). This observation lead to a number of studies which indicated that susceptibility was dependent on immature macrophages which failed to restrict the replication of the virus in vitro (9). These early studies were followed by the studies of Stevens and Cook (10) which showed that macrophages from adult mice were capable of restricting the replication of HSV-1. In the latter studies, the virus replication was aborted before complete progeny virus was made and very little infectious virus was detected after infection.

Other studies showed that a variety of macrophage poisons including silica, carragheenan, trypan blue, and dextran sulfate significantly reduced resistance to an IP infection with HSV-1 or HSV-2 (7,11). Of note was the observation that macrophage poisons failed to augment susceptibility to an intravaginal infection with HSV-2 (11). Further evidence for a role for macrophage in resistance to HSV-1 and HSV-2 comes from experiments in which treatments resulting in activated macrophage function, also augmented resistance significantly (7). Lastly, transfer of macrophages from resistant to susceptible mice has been found to also result in greatly enhanced resistance to HSV-1 and HSV-2 (7).

As a whole these observations appear to offer overwhelming support for a role for macrophages in natural resistance to these virus infections. However, there are difficulties with these various approaches which must be considered. Macrophage poisons may affect mechanisms (such as natural killer cells) other than those intended. Similarly, treatment to augment macrophage function could also affect other systems. Cell transfer experiments are only as good as the purification procedures used to prepare the transfered cells. Such studies were carried out with probable contaminating cells which might also be responsible for resistance. Finally, the studies in the newborn are interesting but fail to take into consideration the large number of immunodeficiencies described in this host.

In conclusion, the macrophage probably plays an important role in resistance to herpesvirus infections. Further studies are required to document this role and the specific mechanism involved.

B. Natural Killer Cells

Natural killer (NK) cells were first described as effectors from normal individuals capable of lysing certain tumor target cells without apparent prior exposure to the targets (12). These cells are now known to spontaneously lyse a variety of tumor targets, virus infected cells, and even some normal targets. These effectors have been under evaluation because of their possible roles in surveillance against malignant adaptation and virus infected cells and their possible role in hematopoietic homeostasis.

The results of our studies of a mouse model of genetic resistance to HSV-1 suggest that NK cell function may be required for resistance to this infection. In these studies adult inbred strains of mice were shown to be genetically resistant or susceptible to IP infection with HSV-1 (6). When the characteristics of resistance to HSV-1 were compared to those of NK function, many similarities were noted. Specifically, most inbred strains of mice with high NK also demonstrated resistance to HSV-1 (13). Resistance to HSV-1 and NK responsiveness are both dominant genetic traits which can be abrogated by macrophage poisons, strontium-89 (^{89}Sr)

and estradiol treatment of mice (14). The studies with ^{89}Sr-treated mice were especially compelling since this treatment converted genetically resistant mice into mice as susceptible to HSV-1 as the genetically most susceptible strains. Such treatment also completely abrogates NK cell function in treated mice.

Studies with both HSV-1 and HSV-2 infected mice have shown that NK function is rapidly augmented in mice soon after infection (15,16). Preliminary studies have also indicated that NK cell function segregated with resistance in backcrossed mice. These results led us to develop an NK assay for evaluation of this function in man (17).

Since our interest in NK was because of its possible role in resistance to HSV-1, an assay utilizing HSV-1 infected fibroblasts was developed. Most studies of human NK function have been carried out with K562 erythroleukemia targets. Since observations with mouse NK cells suggested that there is heterogeneity in that population of cells (18), studies were carried out to determine whether the effectors which lysed HSV-1 infected targets [NK(HSV-1)] were the same as the effectors which lysed the tumor targets [NK(K562)]. Although both of these effector functions were found to be large granular lymphocytes, each function clearly reflected a different subpopulation of cells (19). The effector cells could be distinguished by cold target inhibition and by a variety of monoclonal antibodies to cell surface markers. We have, in addition, found a number of individuals capable of lysing one target but not the other and vice versa. These targets, therefore, detect different effector cell populations.

Earlier studies by Trinchieri et al (20,21) showed that interferon (IFN) was usually made during an NK response to tumor targets or to virus transformed cells. The amount of IFN generated was thought to be sufficient to cause the lysis found with these targets but not with normal cells. These and other results led these investigators to the conclusion that IFN generated during the NK assay was responsible for the cytotoxicity found. A number of studies carried out in our laboratory (22) indicate that although IFN is generated during the normal NK(HSV-1) response, the lysis of target cells is independent of the IFN generated. Specifically, the level of IFN produced during the NK assay failed to correlate with the level of lysis detected. In addition, an anti-IFN α antibody which neutralized all detectable IFN generated during the assay, failed to significantly inhibit lysis of target cells. Lastly, we have found a number of individuals, male homosexuals with severe opportunistic infections, whose peripheral mononuclear cells were unable to generate IFN even though lysis was normal in the same assay. These results clearly indicate that NK(HSV-1) and IFN generation are independent functions probably mediated by different cell populations.

The purpose for developing the NK(HSV-1) assay was to determine whether these effectors might have a role in resistance to herpesvirus infections in man. We have, therefore, evaluated this function in two groups of patients known to have increased susceptibility to herpesvirus infections; i.e. newborns and patients with Wiscott-Aldrich syndrome and a third group comprised of patients with severe herpesvirus infections without malignancy, immunosuppressive therapy, or a known primary cellular immunodeficiency (23). These groups demonstrated NK(HSV-1) responses which were significantly lower than normal and correlated with their susceptibility to infection. These data suggest that NK(HSV-1) function may play a role in resistance to herpes virus infections in man and that severe defects of this function might result in increased susceptibility to infection. In addition to our studies, Sullivan et al (24) have demonstrated low NK(K562) in patients with X-linked lymphoproliferative syndrome. These patients are predisposed to severe infections with various agents including Epstein-Barr virus.

C. Interferon

IFN may participate in the natural resistance to herpesvirus infections in at least three different ways (25). IFN generated at the site of a lesion might protect uninfected cells from infection with the virus and could limit spread of infection from the primary site of inoculation. IFN could also augment NK cell functions, either by differentiating pre-NK cells into mature effectors or by increasing the recycling capacity of effector cells. In addition, the mechanism of IFN's action could be through activation of macrophage function.

Evidence to indicate that IFN generation is required for resistance to HSV-1 was first developed by Gresser et al (26). These investigators treated mice with anti-IFN antiserum and showed that this significantly increased susceptibility to infection. A further indication of a possible role for IFN was derived by Kirchner's group in experiments showing that genetically resistant mice were capable of an early IFN response whereas susceptible strains were not (16). Although these studies suggest a role for IFN in resistance to HSV-1, the mechanism involved has not been determined.

A number of studies have defined patients with congenital or acquired deficiencies of IFN generating capacity (27).

These individuals were evaluated because of the unusually severe nature of the viral, fungal, and bacterial infections that they had.

We have recently studied a group of homosexual men with an acquired immunodeficiency syndrome associated with a variety of opportunistic infections (28). When studied early during their clinical course, these individuals often demonstrated normal mitogen responses and lymphocyte counts but these deteriorated progressively as they became seriously ill. The one consistent correlate of susceptibility to opportunistic infections was a severely diminished capacity of mononuclear cells from these patients to generate IFN in response to HSV-1 infected targets (Lopez, et al, submitted for publication). This deficiency was also detected in three subjects who eventually developed infections two to three months after testing. These data suggest that the diminished capacity to generate IFN might be the primary defect causing increased susceptibility to infection.

CELL MEDIATED IMMUNITY

As noted above, the role of the cell mediated immune (CMI) response will be discussed more completely elsewhere in this book (see Chapter by Nash in this volume). The CMI response is considered here in order to discuss how different defense mechanisms are required for resistance depending on the pathogenesis of the infection. As noted above, the CMI does not appear to play a significant role in resistance to an IP infection with HSV-1. However, when HSV-1 is inoculated intraocularly (10) or subcutaneously (29), the CMI response is absolutely necessary. Thus athymic nude mice inoculated by these routes are highly susceptible to the infections and die 10 to 16 days after inoculation. These results indicate that depending on the pathogenesis of an infection and probably the cellular defense mechanisms which are confronted by the infection, natural resistance mechanisms and cell mediated immunity ply varying role in resistance to the primary infections.

CONCLUDING REMARKS

In all probability, a primary herpesvirus infection induces one aspect or another of the natural resistance system immediately upon invading the susceptible host. This early response is probably required to keep the infection in check so that overwhelming infection does not overtake the host before the cell mediated immune response becomes active. In herpesvirus infections of the peritoneum, infection probably activates a massive response of the natural resistance mechanisms which are sufficient to clear the infection without the requirement of a cell mediated immune response. It is interesting to note that with the IP inoculated mice, the natural resistance mechanisms intercept the progress of HSV-1 and inhibits its travel to the central nervous system where it could become latent. These non-specific mechanisms may thus be important in controlling infections of nerve cells and perhaps of reactivated infections as well.

REFERENCES

1. Nahmias, A.J. and Roizman, B. Infection with herpes simplex viruses 1 and 2. N. Engl. J. Med. 189:667-674, 719-725, 781-789 (1973).
2. Docherty, J.J. and Chapan, M. The latent herpes simplex virus. Bacteriol. Rev. 38:337-55 (1974).
3. Allison, A.C. Interaction of antibodies, complement components, and various cell types in immunity against virus and pyogenic bacteria. Transp. Rev. 19:3-55 (1974).
4. Rawls, W.E. Herpes simplex virus; in Kaplan The Herpesviruses; pp. 291-325 (Academic Press, New York 1973).
5. Schlabach, A.J. Martinez, D., Field, A.K., and Tytell, A. Resistance of C57 mice to primary systemic herpes simplex virus infection, Macrophage dependence and T-cell independence. Infect. Immun. 26:615 (1979).
6. Lopez, C. Genetics of natural resistance to herpesvirus infections in mice. Nature 258:152-53 (1975).
7. Mogensen, S.C. Role of macrophages in natural resistance to virus infections. Microbiol. Rev. 43:1-26 (1979).
8. Andervont, H.B. Activity of herpetic virus in mice. Am. J. Hyg. 14:383-93 (1927).
9. Johnson, R.T. The pathogenesis of herpes virus encephalitis. II. A cellular basis for the development of resistance with age. J. Exp. Med. 120:359-73 (1964).
10. Stevens, J.G., and Cook, M.L. Restriction of herpes simplex virus by macrophages. An analysis of the cell-virus interaction. J. Exp. Med. 133:133 (1971).
11. McGeorge, M.B. and Morahan, P.S.: Comparison of various macrophage-inhibitory agents on vaginal and systemic herpes simplex virus type 2 infections. Infect. Immun. 22:623-26 (1978).
12. Herberman, R.B. and Holden, H.T. Natural cell-mediated immunity. Adv. Cancer Res. 17:305-70 (1978).

13. Lopez, C. Immunological nature of genetic resistance of mice to herpes simplex virus type 1 infection in de The, Henle, and Rapp. Oncogenesis and Herpesviruses; pp. 775-780 (W.H.O. Lyon, France 1978).
14. Lopez, C., Ryshke, R. and Bennett, M. Marrow-dependent cells depleted by ^{89}Sr mediate genetic resistance to herpes simplex virus type 1 infection in mice. Infect. Immun. 28:1028-32 (1980).
15. Amerding, D., Simmon, M., Hammerling, U., Hammerling, G. Rossiter, H. Function, target cell preference and cell surface characteristics of herpes simplex virus type 2 induced non-antigen specific killer cells. Immunobiology 158:347-68 (1981).
16. Engler, H., Zawatzky, R., Goldbach, A., Schroder, C.H., Weyand, C., Hammerling, G.J. and Kirchner, H. Experimental infection of inbred mice with herpes simplex virus. II. Interferon production and activation of natural killer cells in the peritoneal exudate. J. Gen. Virol. 55:25-30 (1981).
17. Ching, C. and Lopez, C. Natural killing of herpes simplex virus type-1 infected target cells: normal human responses and influence of antiviral antibody. Infect. Immun. 26:49-56 (1979).
18. Lust, J.A., Kumar, V., Burton, R.C., Bartlett, S.P. and Bennett, M. Heterogeneity of natural killer cells in the mouse. J. Exp. Med. 154:306-17 (1981).
19. Fitzgerald, P.A., Evans, R. and Lopez, C. Description of cell surface markers on human NK cells using monoclonal antibodies in Resch and Kirchner Mechanisms of Lymphocyte Activation; pp. 595-698 (Elsevier/North Holland, New York 1981).
20. Trinchieri, G. and Santoli, D. Antiviral activity induced by culturing lymphocytes with tumor-derived or virus-transformed cells. Enhancement of human natural killer cell activity by interferon and antagonistic inhibition of susceptibility of target cells to lysis. J. Exp. Med. 147:1299-1312 (1978).
21. Trinchieri, G., Santoli, D., Granato, D. and Perussia, B. Anatagonistic effects of interferons on the cytotoxicity mediated by natural killer cells. Fed. Proc. 40:2705-709 (1981).
22. Fitzgerald, P.A. Von Wussow, P., and Lopez, C. Role of interferon in natural kill of HSV-1 infected fibroblasts. J. Immunol. (in press).
23. Lopez, C., Kirkpatrick, D., Read, S.E., Fitzgerald, P.A., Pitt, J., Pahwa, S., Ching, C. and Smithwick, E.M. Correlation between low natural kill of HSV-1 infected fibroblasts [NK(HSV-1)] and susceptibility to herpesvirus infections. (submitted for publication).

24. Sullivan, J.L., Byron, K.S., Brewster, F.E. and Purtilo, D.T. Deficient natural-killer cell activity in X-linked lymphoproliferative syndrome. Science 210:543-45 (1980).
25. Gresser, I. Commentary: On the varied biologic effects of interferon. Cell Immunol. 34:406-15 (1977).
26. Gresser, I., Tovey, M.G., Maury, C. and Bandu, M.T. Role of interferon in the pathogenesis of virus diseases in mice as demonstrated by the use of anti-interferon serum. II. Studies with herpes simplex virus, Moloney sarcoma, vesicular stomatitis, Newcastle disease, and influenza viruses. J. Exp. Med. 144:1316-23 (1976).
27. Virelizier, J.L. Viral infections in patients with selective disorders of the interferon system. Fifth Int. Congress Virol. p.152 (1981).
28. Siegal, F.P., Lopez, C., Hammer, G.S., Brown, A.E., Kornfield, S.J., Gold, J., Hassett, J., Hirschman, S.Z., Cunningham-Rundles, C., Adelsberg, B.R., Parham, D.M., Siegal, M., Cunningham-Rundles, S. and Armstrong, D. Severe acquired immunodeficiency in male homosexuals, manifested by chronic perianal, ulcerative herpes simplex lesions. N. Engl. J. Med. 305:1439-44 (1981).
29. Nash, A.A., Phelan, J. and Wildy, P. Cell-mediated immunity in herpes simplex virus-infected mice: H-2 mapping of the delayed-type hypersensitivity response and the antiviral T-cell response. J. Immunol. 126:1260 (1981).

CHAPTER 14

CHEMOTHERAPY OF HERPES SIMPLEX VIRUS INFECTIONS

William H. Burns
Rein Saral

Johns Hopkins Oncology Center
Baltimore, Maryland

In the past few decades great strides have been made in the use of chemotherapeutic agents to treat human pathogens. Until recent years, attempts to treat non-ocular herpes simplex virus (HSV) infections have not been successful. Early studies suggested that the pyrimidine nucleoside analogues 5-iodo-2' -deoxyuridine (idoxuridine) and 1-B-D-arabinofuranosyl cytosine (cytarbine) might be effective in the treatment of severe herpes virus infection. However, when evaluated in organized controlled trials it became apparent that they were ineffective (1). Although 9-β-D-arabinofuranosyl adenine (vidarabine) has proven clinical efficacy against HSV infections, the most innovative and exciting development in antiviral chemotherapy for these infections has been the introduction of acyclovir (ACV) into clinical trials. Other promising new agents include E-5-(2-bromovinyl)-2'deoxyuridine (BVdU), phosphonoacetic acid (PAA) and phosphonoformic acid (PFA), the 2'-fluoro-arabinosyl pyrimidine nucleosides (FIAC, FIAU and FMAU), difluoromethylornithine (DFMO) and the interferons.

VIDARABINE

In the early 1970's collaborative studies were initiated to evaluate vidarabine in the treatment of HSV encephalitis and neonatal HSV infection. In vitro studies suggested that this nucleoside derivative had a better therapeutic index than idoxuridine and cytarabine. Twenty-eight patients with biopsy proven HSV infection were treated with either vidarabine or placebo in a randomized double blind study (2). Only 5 of 18 patients treated with vidarabine died

ISBN 0-12-239980-3

compared to 7 of 10 patients treated with placebo ($p=0.03$). This study was discontinued after so few patients had been entered because of the decreased mortality noted in the drug treated group. Of the 13 patients who survived 6 had severe sequelae and 3 of these died 4 to 6 months after treatment. Subsequent to this study patients with HSV encephalitis were treated with vidarabine in an uncontrolled study (3). The results of this study indicated that the drug was most useful in a subpopulation of patients with HSV encephalitis. Individuals under the age of 30 who were treated early were most likely to benefit from treatment. Patients over the age of 30 who began treatment while in semicoma or coma had an extremely poor prognosis with moderate to severe sequelae if they survived. Based on the results of the studies in herpes simplex encephalitis vidarabine has been approved in the United States as therapy for this devastating disease.

Vidarabine has also been evaluated as therapy in neonatal HSV infections. The results of these studies suggest that the drug exerts an antiviral effect but that survivors may experience severe sequelae (4). The drug was most effective in patients who presented with localized central nervous system disease and was less effective in neonates with disseminated disease. Currently there are controlled trials in the United States comparing vidarabine to ACV in the treatment of HSV encephalitis and neonatal HSV infections to determine whether ACV might prove more efficacious and less toxic. Controlled trials of parenteral vidarabine therapy in the treatment of HSV infections in immunocompromised patients have not been reported in the literature. With the advent of ACV these studies will be difficult to perform unless they are directed at treatment of infections with ACV resistant mutants.

INTERFERONS

Interferon has been evaluated as an antiviral agent in HSV infections. Trials reported in the literature have employed human leukocyte interferon supplied by Dr. Cantell in Finland. Patients with trigeminal neuralgia who have surgical decompression of their trigeminal sensory root ganglia predictably reactivate HSV following the procedure. Interferon given as prophylaxis in a randomized, double blind study starting one day prior to the surgical procedure was effective in reducing viral shedding but was not statistically significant in reducing culture positive herpetic lesions (5). In another controlled study interferon was given as prophylaxis of herpes virus infections in renal transplant recipients and in this study HSV infections were not significantly reduced in patients who received interferon (6). Using recombinant DNA technology extremely homogenous interferon preparations are now available for clinical studies. These techniques will provide purified preparations of the multiple α interferons that are encoded for in the human genome and this approach will lead to purified β and γ interferons as well.

In addition, a purified polyclonal interferon preparation derived from a lymphoblastoid cell line is currently available for clinical studies. With the availability of multiple preparations of interferon many studies will be performed to evaluate its role in the treatment of HSV infections. The most important studies will be those directed at treatment of HSV infections in patients with ACV-resistant mutants and studies evaluating combination therapy employing interferon along with ACV or other antiviral agents. Because of drug-related systemic toxicities it will be important in future studies to define the lowest dose of interferon that will inhibit HSV.

ACYCLOVIR

The introduction of this drug heralds a new era in the therapeutics of virus infections. It is the first nucleoside analogue which has specificity for more than one viral encoded enzyme and is therefore far more toxic to HSV than the cell (7). We showed that intravenous ACV was highly effective in the prophylaxis of HSV infections in bone marrow transplant recipients (8). Patients who have latent HSV as determined by serology have a 75% likelihood of reactivating HSV following marrow transplantation. The reactivation occurs predictably 8 days after bone marrow transplantation. In a randomized double blind study, seven of 10 patients who received placebo developed HSV infection while none of the 10 patients who received ACV developed HSV infection ($p=0.003$).

The patients who received ACV also had significant delay in onset of first fever after bone marrow transplantation (9 days versus 6 days, $p=0.03$) when compared to the placebo controls. This study has been confirmed by investigators in England using intravenous ACV (9) and in the United States using oral ACV (10). In our study ACV prophylaxis did not affect latent virus. Five of 10 patients developed HSV infections after cessation of ACV and 2 developed viral shedding. These infections were mild, unlike the HSV infections encountered early after transplantation which historically were associated with a 10% mortality in seropositive patients.

Studies utilizing intravenous ACV in the treatment of reactivated HSV infections in immunocompromised hosts (11) and primary genital herpes (12) have also produced positive results and the drug is currently approved in the United States for these infections. Acyclovir is also available as a topical drug and is approved for primary genital HSV infection (13) and reactivated HSV infection in the immunocompromised host (14). Several studies have been done evaluating the oral formulation. As noted, oral ACV was effective prophylaxis in preventing reactivation of HSV in bone marrow transplant recipients (10) and has also been shown to be effective in the treatment of primary genital herpes but less so in recurrent disease (15).

LATENCY

Some viruses (e.g., influenza virus) have evolved mechanisms for maintaining high recombination/mutation rates to evade the immune system by clothing themselves in new antigens and thus ensure successful reinfection and spread. Herpesviruses have evolved differently, adapting themselves to establish latent infections in particular cell types during primary infections with subsequent episodes of reactivation and spread to new hosts. After decades of speculation and experimentation, the hypotheses of Goodpasture are firmly established and most investigators agree that HSV and VZV establish latent infections in sensory ganglia (16) and to a lesser extent the CNS (17-19). The molecular biology of latency is much less clear. Using electron microscopy, Baringer and Swoveland found small numbers of virus particles in scattered ganglionic cells (20). However, viral antigens are not found in the ganglia and viral TK activity in the ganglia soon becomes undetectable following inoculation of mice (21) and guinea pigs (22). Nucleic acid hybridization studies indicate that although viral DNA is present in the ganglia many weeks after infectious virus is gone, viral RNA transcription cannot be detected (19). The indications are, therefore, that the viral genome is primarily in a quiescent state, nonproductive of viral products. This conclusion is strengthened by the inability to eliminate the latent state clinically by prolonged treatment with effective antiviral drugs. Furthermore, there has been little success in experimental models in eradicating latency by treatment with a number of agents during reactivated infection both in vitro (23-25) and in vivo (26,27). However, ACV, BVdU and PAA did appear effective in preventing the reactivation process in vitro as long as the drug was present in the culture medium of explanted ganglia (23-25,28).

RESISTANCE

Although HSV is regarded as a genetically rather stable virus, restriction enzyme analyses (REA) demonstrate moderate heterogeneity among clinical isolates and laboratory stock virus. By REA assessment, HSV is less heterogeneous than CMV but more so than VZV. Heterogeneity among HSV clinical isolates has also been observed in susceptibility to antiviral agents (29) and stocks of cloned isolates of HSV appear to contain thymidine kinase (TK) mutants with a frequency of 0.1 to 1 percent (30,31). Early concern for the emergence of drug-resistant HSV was confined to the one clearly successful treatment setting - herpetic keratitis. High concentrations of TFT, IUdR and vidarabine could be achieved in ocular tissues following topical administration and reports of resistant virus began to appear (32).

With increasing topical and systemic use of effective antiviral agents, one anticipates that the number of resistant isolates will rise, but the extent to which such mutants will present clinical problems similar to those encountered with antibiotic-resistant bacteria is not yet known. Two virus-specific enzymes (TK and DNA polymerase) are involved in the antiviral effect of ACV against HSV, and laboratory investigations have clearly demonstrated that resistant virus can result from mutations in either gene (33-36). Most resistant virus isolates have deficient TK activity, probably reflecting a higher proportion of lethal mutations in the polymerase gene than in the less crucial TK gene. The second class of ACV-resistant mutants are the DNA polymerase mutants. Most of them are coresistant to PAA, implying that the polymerase has altered binding of both PAA and acyclo-GTP. One DNA polymerase mutant retains sensitivity to vidarabine (37). The growing collection of drug-resistant DNA polymerase mutants with varying patterns of drug sensitivity provides an opportunity for a genetic analysis of this important enzyme and its nucleotide binding site(s). These studies will also provide a rational basis for choosing non-crossresistant drugs as similar mutants are encountered clinically.

The behavior of these ACV-resistant mutants has been examined in mouse models. Neural tissue is very low in cellular TK activity and it is interesting to note that the herpesviruses that assume latent states in neuronal cells

(HSV and VZV) encode for TK. One can speculate that the loss of TK activity would make it difficult for the virus to replicate or establish latency in such cells, and this is borne out of pathogenicity studies in mice. Although both classes of mutants replicate well in fibroblasts in vitro, replication of TK^- mutants is modestly reduced in the skin of mice and markedly reduced after intracrebral inoculation (38-40). The LD50 for the TK^- mutants is 100-1000 greater than that for wild type virus or DNA polymerase mutants. Similarly, larger inocula of TK^- mutants are required to establish latency. The animal models thus predict that ACV-resistant TK^- mutants will be inherently less neurovirulent than wild type HSV.

SPECULATION

With the above background one can speculate on the clinical significance of resistant mutants and possible approaches to the problem. First, by far the most frequent ACV-resistant mutants to emerge in the laboratory and clinically have been strains that have lost the ability to induce TK. Fortunately, this is the class of mutants with decreased cutaneous and neurovirulence. Although cutaneous and visceral lesions may persist despite ACV therapy in the individual infected with these strains, these strains are unlikely to produce encephalitis and are at a disadvantage for establishing latency. This latter point is particularly important from a public health viewpoint since the reservoir of HSV is the latent virus which episodically activates in the ganglia, replicates in the skin and mucous membranes, and is spread to non-immune individuals. One would predict that few if any TK^- strains can participate in this life cycle. A patient reported by Sibrack and her colleagues illustrates this point (41). The patient had a chronic immunodeficiency syndrome and recurrent HSV infections and underwent repeated ACV treatments. He died of bacterial pneumonia and was found to have resistant virus in multiple organs at autopsy. Although the cerebrospinal fluid was positive for the resistant strain, cultures of the brain produced no virus. Presumably, TK^- virus could replicate in the meninges but not the nueronal tissue poor in cellular TK. The difficulty TK^- virus has in establishing latency is demonstrated by another patient we recently studied. This patient developed oral HSV infection with wild type virus prior to treatment with ACV. Resistant TK^- virus was then isolated while on therapy and later virus excretion ceased. After 10 weeks of no ACV therapy and no virus shedding, the patient had a reactivated oral HSV infection from which only wild type virus could be isolated.

The second point is that the resistant mutants likely to be most dangerous are of two types: 1) mutants with altered TK resulting in decreased phosphorlyation of ACV (or other nucleoside analogs) but which retain the ability to phosphorylate thymidine, and 2) DNA polymerase mutants with normal TK activity. These strains should be capable of establishing latency, exhibit neurovirulence like that of wild-type virus, and thus enter the reservoir and participate in the classical HSV life-cycle in the face of ACV and similar-acting drugs. An example of the former type of mutant is the laboratory isolate reported by Darby (42). This isolate phosphorylates thymidine normally but has little affinity for ACV. Examples of laboratory-derived DNA polymerase mutants have been reported (26,35,36). Neither of these more dangerous types of mutants has been observed clinically, but with the increasing use of ACV it is only a question of time before mutants of these last 2 classes emerge and become major public health problems.

Therapeutic strategies can increasingly be formulated on a growing body of knowledge concerning the behavior of the mutants and mechanisms of action of available antiviral agents. First, indiscriminate use of ACV and like drugs should be strongly condemned. Chronic administration of the drug at times of high virus load and in ways that are only partially successful in preventing viral replication are most likely to result in the appearance of resistant strains. ACV and similar drugs should only be used in situations where the virus infection is accompanied by significant morbidity and mortality. It should not be used topically in recurrent genital herpes infections since controlled studies do not indicate a significant clinical benefit. Second, although clinical infectious disease experience counsels against most prophylactic usage of antibiotics, prophylactic use of ACV is justified in well-defined, high risk patient populations with expected high incidence of infection accompanied by significant morbidity and mortality during a specific time period. This recommendation recognizes and takes advantage of the unique host-virus relationship of the latent state. It results in effective restriction of viral DNA replication while the viral genomic load is at an absolute minimum, thus limiting the virus population available for mutation/ selection. It is consistent with the in vitro studies mentioned above (23-25). Our ACV prophylactic study of HSV infection in bone marrow transplant patients (8) consisted of only 20 patients, but our subsequent experience has reinforced our initial conclusion that prophylactic use of ACV in such a population can completely prevent HSV reactivation and clinical infection, and that resistant virus is more likely to occur on treatment of patients with established infection and an abundant load of replicating virus. An analogy may be made to INH and tuberculosis where treatment following a relatively small inoculum of mycobaterium is successful but with large inocula treatment is associated with the development of resistance.

We have never isolated resistant virus from high risk patients being treated prophylactically with ACV, but have done so in six patients treated for established infection. Two of the isolates have been previously reported to be TK^- mutants (43). The four recent isolates also have altered TK activity and all are co-resistant to BVdU. Three of the four isolates are sensitive to FIAC, FIAU and FMAU - all of which require phosphorylation by the HSV TK for their antiviral effects. This implies that the viral TK of these mutants retain the ability to phosphorylate these compound while having lost their affinity for ACV and BVdU. One resistant isolate, also a TK^- mutant, is resistant to the fluoro-arabinosyl compounds. All six resistant isolates are sensitive to PAA and interferon. Clearly, as ACV-resistant strains of HSV are increasingly encountered it will be important to screen them for resistance patterns to the available antiviral agents to determine further treatment of individual patients.

New therapeutic strategies will probably involve the use of multiple agents with additive or synergistic antiviral activity. It has been reported that various combinations of vidarabine, BVdU, TFT, PFA, interferon and ACV have combined additive or synergistic effects against HSV (44-46). Further investigations of the efficacy and toxicities of drug combinations are needed before clinical trials of these agents are undertaken. As HSV mutants emerge that are resistant to all antiviral agents which act at the DNA polymerase level, interferon and DFMO may play important therapeutic roles. DFMO is an inhibitor of ornithine decarboxylase and ultimately polyamine synthesis, the latter apparently required to provide a proper "scaffolding" for the viral DNA. It has in vitro activity against several viruses, including HSV (47), and toxicology data is available from phase I trials of the drug as an anti-tumor agent.

Clearly the next decade will be an exciting one with the entry of several candidate antivirals into clinical trials. As noted previously, ACV is being compared to vidarabine in HSV encephalitis and neonatal HSV infection. Other studies with HSV infections will have to accept the results of clinical studies with ACV as the yardstick of success. Although the goal to prevent or abolish latency is most noble, this will probably not be possible with current and future antiviral agents. Ultimately, public health control of HSV infections will require development of an effective and safe vaccine and immunization of all persons prior to exposure to the virus. This has been the case for all other virus diseases that have been brought under control (variola, poliomyelitis, rubeola, etc.) and will be especially true for the herpesviruses with their propensity to develop latent infections.

REFERENCES

1. Boston Interhospital Virus Study Group and the NIAID-Sponsored Cooperative Antiviral Clinical Study, 1975. Failure of high dose 5-iodo-2'-deoxyuridine in the therapy of herpes simplex virus encephalitis. N.Engl.J.Med. 292:599-603.
2. Whitley,R.J., Soong,S.-J., Dolin,R., Galasso,G.J., Chien,L.T., Alford,C.A., and the Collaborative Study Group, 1977. Adenine arabinoside therapy of biopsy-proved herpes simplex encephalitis: NIAID Collaborative Antiviral Study. N.Engl.J.Med. 297:289-294.
3. Whitley,R.J., Soong,S.-J., Hirsch,M.S., Karchmer,A.W., Dolin,R., Galasso,G., Dunnick,J.K., Alford,C.A., and the NIAID Collaborative Antiviral Study Group, 1981. Herpes simplex encephalitis: Vidarabine therapy and diagnostic problems. N.Engl.J.Med. 304:313-318.
4. Whitley,R.J., Nahmias,A.S., Soong,S.-J., Galasso,G.G., Fleming,C.L., and Alford,C.A., 1980. Vidarabine therapy of neonatal herpes simplex virus infection. Pediatrics. 66:495-501.
5. Pazin,G.J., Armstrong,J.A., Lam,M.T., Tarr,G.C., Jannetta,P.J., and Ho, M., 1979. Prevention of reactivated herpes simplex infection by human leukocyte interferon after operation on the trigeminal root. N.Engl.J.Med. 301:225-30.
6. Cheeseman,S.H., Rubin,R.H., Stewart,J.A., Tokkoff-Rubin, N.E., Cosimi,A.B., Cantell,K., Gilbert,J., Winkle,S., Herrin,J.T., Black,P.L., Russell,P.S., and Hirsch,M.S., 1979. Controlled clinical trial of prophylactic human leukocyte interferon in renal transplantation: effects on cytomegalovirus and herpes simplex virus infections. N.Engl.J.Med. 300:1345-1349.
7. Elion,G.B., Furman,P.A., Fyfe,J.A., deMiranda,P., Beauchamp,L., and Schaeffer,H.J. 1977. Selectivity of action of an antiherpetic agent, 9-(2-hydroxyethoxymethyl) guanine. Proc.Natl.Acad.Sci. USA. 74:5716-5720.

8. Saral,R., Burns,W.H., Laskin,O.L., Santos,G.W., and Lietman,P.S. 1981. Acyclovir prophylaxis of herpes simplex virus infections: A randomized, double blind, controlled trial in bone marrow transplant recipients. N.Engl.J.Med. 305:63-67.
9. Hann,I.M., Prentice,H.G., Blacklock,H.A., Ross,M., Brigden,D., Clark,A., Burke,C., Noone,P., and Keaney,M. 1982. Acyclovir prophylaxis of herpes virus infections in severely immunocompromised patients. A randomised double-blind controlled trial. Exp. Hematol. 10 (10):2-4.
10. Wade,J.C., Newton,B., Flournoy,N., and Meyers,J.D., 1982. Oral acyclovir prophylaxis of herpes simplex virus infections after marrow transplant. Intersci.Conf.Antimicrob. Ag.Chrmother. 98.
11. Meyers,J.E., Wade,J.C., Mitchell,C.D., Saral,R., Lietman,P.S., Durack,D.T., Levin,M.J., Sergreti,A.C. and Balfour,H.H., 1982. Multicenter collaborative trial of intravenous acyclovir for treatment of mucocutaneous herpes simplex virus infection in the immunocompromised host. Am.J.Med.Acyclovir Symposium, July 20:229-235.
12. Mindel,A., Adler,M.W., Sutherland,S., Fiddian,A.P., 1982. Intravenous acyclovir treatment for primary genital herpes. Lancet i:697-700.
13. Corey,L., Nahmias,A.J., Guinan,M.E., Benedetti,J.K., Critchlow,C.W., and Holmes,K.K., 1982. A trial of topical acyclovir in genital herpes simplex virus infections. N.Engl.J.Med. 306:1313-1319.
14. Whitley,R., Barton,N., Collins,E., Whelchel,J., Diethelm,A.G., 1982. Mucocutaneous herpes simplex virus infections in immunocompromised patients. A model for evaluation of topical antiviral agents. Am.J.Med. Acyclovir Symposium, July 20:-236-240.
15. Nilsen,A.E., Aasen,T., Halsos,A.M., Kinge,B.R., Tjotta,E.A.L., Wikstrom,K. and Fiddian,A.P., 1982. Efficacy of oral acyclovir in the treatment of initial and recurrent genital herpes. Lancet ii:571-573.
16. Stevens,J.G., 1975. Latent herpes simplex virus and the nervous system. Curr.Top.Microbiol.Immunol. 70:31-50.
17. Knotts,F.B., Cook,M.L., and Stevens,J.E. 1973. Latent herpes simplex virus in the central nervous systems of rabbits and mice. J.Exp.Med. 138:740-744.
18. Cook,M.L., and Stevens,J.G. 1976. Latent hepetic infections following experimental viraemia. J.Gen.Virol. 31:75-80.
19. Puga,A., Rosenthal,J.D., Openshaw,H., and Notkins,A.L., 1978. Herpes simplex virus DNA and mRNA sequences in acutely and chronically infected trigeminal ganglia of mice. Virology, 89:102-111.

20. Baringer,J.R., and Swoveland,P., 1973. Recovery of herpes simplex virus from human trigeminal ganglions. N.Engl.J.Med. 288:649-650.
21. Yamamoto,H., Walz,M.A., and Notkins,A.L., 1977. Viral-specific thymidine dinase in sensory ganglia of mice infected with herpes simplex virus. Virology 76:866-869.
22. Fong,B.S., and Scriba,M., 1980. Use of I-125 deoxycytidine to detect herpes simplex virus-specific thymidine kinase in tissues of latently infected guinea pigs. J.Virol. 34:644-649.
23. Wohlenberg,C., Openshaw,H., and Notkins,A.L. 1979. In vitro system for studying the efficacy of antiviral agents in preventing the reactivation of latent herpes simplex virus. Antimicrob. Ag. Chemother. 15:625-627.
24. Klein,R.J., DeStefano,E., Friedman-Kien,A.E., Brady,E., 1981. Effect of acyclovir on latent herpes simplex virus infections in trigeminal ganglia of mice. Antimicrob. Ag. Chemother. 19:937-939.
25. Park,N.-H., Pavan-Langston,D., DeClercq,E., 1982. Effect of acyclovir, bromovinyldeoxyuridine, vidarabine, and L-lysine on latent ganglionic herpes simplex virus in vitro. Am.J.Med. Acyclovir Symposium, July 20:151-154.
26. Field,H.J., Bell,S.E., Elion,G.B., Nash,A.A., and Wildy,P. 1979. Effect of acycloguanosine treatment on acute and latent herpes simplex infections in mice. Antimicrob. Ag. Chemother. 15:554-561.
27. Blyth,W.A., Harbour,D.A., and Hill,T.J., 1980. Effect of acyclovir on recurrence of herpes simplex skin lesions in mice. J.Gen.Virol. 48:417-419.
28. Klein,R.J., 1982. Treatment of experimental latent herpes simplex virus infections with acyclovir and other antiviral compounds. Am.J.Med.Acyclovir Symposium, July 20:138-142.
29. Smith,K.D., Kennell,W.L., Poirier,R.H., and Lynd,F.T., 1980. In vitro and in vivo resistance of herpes simplex virus to 9-(2-hydroxyethoxymethyl) guanine (acyloguanosine). Antimicrob.Ag.Chemother. 17:144-150.
30. Hall,J.D., and Almy,R.E., 1982. Evidence for control of herpes simplex virus mutagenesis by the viral DNA polymerase. Virology 116:535-543.
31. Field,H.J., Larder,B.A., and Darby,G., 1982. Isolation and characterization of acyclovir-resistant strains of herpes simplex virus. Am.J.Med.Acyclovir Symposium, July 20:369-371.
32. Hirano,A., Yumura,K., Kurimura,T., Katsumoto,T., and Moriyama,H., 1979. Analysis of herpes simplex virus isolated from patients with recurrent herpes keratits exhibiting "treatment-resistance" to

5-iodo-2'-deoxyuridine. Acta-Virol. (PRAHA) 23(3):226-230.

33. Crumpacker,C.S., Chartrand,P., Subak-Sharpe,J.H., and Wilke,N.M., 1980. Resistance of herpes simplex virus to acycloguanosine-genetic and physical analysis. Virol. 105:171-184.
34. Field,H.J., Darby,G., and Wildy,P. 1980. Isolation and characterization of acyclovir-resistant mutants of herpes simplex virus. J.Gen.Virol. 49:115-124.
35. Coen,D.M., and Schaffer, P.A. 1980. Two distinct loci confer resistance to acycloguanosine in herpes simplex virus type 1. Proc. Natl. Acad. Sci. USA. 77:2265-2269.
36. Schnipper,L.E. and Crumpacker,C.S. 1980. Resistance of herpes simplex virus to acycloguanosine: Role of viral thymidine kinase and DNA polymerase loci. Proc. Natl. Acad. Sci. USA. 77:2270-2273.
37. Coen,D.M., Furman,P.A., Gelep,P.T., and Schaffer,P.H., 1982. Mutations in the herpes simplex virus DNA polymerase gene can confer resistance to 9-beta-D-arabinofuranosyladenine. J.Virol. 41:909-918.
38. Field,H.J., and Darby,G., 1980. Pathogenicity in mice of strains of herpes simplex virus which are resistant to acyclovir in vitro and in vivo. Antimicrob. Ag. Chemother. 17:209-216.
39. Field,H.J., and Wildy,P. 1978. The pathogenicity of thymidine kinase-deficient mutants of herpes simplex virus in mice. J. Hyg. 81:267-277.
40. Sibrack,C.D., McLaren,C., and Barry,D.W. 1982. Disease and latency characteristics of clinical herpes simplex virus isolates after acyclovir therapy. Am. J. Med. Acyclovir Symposium, July 20:372-375.
41. Sibrack,C.D., Gutman,L.T., Wilfert,C.M., McLaren,C., St.Clair,M.H., Keller,P.M., and Barry,D.W. 1982. Pathogenicity of acyclovir-resistant herpes simplex virus type 1 from an immunodeficient child. J.Inf. Dis. 146:673-682.
42. Darby,G., Field,H.J., and Salsibury,S.A., 1981. Altered substrate specificity of herpes simplex virus thymidine kinase confers acyclovir-resistance. Nature. 289:81-83.
43. Burns,W.H., Santos,G.W., Saral, R., Laskin,O.L., and Lietman,P.S., McLaren,C., Barry,D.W., 1982. Isolation and characterization of resistant herpes simplex virus after acyclovir therapy. Lancet i:421-423.
44. Levin,M.J., and Leary,P.L. 1981. Inhibition of human herpesviruses by combinations of acyclovir and human leukocyte interferon. Infec. Immun. 32:995-999.
45. Schinazi,R.F., Peters,J., Williams,C.C., Chance,D. and Nahmias,A.J., 1982. Effect of combinations of acyclovir with vidarabine or its 5'-monophosphate on herpes simplex

viruses in cell culture and in mice. Antimicrob. Ag. Chemother. 2:499-507.
46. Schinazi,R.F., and Nahmias,A.J., 1982. Different in vitro effects of dual combinations of anti-herpes simplex virus compounds. Am.J.Med.Acyclovir Symposium, July 20:40-48.
47. Tuomi,K., Mantyjarvi,R., and Raina,A., 1980. Inhibition of Semliki forest and herpes simplex virus production in difluoromethylornithine-treated cells: reversal by polyamines. EIs/H.H. Biomed. Press. 121:292-294.

IV

CYTOMEGALOVIRUS

CHAPTER 15

THE NATURE OF MATERNAL CYTOMEGALOVIRUS INFECTION AND ITS CONSEQUENCES FOR THE INFANT[1]

Sergio Stagno, Robert F. Pass,
Meyer E. Dworsky, and Charles A. Alford

Departments of Pediatrics and Microbiology
University of Alabama
School of Medicine.
Birmingham, Alabama

INTRODUCTION

Despite intense study our understanding of cytomegalovirus (CMV) infections is still fragmentary. Critical gaps in knowledge are especially important with respect to the pathogenesis of prenatal CMV infection. In this review we will focus on some of the newer and more relevant findings on CMV infection during pregnancy with particular emphasis on the relation that exists between maternal immunity, intra and extrauterine transmission of virus and virulence of infection in the offspring.

CMV is unquestionably the leading cause of congenital viral infection with a prevalence ranging between 0.4 and 2.3 percent of all live births (1). It has been estimated that in the United States alone, approximately 30,000 infants are born each year with congenital CMV infection and a conservative figure suggests that between 2700 and 7600 of these infants are at risk of developmental abnormalities (2) (Table 1). Nearly a decade ago Weller concluded that the social toll attributable to congenital CMV infection far exceeds that produced by rubella virus (3). CMV is also transmitted from mother to infant during the early months of life. This occurs either at delivery from contact with an

[1]This work is supported by grants from the National Institute of Child Health and Human Development #HD10699 and from the General Clinical Research Center #5 MO1 RR32.

ISBN 0-12-239980-3

infected genital tract (natal CMV infection) or by ingestion of infected breast milk (2). The disease spectrum of natal and perinatal CMV infections has not been well defined. Although these infections are clearly less serious than congenital infections, it is yet unclear what proportion of infected infants develop acute disease and how many go on to develop delayed complications.

TABLE 1. Public Health Impact of Congenital CMV Infection in the USA

	ESTIMATED FIGURE
No. of live births per year in U.S.A.	3,000,000
Rate of congenital CMV infection (average)	1%
No. of infected infants	30,000
Symptomatic at birth (5-10%)	1,500 - 3,000
Fatal Disease (î 20)	300 - 600
No. with sequelae (90% of survivors)	1,080 - 2,160
Asymptomatic at birth (90 - 95%)	27,000 -28,500
No. with late sequelae (5-17%)	1,350 - 4,845
Total No. with sequelae of fatal outcome	2,730 - 7,605

Reproduced with permission from Stagno et al., Clinical Obstetrics and Gynecology, Knox, G.E. (ed), 1982, pp 563-576.

EPIDEMIOLOGIC BACKGROUND

CMV is a member of the herpesvirus family and has been found in all populations thus far tested (4). CMV maintains a delicately balanced parasitic relationship with the human host that is probably the result of longstanding coevolution. Few individuals escape infection during their lifetime; however, the age of acquisition differs in various geographic and socioeconomic settings. As with the other viruses of this family despite the development of a vigorous immune response, viral shedding after a primary infection normally persists for months, even years, until the infection eventually becomes latent. Even then, the latent state may be interrupted by periodic bouts of reactivation. In the vast majority of cases, CMV infection are subclinical including those acquired in utero and at or shortly after delivery, so that infected individuals remain active and continue to expose other susceptible people. In addition to horizontal transmission, CMV has the ability to disseminate through the placenta.

TABLE 2. Incidence of Congenital CMV Infection According to Rate of Maternal Immunity

LOCATION	NO. INFANTS STUDIED	% CONGENITAL CMV INFECTION	RATE MATERNAL IMMUNITY
Manchester, England	6,051	0.24	25%
Aarhus-Viborg, Denmark, 1979	3,060	0.4	52%
Hamilton, Canada, 1980	15,212	0.42	44%
Halifax, Canada, 1975	542	0.55	37%
Birmingham, AL (Upper Socioec.),1981	2,698	0.6	60%
Houston, TX (Upper Socioec.),1980	461	0.6	50%
London, England,1973	720	0.69	58%
Houston, TX (Low Socioec.), 1980	461	1.2	83%
Abidjam, Ivory Coast, 1978	2,032	1.38	100%
Sendai, Japan, 1970	132	1.4	83%
Santiago, Chile, 1978	118	1.7	98%
Helsinski, Finland, 1977	200	2.0	85%
Birmingham, AL (Low Socioec.),1980	1,412	2.2	85%

Reproduced with permission from Stagno et al, Clinical Obstetrics and Gynecology, Knox, G.E. (ed), 1982, pp 563-576.

Congenital CMV infection is present in approximately one percent of all newborn infants but as illustrated in Table 2, the incidence is quite variable among different populations (5-14). Contrary to what might have been expected, there is a direct relationship between the incidence of congenital CMV infection and the rate of maternal seropositivity. This phenomenon is due to the fact that virus can be transmitted to the fetus after reactivation of latent infection as well as after primary maternal CMV infections (2).

During the first year of life an additional large number of infants become infected as a result of maternal-infant transmission (15,16). By the end of the first year of life between ten and perhaps 40 percent of infants are excreting virus into the urine. The rate of acquisition of CMV during first year of life is influenced by the rate of seropositivity of the mothers and the prevalence of breast feeding. Probably other factors such as race and socioeconomic background may also operate by as yet unknown mechanisms. In premature infants who require prolonged and intensive medical care blood transfusions are an important iatrogenic cause of CMV infection (17).

Acquisition of CMV infection beyond early infancy is gradual. Seroepidemiologic studies indicate that the incidence of infection is inversely related to socioeconomic status. Although data are still limited, there is good reason to believe that horizontal transmission requires rather intimate contact (18). A unique feature of CMV infection is persistent or intermittent excretion of virus in urine, milk, saliva, semen, cervical secretions, stools, and tears. Children with congenitally, natally or postnatally acquired infections shed virus into urine and saliva for years (19). Close contact between these infected young children and uninfected playmates, as may occur in day care centers and boarding schools, is probably the most important factor responsible for the earlier and more rapid acquisition of infection (20). It is reasonable to assume that exposure to infected saliva and urine directly or through fomites is probably the route by which postnatal primary CMV infections are acquired. Although the presence of CMV in oropharyngeal secretions suggests the possibility of respiratory spread, proof for airborn transmission is still lacking. In general, in developing countries the majority of the population has acquired CMV before reaching
puberty while in developed countries the infection is acquired at a lower rate. In adolescents and young adults, the presence and persistence of CMV in saliva, cervical secretions, and semen indicates the infection may be spread by kissing and sexual contact. Evidence exists for the direct transmission of virus with blood products and transplant of organs (17,21). With blood transfusions, the risk of infection is directly related to the number of blood donors and the amount of blood transfused.

THE NATURE OF CMV INFECTION IN PREGNANT WOMEN

Our understanding of the natural history of CMV infections during pregnancy is far from complete. There is no evidence that pregnancy per se increases the risk of acquiring CMV infection; however, during gestation there are some profound modifications of the viral host relationships that result in fluctuating rates of reactivation of endogenous CMV.

Unlike congenital rubella and toxoplasmosis congenital CMV infection frequently occurs in the face of substantial humoral immunity as a result of recurrent infections (most likely reactivations of latent virus as opposed to reinfection with a different strain). Thus, maternal immunity does not always provide enough protection against future intrauterine transmissions. Far from being a rare event congenital infection resulting from recurrent CMV infection has been shown to be quite common especially in highly immune populations (12,14). The initial clue was provided by three reports describing instances of congenital CMV infections in consecutive pregnancies (22,24). However, the most convincing evidence came from a prospective study of women known to be seroimmune before conception (14). As illustrated in Table 3 the rate of congenital CMV infection in the general delivery population was 2.2 percent. The incidence of congenital infection among 541 infants born to seropositive women was a close 1.9 percent.

TABLE 3. Incidence of Congenital CMV Infection in Low Income Population

	Total	No. Infected (%)
Incidence in general infant population	1,412	31 (2.2)
Incidence with recurrent maternal infection		
previously seropositive	457	8 (1.8)
prior CMV excretion	58	1 (1.7)
prior intrauterine transmission	26	1 (3.8)
	541	10 (1.9)

Reproduced with permission from Stagno et al., Clinical Obstetrics and Gynecology, Knox, G.E., (ed), 1982, pp 563-576.

Clearly, the ten cases illustrated here cannot have been infected as a result of primary maternal CMV infections since their mothers had experienced CMV infections from one to several years before this, their last studied pregnancy. Shortly after our studies were published, Schopfer et al found that in an Ivory Coast population in which virtually all inhabitants are infected in childhood, the prevalence of congenital CMV infection was 1.4 percent (12). More recently, we have obtained similar results in a highly immune Chilean population (25). These observations support the belief that reactivation of latent virus is more important in the genesis of congenital infection in highly immune populations than is primary maternal infection. This unique characteristic of CMV probably accounts for the inordinately high rates of intrauterine infections with this virus incomparison with other microbial agents.

This remarkable phenomenon of intrauterine transmission despite maternal immunity has been attributed to reactivation of endogenous virus, but the possibility of reinfection by an exogenous strain of virus cannot be excluded (10,14,26). To better understand the relative importance of these two mechanisms as causes for intrauterine and perinatal transmission we used restriction endonuclease enzymes to analyze the genetic homology of strains of CMV isolated from mother-baby pairs or repeatedly from the same women (26). Strains of CMV obtained from unrelated persons were all genetically different. This observation is consistent with the results reported by Huang and colleagues who have examined more than 100 strains. However, the viruses recovered from related individuals (mother-baby pairs) or repeatedly from the same individual were most often identical. In some cases, the intervals separating the viral isolations varied from one to six years. Of particular interest is the observation that the viruses isolated from each of three pairs of congenitally infected siblings were genetically identical (14,26). In two of these three pairs the first born baby was severely affected while the second born sibling was subclinically infected, suggesting that virulence is not strain dependent and that other factors, probably, maternal immunity in some way attenuated the fetal infection. Clearly then, reactivation of latent virus appears as the dominant mechanism responsible for recurrent maternal CMV infection as well as intrauterine transmission in immune women. Reinfection with a different strain appears to be less common. However, until a much larger number of strains can be studied it would be inappropriate to conclude that reinfections have an insignificant role, particularly in maternal reinfection.

Even though maternal immunity cannot completely eliminate transmission of CMV to the fetus it may still have a beneficial effect by reducing the virulence of infection in the offspring. Defining this possibility is of great importance for the design of appropriate control measures including the development of vaccines. In order to better characterize the relative roles of primary and recurrent maternal CMV infections in the pathogenesis of congenital involvements we initiated a prospective study in two populations of different socioeconomic background living in the same urban setting [27]. Pregnant women from the middle income or upper income group differed significantly from those in the low income groups ($P < 0.001$) in the following ways. They were more serosusceptible to CMV (45 percent versus 18 percent). They were also older (mean age 26.5 versus 22.6 years), predominantly white (85 percent versus nine percent), and more often married (99 percent versus 42 percent). Their first prenatal visit occurred earlier (mean gestational age, 9.1 versus 12.7 weeks). As summarized in Table 4, the overall incidence of congenital infection, calculated irrespective of the serologic status of the mother, was significantly higher (1.6 versus 0.6 percent, $P < 0.001$) in the low income group.

TABLE 4. Congenital CMV Infection and Maternal Immune Status

	Middle-Upper Socioeconomic Background	Low Socioeconomic Background	
Rate of Congenital CMV Infection	16/2698 (0.6%)*	16/1014(1.6%)	($p < 0.001$)
Initially Seronegative Mothers			
Primary gestational CMV infection (seroconversions)	17/1203 (1.4%)	4/179 (2.2%)	($p = 0.4$)
Rate of intrauterine infection	8/17 (47%)	3/4 (75%)	
Risk of congenital infection for seronegative mothers	8/1203 (0.7%)	3/179 (1.6%)	($p = 0.15$)
Initially Seropositive Mothers			
Risk of congenital CMV infection	7/1495 (0.5%)	13/835 (1.5%)	($p = 0.026$)

*Includes a set of twins.

Reproduced with permission from Stagno et al., N Engl J Med, 1982:306:945.

There was no evidence of a significant difference in the incidence of primary CMV infection in susceptible women in the two groups (P = 0.4). The incidence was 1.4 percent in the upper income group and 2.2 percent in the low income group. However, because there were nearly three times as many serosusceptible patients in the higher socioeconomic group, the actual risk of primary gestational infection in this group was significantly higher than that found in the cohort with a low socioeconomic background. Consequently, more congenital infections (50 percent [eight of 16]) were due to primary infection in the higher income group than in the lower income group (18 percent (three of 16)). The obvious corollary of these findings is that intrauterine infection more often follows recurrent maternal infection in the economically disadvantaged (82 percent versus 50 percent). For reasons that are unknown at present, intrauterine infection occurs more often in seroimmune women from the lower income sector than in those from the higher income brackets. Perhaps factors such as crowding, earlier age at initial infection, or host genetic factors may play a part in these discrepant transmission rates. Nevertheless, the data verify previous suggestions that on a worldwide basis congenital CMV infection more often results from recurrent maternal infection, certainly in developing nations and probably in developed countries.

In CMV infection, as in other virus infections during pregnancy, there appears to be some innate barrier against vertical transmission. As summarized in Table 4 the rate of intrauterine transmission was 75 percent (three of four) in the low income group and 47 percent (eight of 17) in the higher income group [27]. Although the rates of intrauterine transmission and the overall risk of congenital infection after the occurrence of primary infection were apparently higher in the low income group they were not significantly different between the groups. Three previous studies had also observed this phenomenon of protection against vertical transmission [11,28,29]. Combining these studies and ours a total of 59 primary infections which occurred during pregnancy resulted in only 24 episodes of congenital infection (42 percent). Although information is still fragmentary it appears that gestational age does not influence the rate of intrauterine infection following primary infection.

Although maternal immunity is an incomplete barrier against vertical transmission, it appears to reduce the virulence of the fetal infection [27]. In our studies, 33 infected infants born to women who had primary CMV infection and 27 infected infants born to mothers who were seropositive at the beginning of their pregnancy were clinically evaluated during the neonatal period. Only five infants had signs and symptoms compatible with congenital cytomegalovirus infection, which was clinically apparent in the nursery. All five were infected after primary maternal CMV infection (five of 33 [15 percent] versus none of 27; P = .035). Three of these symptomatic infants had hepatosplenomegaly and jaundice with direct hyperbilirubinemia; one of them also had petechiae with thrombocytopenia. In addition to these symptoms the other two infants had evidence of central-nervous system damage, which was characterized by hydrocephalus, chorioretinitis, and optic atrophy in one infant and by microephaly in the other. Of the two infants with severe disease, one died at one year of age and the other survived with profound psychomotor retardation. None of the three patients with milder infection had late complications. It should be noted that primary maternal infection does not inevitably lead to virulent fetal infection. In fact, most of the infants (85 percent) born after such infections in this study had subclinical involvement [27]. We also have evidence that infants in this group, as compared with babies born after recurrent maternal infection, are exposed to increased antigenic stimulation in utero as reflected by higher levels of fetal IgM production and increased levels of virus excretion in the early months of life. Because of the small number of cases in which the type of maternal infection has been related to the outcome of the fetal infection and because of the relatively short observation periods, we cannot exclude the possibility that severe fetal infection may occasionally result from recurrent maternal infection. Indeed, one such case has been reported [30].

VIROLOGIC AND IMMUNOLOGIC EVENTS DURING PREGNANCY

Several studies have reported that virus can be shed at variable rates from single or multiple sites following primary or recurrent infections in females whether pregnant or not. Sites of excretion include the genital tract, urinary tract, pharynx, and breast. Table 5 summarizes the prevalence of viral shedding according to site and pregnant status in our low income population [2].

TABLE 5. Rate of CMV Excretion by Site in Pregnant and Nonpregnant Women of Low Socioeconomic Background in Birmingham, Alabama

Site	Pregnant No. +/Total (%)	Nonpregnant No. +/Total (%)
Cervix	134/1552 (8.6)	43/398 (10.8)
Urine	27/684 (3.9)	6/230 (2.6)
Throat	10/562 (1.8)	
Amniotic Fluid[1]	0/37 (0)	
Buffy Coat[1]	2/108 (1.8)	
Milk[2]	51/353 (14.4)	

[1]Specimens collected from women excreting CMV in other sites.
[2]Immediate post partum.
Reproduced with permission from Stagno et al., Clinical Obstetrics and Gynecology, Knox, G.E. (ed), 1982, pp 563-576.

In pregnant women, virus was excreted most commonly from the cervix (8.6 percent) and in decreasing order from the urinary tract (3.9 percent), and the throat (1.8 percent). From women shedding in other sites we examined 37 specimens of amniotic fluid and the buffy coats of 108 specimens of heparinized blood. CMV was isolated twice from buffy coats but not from amniotic fluids. In the immediate postpartum period viral shedding into breast milk occurred in 14.4 percent of the patients. Cervical and urinary tract shedding in nonpregnant women are comparable with those found in pregnant cohorts of similar demographic and socioeconomic characteristics [2,31]. The groups of pregnant and nonpregnant women studied by us attended the same public health clinic, were of low socioeconomic background, and were matched for age, race, marital status, and the history of previous Neisseria gonorrheae infection [31]. Most other studies of nonpregnant women have been done at sexually transmitted disease clinics and have not included pregnant women of similar socioeconomic backgrounds [32-34]. In these studies, rates of cervical shedding ranged from 5.2 percent for nonpregnant women drawn from private practice or family planning clinics to 24.5 percent among women attending a sexually-transmitted-disease clinic.

Pregnancy per se has no discernible effect on the overall prevalence of viral shedding. However, gestational age has a significant influence on the rate of cervical CMV excretion. In four studies which included nearly 2,000 women of various ethnic and socioeconomic backgrounds the rate of cervical excretion increased from an average of 2.6 percent in the first trimester to 7.6 percent near term [31,35-37]. This phenomenon was initially interpreted as an indication that pregnancy enhances productive CMV infection in the genital tract [36]. It was assumed that the lower rate seen during the first trimester was similar to the frequency in the nonpregnant state. Our study included a group of nonpregnant control women and their rate of excretion was identical to that found in pregnant women near term, and pregnant women who shed virus near term were seropositive before the onset of excretion. We concluded that productive CMV infection is significantly suppressed in early gestation and, as the suppressive effect wanes with advancing pregnancy, viral shedding resulting from reactivations steadily increases. It has been speculated that this phenomenon may have teleological significance for the protection of the fetus from viral infection during the critical early months of gestation [10].

In order to determine whether pregnancy hormones might be the mediators of the suppression of viral shedding in early gestation, Knox et al did in vitro studies in our laboratory [38]. Although none of the hormones usually associated with pregnancy changes had any effect on the growth of CMV in vitro, a peptide hormone, epidermal growth factor (EGF), was shown to suppress CMV replication while enhancing the growth of human fibroblasts in culture. Estradiol, a hormone which increases in late gestation, reduced the suppressive effect of EGF on CMV replication without altering the mitogenic properties of EGF [10]. Thus, naturally occurring hormones can directly alter the growth of CMV and be modulated by other hormones, simultaneously. Whether in vitro findings can be extrapolated to the in vivo suppression of CMV replication in early gestation is certainly not definitive.

Age can also influence recurrent CMV shedding in the genital and urinary tract of women [39]. Viral shedding is inversely related to age after puberty. In our low socioeconomic group, the prevalence of CMV excretion in the genital tract fell from a high level of 15 percent in girls between 11 and 14 years of age to undetectable levels in women of 31 years or older. From a peak of about eight percent in the younger group, urinary excretion fell to zero in women 26 years and older. No CMV excretion occurred from either site in post menopausal women.

The role of maternal immunity in the pathogenesis of congenital CMV infection is not well understood. The transient depression of cellular immune responses to CMV antigens during the second and third trimesters may be yet another peculiar aspect of the relationship between CMV and the pregnant human host [40-43]. Gehrz and collaborators described this phenomenon in a small group of seropositive pregnant women and showed that depressed CMV-specific lymphocyte proliferative responses returned to levels found in early pregnancy by 90-120 days postpartum [43]. In a prospective study of seropositive pregnant and nonpregnant women, Pass and collaborators in our laboratory, did not corroborate these findings using the lymphocyte blastogenic response to CMV, herpes simplex and phytohemagglutinin antigens [44]. In both studies there was no generalized depression of cellular immunity since numbers of T lymphocytes, T-cell proliferative responses to other mitogens, and serum antibody titers remained unchanged during the study period [43-44]. It is interesting to note that none of the mothers studied by Gehrz shed virus during the period of depressed cellular immune response, nor did they transmit the infection to their infants [43]. The reasons for their change in blastogenic response have not been defined but immunosuppressive factors such as IgG alloantibodies, alpha fetoprotein, and human chorionic gonadotropin have been incriminated during pregnancy [43]. It has also been suggested that mothers of infants with congenital CMV infection may have impaired cellular immune responses which in some cases last several years [41,42]. Again, the defect appears to be specific for CMV since blastogenic responses to other antigens like herpes simplex virus remain normal. The implications of these observations is that a defect or cell mediated immunity may increase the likelihood of transplacental transmission. However, before a causal relationship is accepted a carefully done study among mothers with documented primary and recurrent infection who do and do not transmit virus in utero will be required [42]. Whatever the nature of the suppression of the blastogenic response to CMV may be, it is quite clear that the defect does not involve humoral immunity. Actually, there is no correlation between the height the antibody response and the presence, absence, or magnitude of the blastogenic response to CMV [42].

DEFINING RISK OF INTRAUTERINE TRANSMISSION

Pre-existing maternal immunity does not prevent the virus from reactivating and, more important cannot reliably prevent intrauterine infection. Although CMV excretion is a relatively common event during and after pregnancy, several studies have demonstrated that the simple isolation of virus during pregnancy whether from cervix, urine, or both is also a poor indicator of the risk of intrauterine infection

[11,15,45]. At present, it is impossible to define by serologic or virologic means which patient may undergo reactivations of CMV infections, nor is it possible to define the time of intrauterine transmission with such reactivations of maternal infection [2]. The sites from which CMV reactivates to produce congenital infection are not known, but may well be inaccessible to sampling during pregnancy. With primary CMV infections, the risk of transmission to the fetus is more predictable, occurring in approximately 40 percent of cases (range 25 to 75 percent) [2,11,27,28,29]. Since primary infections are usually asymptomatic, the diagnosis must be confirmed by the appearance of de novo antibodies in convalescent sera (seroconversion). However, because prenatal care usually begins between eight and 14 weeks of pregnancy, localizing a primary infection to the first trimester is nearly impossible with conventional serology. This is unfortunate since it is assumed, by analogy with rubella and toxoplasma, that CMV many produce its most severe effects on the fetus as a result of infections occurring early in pregnancy [46]. In search for a more reliable marker to detect primary CMV infections, particularly those that are subclinical, a serologic test should meet the following criteria. It should be able to measure a type of antibody that is detectable only during the acute phase of primary infection in all or most patients, irrespective of whether the infection is asymptomatic or subclinical. The antibodies measured by this ideal test should decline after the acute phase of the infection to become undetectable within a few months. Finally, and most important, this test must fail to detect antibodies when recurrent CMV infections occur during pregnancy. With these criteria in mind several tests have been evaluated. One that received attention was the immunofluorescent test (IF) to detect antibodies to CMV induced early antigens. Results fell short of expectations [47]. This test is not a good marker of recent primary CMV infection in pregnant women because sera examined months and even years after acquisition still reacted with early CMV antigens. Moreover, the fluctuations in antibody titers which occurred in some patients over time could not be temporally related to the onset of a recurrence of CMV infection. Thus, this antibody assay is not even a good marker for the onset of reactivations.

Infections with rubella [48], Epstein-Barr [49], and Hepatitis A [50] viruses can now be diagnosed by testing single sera for the presence of virus-specific IgM antibodies. For the purpose of detecting IgM antibodies in primary CMV infections, many different techniques have been described in recent years, including IF [51-53], enzyme linked immunosorbent assay [54-57], immunoperoxidase staining [58], radioimmunoassay (RIA) [59,60], indirect hemagglutination [61], and latex agglutination [62]. Unfortunately for most of these tests the evaluation has been inadequate. For instance few studies included sera from patients with well characterized primary and recurrent CMV infections. Of all tests available RIA appears to be the most reliable because in normal hosts including pregnant women positive results for IgM antibodies occur only during the acute phase of primary infections and not with reactivations [46]. With this test serum specific IgM antibodies can be detected in nearly 90 percent of pregnant women with primary CMV infections, and the antibody response persists for up to four months. Other procedures, particularly the IF-IgM test, do not discriminate well between acute infections and recurrent episodes of infection [46]. In our experience no less than 18 percent of the serum samples from patients with recurrent infections react in the IF-IgM assay. These reactions are not restricted to low titer responses and still occur after rheumatoid factors are removed. The reason for these reactions are unknown but the problem also occurs in umbilical cord serum. The results of the IgM RIA indicate it is possible to diagnose primary infections in the first trimester of pregnancy by simply testing a single serum sample for IgM antibodies [46]. The fact that with the RIA test IgM antibodies persist for approximately four months make it ideal to test women at the first prenatal visit which occurs at an average of nine to 14 weeks gestation.

Betts and colleagues have recently described a cytolytic antibody assay that is mediated by an IgM antibody which in the presence of complement can lyse CMV infected target cells [63]. This antibody is detectable for one to three months in the sera of patients with community-acquired CMV infection and in the sera of renal transplant recipients with primary CMV infection. The cytolytic antibody assay has not been evaluated in pregnant women but appears to meet the criteria of a good serologic marker of recent primary CMV infection in pregnant women.

It is also difficult to investigate if the fetus has been invaded following the viremic phase of either primary or recurrent maternal infections. In a few instances CMV has been isolated from amniotic fluid obtained by amniocentesis. In three cases CMV infection was suspected on the basis of maternal symptoms (mononucleosis like illness early in pregnancy) or insufficient fetal growth and the fetuses were not only infected but affected [64-67]. However, in our personal experience and in a case reported by Hayes et al [68], four women who acquired CMV in early pregnancy (three were symptomatic) virus was not isolated from amniotic fluid even though shortly thereafter CMV was isolated from fetal or placental tissue or both. Although isolation of CMV from amniotic fluid is a strong suggestion of fetal infection, clearly, failure to isolate virus is not enough evidence to rule it out. Until more data are available the diagnostic value of amniocentesis remains uncertain.

MATERNAL CMV EXCRETION AND PERINATAL TRANSMISSION

In contrast to the generally poor correlation that exists between CMV excretion during pregnancy and fetal infection, there is a close association between maternal shedding and transmission to the offspring either at delivery or during the first months of life [16]. In Table 6 the efficiency of transmission to the offspring is compared for the various sites of maternal excretion in a population of low socioeconomic background.

TABLE 6. Association between Maternal Excretion of CMV from Various Sites and Subsequent Infection of the Infant

Only Site of Maternal Excretion	No. of Infants Infected/ No. Exposed*
Breast milk	
Breast milk	19/30 (63)
Bottle-fed infant	0/9 (0)
Cervix	
Third trimester and postpartum	8/14 (57)
Third trimester	18/68 (26)
First and second trimester	1/8 (12)
Urine+	0/11 (0)
Saliva#	0/15 (0)
Nonexcreting women	
Bottle-fed infant	0/125 (0)
Breast-fed infant	1/11 (9)

*Figures in parentheses denote percentages.
+Late third trimester.
#Excretion one day postpartum.
Reproduced with permission from Stagno et al., N Engl J Med, 1980, 302:1073.

Of course, in this study congenital CMV infections had been previously excluded in all infants by means of urine cultures done within the first week of life. The two most efficient routes of transmission were infected breast milk, which resulted in 63 percent rate of perinatal infection, and the infected genital tract particularly in late gestation, which was associated with transmission in 57 percent of the cases (natal infection). Viral shedding from the pharynx and urinary tract of the mother late in gestation and during the first months postpartum hs not been associated with natal or postnatal infections in our study population but, because of small numbers of infants examined to date, a lesser role for these two sources cannot yet be excluded. Natal and breast milk transmission appear to be the most important routes for perinatal CMV acquisition given the high rate of excretion and the efficiency of transmission from these sources. There is considerable variability in perinatal transmission of CMV throughout the world [16]. The age of the mother and their prior experience with CMV, which in turn influence the frequency of viral excretion into the genital tract and breast milk, are certainly important factors. Younger seropositive women who breast feed are at a greater risk for transmitting virus in early infance, especially in lower socioeconomic groups. It is remarkable that in Japan, Guatemala, Finland and Thailand, where the rates of CMV excretion within the first year of life are extremely high (39 to 56 percent), the practice of breast feeding is almost universal, and the majority of women of childbearing age are seroimmune for CMV [16].

The incubation period of CMV infection acquired during the perinatal period ranges between four and 12 weeks (average eight weeks) [15]. Although the quantity of virus excreted by infants with perinatal infection is less than that seen with intrauterine acquisition, the infection is also of a chronic nature with viral shedding persisting for years [19]. CMV infection acquired in the neonatal period occasionally results in clinical illness. In our preliminary experience approximately five to ten percent of infants infected through these routes have developed a rather distinct pneumonitis syndrome which in some cases required their hospitalization [69].

REFERENCES

1. Stagno S, Pass RF, Alford CA: Perinatal infections and maldevelopment. In: The Fetus and the Newborn, Bloom AD and James LS (eds). Alan R. Liss, Inc. (New York), 1981, pp 31-50.
2. Stagno S, Pass RF, Dworsky ME, Alford CA: Maternal cytomegalovirus infection and perinatal transmission.

In: Clinical Obstetrics and Gynecology, Knox GE (ed). J.B. Lippincott Co. (Philadelphia), in press, 1982.
3. Weller TH: The cytomegaloviruses: ubiquitous agents with protean clinical manifestations. N Eng J Med 285:203, 267, 1971.
4. Gold E, Nankervis GA: Cytomegalovirus. In: Viral Infections of Humans, Evans AF (ed). Plenum Medical Book Company (New York), 1976, pp 143-161.
5. MacDonald H, Tobin JO'H: Congenital cytomegalovirus infection: a collaborative study on epidemiological, clinical and laboratory findings. Develop Med Child Neurol 20:471, 1978.
6. Andersen HK, Brostrom K, Hansen KB, Leerhoy J, Pedersen M, Osterballe O, Felsager U, Mogensen S: A prospective study on the incidence and significance of congenital cytomegalovirus infection. Acta Paediatr Scand 68:329, 1979.
7. Larke BRP, Wheatley E, Saigal S, Chernesky MA: Congenital cytomegalovirus infection in an urban Canadian community. J Infect Dis 142:647, 1980.
8. Embil JA, MacDonald JM, Scott KE: Survey of a neonatal population for the prevalence of cytomegalovirus. Scand J Infect Dis 7:165, 1975.
9. Montgomery JR, Mason Jr EO, Williamson AP, Desmond MM, South MA: Prospective study of congenital cytomegalovirus infection. South Med J 73:590, 1980.
10. Alford CA, Stagno S, Pass RF: Natural history of perinatal cytomegalovirus infection. In: Perinatal Infections, Ciba Foundation Symposium. Excerpta Medica (Amsterdam), 1980, pp 125-147.
11. Stern H, Tucker SM: Prospective study of cytomegalovirus infection in pregnancy. Br Med J 2:268, 1973.
12. Schopfer K, Laube E, Kreck U: Congenital cytomegalovirus infection in newborn infants of mothers infected before pregnancy. Arch Dis Child 53:536, 1978.
13. Granstrom ML, Leinikki P, Santavuori P, Pettay O: Perinatal cytomegalovirus infection in man. Arch Dis Child 52:354, 1977.
14. Stagno S, Reynolds DW, Huang ES, Thames S, Smith RJ, Alford CA: Congenital cytomegalovirus infection: occurrence in an immune population. N Engl J Med 296:1254, 1977.
15. Reynolds DW, Stagno S, Hosty TS, Tiller M, Alford CA: Maternal cytomegalovirus excretion and perinatal infection. N Engl J Med 289:1, 1973.
16. Stagno S, Reynolds DW, Pass RF, Alford CA: Breast milk and the risk of cytomegalovirus infection. N Engl J Med 302:1073, 1980.

17. Yeager AS: Transfusion-acquired cytomegalovirus infection in newborn infants. Am J Dis Child 128:478, 1974.
18. Hanshaw JB, Dudgeon JA: Viral Diseases of the Fetus and Newborn. W.B. Saunders Co. (Philadelphia), 1978.
19. Stagno S, Reynolds DW, Tsiantos A, Fuccillo DA, Long W, Alford CA: Comparative serial virologic and serologic studies of symptomatic and subclinical congenitally and natally acquired cytomegalovirus infections. J Infect Dis 132:568, 1975.
20. Pass RF, August AM, Dworsky ME, Reynolds DW: Cytomegalovirus infection in a day care center. Program Issue APS/SPR, Pediatr Res, 16:248A, 1982 (Abstract #1014).
21. Ho M, Suwansirikul S, Dowling JN, Youngblood LA, Armstrong JA: The transplanted kidney as a source of cytomegalovirus infection. N Engl J Med 293:1109, 1975.
22. Embil JA, Ozere RL, Haldane EV: Congenital cytomegalovirus infection in two siblings from consecutive pregnancies. J Pediatr 77:417, 1970.
23. Krech U, Konjajev Z, Jung M: Congenital cytomegalovirus infection in siblings from consecutive pregnancies. Helv Paediatr Acta 26:355, 1971.
24. Stagno S, Reynolds DW, Lakeman A, Charamella LJ, Alford CA: Congenital cytomegalovirus infection: consecutive occurrence due to viruses with similar antigenic compositions. Pediatrics 52:788, 1973.
25. Stagno S, Torres J, Dworsky ME, Mesa T, Hirsh T: Prevalence and importance of congenital cytomegalovirus infection in three different populations. J. Pediatr, in press, 1982.
26. Huang E-S, Alford CA, Reynolds DW, Stagno S, Pass RF: Molecular epidemiology of cytomegalovirus infections in women and their infants. N Engl J Med 303:958, 1980.
27. Stagno S, Pass RF, Dworsky ME, Henderson RE, Moore EG, Walton PD, Alford CA: Congenital cytomegalovirus infection: the relative importance of primary and recurrent maternal infection. N Engl J Med 306:945, 1982.
28. Griffiths PD, Campbell-Benzie A: A prospective study of cytomegalovirus infection in pregnant women. Br J Obstet Gynaecol 87:308, 1980.
29. Grant S, Edmond E, Syme J: A prospective study of cytomegalovirus infection in pregnancy. I. Laboratory evidence of congenital infection following maternal primary and reactivated infection. J Infect 3:24, 1981.
30. Ahlfors K, Harris S, Ivarsson S, Svanberg L: Secondary maternal cytomegalovirus infection causing symptomatic congenital infection. N Engl J Med 305:284, 1981.

31. Stagno S, Reynold D, Tsiantos A, Fuccillo DA, Smith RJ, Tiller M, Alford CA: Cervical cytomegalovirus excretion in pregnant and nonpregnant women: suppression in early gestation. J Infect Dis 131:522, 1975.
32. Willmott FE: Cytomegalovirus in femal patients attending a VD clinic. Br J Vener Dis 51:278, 1975.
33. Jordan MC, Rousseau WE, Noble GR, Stewart JA, Chin TDY: Association of cervical cytomegalovirus with venereal disease. N Engl J Med 288:932, 1973.
34. Gump DW, Horton EL, Phillips CA, Mead PB, Forsyth BR: Contraception and cervical colonization with mycoplasmas and infection with cytomegalovirus. Fertil Steril 26:1135, 1975.
35. Foy HM, Kenny GE. Wentworth BB, Johnson WL, Grayston JT: Isolation of mycoplasma hominis T-strains, and cytomegalovirus from the cervix of pregnant women. Am J Obstet Gynecol 106:635, 1970.
36. Numazaki Y, Yano N, Morizuka T, Takai S, Ishida N: Primary infection with human cytomegalovirus: virus isolation from healthy infants and pregnant women. Am J Epidemiol 91:410, 1970.
37. Montgomery R, Youngblood L, Medearis Jr, DN: Recovery of cytomegalovirus from the cervix in pregnancy. Pediatrics 49:524, 1972.
38. Knox GE, Reynolds DW, Cohen S, Alford CA: Alteration of the growth of cytomegalovirus and herpes simplex virus type 1 by epidermal growth factor, a contaminant of crude human chorionic gonadotropin preparations. J. Clin Invest 61:1635, 1978.
39. Knox GE, Pass RF, Reynolds DW, Stagno S, Alford CA: Comparative prevalence of subclinical cytomegalovirus and herpes simplex virus infections in the genital urinary tracts of low-income, urban women. J Infect Dis 140:419, 1979.
40. Gehrz RC, Marker SC, Knorr SO, Kalis JM, Balfour HH: Specific cell-mediated immune defect in active cytomegalovirus infection of young children and their mothers. Lancet 2:844, 1977.
41. Starr SE, Tolpin MD, Friedman HM, Paucker K, Plotkin SA: Impaired cellular immunity to cytomegalovirus in congenitally infected children and their mothers. J. Infect Dis 140:500, 1979.
42. Reynolds DW, Dean PH, Pass RF, Alford CA: Specific cell-mediated immunity in children with congenital and neonatal cytomegalovirus infection infection and their mothers. J Infect Dis 140:493, 1979.
43. Gehrz RC, Christianson WR, Linner KM, Conroy MM, McCue, SA, Balfour HH Jr: Cytomegalovirus-specific humoral and

cellular immune response in human pregnancy. J Infect Dis 143:391, 1981.
44. Pass RF, Dworsky ME: Personal communication.
45. Nankervis A, Kumar ML, Gold E: Primary infection with cytomegalovirus during pregnancy. Pediatr Res 8:487, 1974.
46. Griffiths PD, Stagno S, Pass RF, Smith RJ, Alford CA Jr: Infection with cytomegalovirus during pregnancy: specific IgM antibodies as a marker of recent primary infection. J Infect Dis 145:647, 1982.
47. Griffiths PD, Stagno S, Reynolds DW, Alford CA: A longitudinal study of the serological and virological status of 18 women infected with cytomegalovirus. Arch Virol 58:111, 1978.
48. Pattison JR, Dane DS, Mace JE: Persistence of specific IgM after natural infection with rubella virus. Lancet 1:185, 1975.
49. Henle W, Henle GE, Horwitz CA: Epstein-Barr virus specific diagnostic tests in infectious mononucleosis. Hum Pathol 5:551, 1974.
50. Lemon SM, Brown CD, Brooks DS, Simms TE, Bancroft WH: Specific immunoglobulin M response to hepatitis A virus determined by solid-phase radioimmunoassay. Infect Immun 28:927, 1980.
51. Schmitz H, Kampa D, Doerr HW, Luthardt T, Hillemanns HG, Wurtele A: IgM antibodies to cytomegalovirus during pregnancy. Arch Virol 53:177, 1977.
52. DeSilva LM, Kampfner GL, Lister CM, Tobin JO'H: Identification of pregnancies at risk from cytomegalovirus infection. J Hyg (Camb) 79:347, 1977.
53. Hekker AC, Brand-Saathof B, Vis J, Meijers RC: Indirect immunofluorescence test for detection of IgM antibodies to cytomegalovirus. J Infect Dis 140:596, 1979.
54. Schmitz H, Doerr HW, Kampa D, Vogt A: Solid-phase enzyme immunoassay for immunoglobulin M antibodies to cytomegalovirus. J Clin Microbiol 5:629, 1977.
55. Cappel R, de Cuyper F, de Braekkeleer J: Rapid detection of IgG and IgM antibodies for cytomegalovirus by the enzyme linked immunosorbent assay (ELISA). Arch Virol 58:253, 1978.
56. Krishna RV, Meurman OH, Ziegler T, Krech UH: Solid-phase enzyme immunoassay for determination of antibodies to cytomegalovirus. J Clin Microbiol 12:46, 1980.
57. van Loon AM, Heessen FWA, van der Logt JThM, van der Veen J: Direct enzyme-linked immunosorbent assay that uses peroxidase-labelled antigen for determination of immunoglobulin M antibody to cytomegalovirus. J Clin Microbiol 13:416, 1981.

58. Gerna G, Chambers RW: Rapid detection of human cytomegalovirus and herpes virus hominis IgM antibody by the immunoperoxidase technique. Intervirology 8:257, 1977.
59. Knez V, Stewart JA, Ziegler DW: Cytomegalovirus specific IgM and IgG response in humans studied by radioimmunoassay. J Immunol 117:2006, 1976.
60. Torfason EG, Kallander C, Halonen P: Solid-phase radioimmunoassay of serum IgG, IgM and IgA antibodies to cytomegalovirus. J Med Virol 7:85, 1981.
61. Cremer NE, Hoffman M, Lennette EH: Analysis of antibody assay methods and classes of viral antibodies in serodiagnosis of cytomegalovirus infection. J Clin Microbiol 8:153, 1978.
62. Schmidt WAK, Klein M: A new method for the determination of virus specific IgG and IgM antibodies. Arch Virol 66:67, 1980.
63. Betts RF, Schmidt SG: Cytolytic IgM antibody to cytomegalovirus in primary cytomegalovirus infection in humans. J Infect Dis 143:821, 1981.
64. Davis JE, Tweed GV, Steward JA, Bernstein MT, Miller GL, Gravelle CR, Chin TDY: Cytomegalovirus mononucleosis in a first trimester pregnant female with transmission to the fetus. Pediatrics 48:200, 1971.
65. French MLV, Thompson JF, White A: Cytomegalovirus viremia with transmission from mother to fetus. Ann Intern Med 86:748, 1977.
66. Huikeshoven FJM, Wallenburg HCS, Jahoda MGJ: Diagnosis of severe fetal cytomegalovirus infection from amniotic fluid in the third trimester of pregnancy. Am J Obstet Gynecol 142:1053, 1982.
67. Yambao TJ, Clark D, Weiner L, Aubry RH: Isolation of cytomegalovirus from the amniotic fluid during the third trimester. Am J Obstet Gynecol 142:937, 1982.
68. Hayes K, Gibas H: Placental cytomegalovirus infection without fetal involvement following primary infection in pregnancy. J Pediatr 79:401, 1971.
69. Stagno S, Brasfield DM, Brown MB, Cassell GH, Pifer LL, Whitley RJ, Tiller RE: Infant pneumonitis associated with cytomegalovirus, chlamydia, pneumocystis, and ureaplasma - a prospective study. Pediatrics 68:322, 1981.

CHAPTER 16

CELL MEDIATED IMMUNITY TO HUMAN CYTOMEGALOVIRUS

Alain H. Rook

Gerald V. Quinnan, Jr.

Division of Virology
Office of Biologics
National Center for Drugs and Biologics
Food and Drug Administration
Bethesda, Maryland 20205

INTRODUCTION

Cytomegalovirus (CMV) infects most normal individuals during their lifetime, but the consequences of such infections are usually minimal. In contrast, there is a high frequency of serious infections among those with immature or depressed immune systems. Both B and T effector cells undoubtedly contribute immune functions in virus infections. In CMV infections the weight of evidence suggests that the effects of cellular components are ordinarily of greater significance than humoral components of the immune system.

Sixty to 90 percent of kidney transplant recipients develop CMV infection (1) with mortality rates in this population estimated to be as high as 10 percent (2). The incidence of CMV pneumonia among bone marrow allograft recipients is greater than 20 percent with mortality in excess of 80 percent (3). Perinatal infection occurs in approximately 5 percent of infants (4), and may be complicated by serious interstitial pneumonitis, especially in premature infants (5). In each of these groups the importance of the cellular immune system in recovery from CMV infection is typified by the observation that they may be vulnerable to persistent or fatal infection despite the presence of circulating antibodies to CMV. A few of the types of evidence that support this interpretation of available data are listed in Table 1.

ISBN 0-12-239980-3

TABLE 1. Evidence for the Importance of Cell Mediated Immunity in Recovery from CMV Infection

1. High susceptibility of T cell deficient nude mice	(Starr & Allison, 1977)
2. Increased susceptibility to murine CMV in NK cell deficient beige mice	(Shellam et al., 1981)
3. Reactivation and dissemination of CMV in latently infected mice by immunosuppression with cyclophosphamide	(Mayo et al., 1977)
4. High frequency of severe infection in transplant recipients, cancer patients and infants	(Betts et al., 1977; Neiman et al., 1980; Stagno et al., 1975; Arvin et al., 1980)

Data from animal studies provide additional evidence of the prominent role of cell-mediated immunity (CMI) in limiting the in-vivo spread of CMV. A variety of specific defects in CMI predispose to adverse effects of CMV infection. For example, athymic mice are exquisitely susceptible to murine CMV (6). Starr, et al. found that lethal infection resulted from as few as 1 to 10 plaque forming units (PFU) in nude mice compared to 10^5-10^6 PFU in normal mice. Moreover, reconstitution of nude mice with spleen cells from CMV-immune euthymic littermates conferred protection that was abrogated by prior treatment of the spleen cells with anti-thy 1.2 serum and complement (7). Beige mice possess a different genetic defect in CMI which involves depressed natural killer (NK) cell activity. Shellam and colleagues (8) have demonstrated that beige mice also have a heightened susceptibility to murine CMV infection, and that susceptibility of a number of strains of mice with normal immune systems is inversely proportional to their splenic NK cell activity (9). These studies indicate that deficiencies in various cellular functions may result in the inability of the host immune system to control replication of CMV in-vivo.

In individuals with depressed immunity the manifestations of CMV infection are diverse. Mild illness may consist of fever with atypical lymphocytosis, leukopenia, thrombocytopenia, and elevated serum transaminase levels. More significant manifestations are interstitial pneumonitis, hepatitis, hemorrhagic gastroenteritis, encephalitis, myocarditis, chorioretinitis, and secondary infedtions with opportunistic organisms (10). Fatal disease and the more severe manifestations of infection are related to impairment of certain specific cellular functions. The extent to which these cellular defects correlate with severity of disease and recovery undoubtedly reflects the relative importance of CMI in CMV, compared to other virus infections. Because changes in specific functions relate to marked differences in disease manifestations, CMV infections provide a useful model for study of the mechanisms whereby CMI exerts antiviral effects. We will review here our current understanding of the role of CMI and propose areas where further study may define methods for therapy of infections with this virus.

LYMPHOCYTE BLASTOGENESIS

The most widely used measure of CMI to CMV has been the lymphocyte transformation or blastogenesis assay. Lymphocytes from normal immune individuals proliferate when stimulated with CMV antigen (11). While lymphocytes from non-immune subjects generally do not respond there is no correlation between the magnitude of the blastogenic response and levels of antibody to CMV in the serum of immune individuals (12). This response to CMV is specific in that cross-reactivity with other herpes viruses is not observed (11). However, such cross-reactivity is commonly observed between many different strains of CMV, with some laboratory strains, such as AD 169, being broadly reactive. The capacity of lymphocytes to proliferate in vitro in response to CMV antigens usually does not occur until 1-2 months after infection (13).

The ability of lymphocytes to proliferate in response to CMV antigens in vitro does not appear to correlate with the ability of individual transplant patients to recover from CMV infection, since it develops only after recovery from primary infection, sometimes after many months (14,15). However, lymphocyte recruitment is an essential component of effector B and T cell development and factors which inhibit this process must have an impact on the effectiveness of the immune response in vivo. Renal transplant recipients treated with antithymocyte globulin have greater depression of responses to phytohemagglutinin and CMV antigens and are at greater risk of serious complications from CMV infections than patients who do not receive this drug (16). Individuals with malignancies also may have suppressed blastogenesis and enhanced susceptibility to deleterious effects on CMV infection (17). Women who have recently given birth to congenitally infected infants have been reported in one study to have absence of CMV-specific in vitro proliferation responses (18). This may be explained by enhanced suppressor cell activity which is a physiologic effect of pregnancy and which might be manifest in some cases of CMV infection as an inability to mount a sufficient cellular response to prevent maternal-fetal transmission (19).

TABLE 2. Evidence for the Immunosuppressive Effect of CMV

1.	Highly frequency of superinfection	(Rand et al., 1978)
2.	Depressed lymphocyte responsiveness to mitogens and antigens	(Levin et al., 1979)
3.	Delayed skin allograft rejection	(Howard et al., 1974)
4.	Decreased antibody response to sheep erythrocytes	(Howard & Najarian, 1974)

Infection with CMV itself exerts an immunosuppressive effect (Table 2). Lymphocyte transformation responses to concanavalin-A and pokeweed mitogen are depressed as are responses to certain other antigens which were capable of evoking blastogenesis prior to infection (20). In addition, transplant patients with CMV infection appear predisposed to serious infections with other opportunistic agents (21). The interpretation that this predisposition results from CMV infection is supported by animal studies which have shown that CMV infection of immunocompetent mice is associated with enhanced susceptibility to these same agents (22,23). Other evidence of immune inhibition by CMV includes depressed responses to challenge with a second antigen (24) and suppression of lymphocyte proliferation by CMV infected macrophages (25). The recently described acquired immunodeficiency syndrome of homosexuals may be, in part, the result of CMV infection (26,27,33).

TABLE 3. Mechanisms of Immunosuppression by CMV

1.	Direct effect of the virus	(Booss & Wheelock, 1977)
2.	Monocyte dysfunction	(Carney et al, 1981)
3.	Alterations in immuno-regulatory T-cell subsets	(Carney et al., 1981)

The immunosuppressive effect of CMV infection might occur by a variety of mechanisms (Table 3). Booss and Wheelock found that CMV might have a direct effect on responding lymphocytes since addition of the virus to stimulated cultures inhibited their response (28). Alternatively, they also found that serum from infected mice contained a soluble suppressor substance (29). Other workers have found that peripheral blood from individuals with CMV-mononucleosis contains adherent suppressor cells (30) and that CMV-infected leukocytes can inhibit proliferation of autologous, mitogen-stimulated lymphocytes (25). Macrophages could function as suppressor cells or their capacity to release necessary lymphokines could be inhibited by exposure to virus. Finally, a suppressor T cell response and reduction in numbers of helper T cells have been observed in transplant patients and otherwise healthy individuals with CMV infection (31,32,49).

In as much as the in vitro proliferation response reflects the capacity for activation and recruitment of immune or non-immune lymphocytes, and the implied components of those processes, including lymphokine production and responsiveness of appropriate cell types (34,35), its integrity must be a determinant of the effector cell maturation process.

IMMUNOREGULATION

The lymphokine dependent events measured in blastogenesis assays are modulated by specific and non-specific immunoregulatory cells and soluble factors. The information available regarding the nature of immunoregulatory functions in CMV infection was reviewed briefly above in the context of virus induced immunosuppression. One circumstance where profound alterations in immunoregulatory phenomena have been consistently observed is the acquired immunodeficiency syndrome of homosexuals (26,27,33). Perhaps excessive suppressor cell activity underlies their remarkable susceptibility to all infections, including CMV. Undoubtedly, appropriate regulation of effector cell activity is critical in all virus infections and more research on these responses in CMV infection is needed.

CYTOTOXIC LYMPHOCYTES

Cell-mediated cytotoxicity is regarded as a potentially

important function in virus infections, since killing of infected cells prior to formation of intact virions could interrupt the spread of virus from cell-to-cell. There are three types of effector mechanisms which are known to mediate killing of CMV-infected cells. The effector lymphocytes involved are cytotoxic T lymphocytes (Tc), natural killer cells (NKC) and antibody-dependent killer (K) cells. In a murine model the earliest of these responses, occuring 3-5 days after virus inoculation, is that mediated by NKC (36). The rise in NKC activity is preceded by a rise in serum interferon (37). From approximately day 6 to 21 of infection, virus-specific Tc cells are present in spleens and peripheral blood (38,39). Beginning about day 10, and persisting for many months, antibody with the capacity to arm K cells to mediate antibody-dependent cell mediated cytotoxicity (ADCC) is present in serum of mice (40).

TABLE 4. Characteristics of Different Types of Effector Cells Mediating Virus Specific Cytotoxicity

	CTL	NK	ADCC
HLA-Restriction	+	-	-
Sheep Erythrocyte Rosette Formation	+	-	-
Fc Receptor	-	+	+
T-Cell Antigen (OKT 3)	+	-	-
Nylon Wool Adherence	-	-	-
Antibody Dependence	-	-	+

The responses that occur in humans have many similarities to those observed in the murine model. Some properties of human lymphocytes which differentiate the three types of cytotoxic effects are summarized in Table 4. These properties fall into three categories: cell surface markers, HLA-restriction, and antigenic specificity (41,42). Tc cells form rosettes with sheep erythrocytes at 29-37°C (41). The converse findings characterize the surfaces of NKC and K cells. The restriction of killing to virus-infected target cells with which the effector cells share HLA antigens is also unique to Tc cells. The nature of the T cell receptor which restricts their activity in this fashion is unknown, but HLA-restriction (or H-2 restriction in the mouse) does appear to be a property common to human Tc directed against a number of viruses (43-46). The Tc cell receptor is also specific for antigens of the infecting virus. NKC may kill CMV-infected diploid fibroblasts to a greater degree than uninfected fibroblasts (47), but they also kill other cell types, most notably lymphoid tumor cells. Apparent virus-specificity of NKC may result from greater sensitivity of infected than uninfected target cells to their cytotoxic effect, or activation of the NKC by virus-induced interferon. K cells derive their antigen specificity through antiviral antibodies which sensitize target cells or arm the K cells through their Fc-receptor. Non-virus specific cytotoxicity assays using tumor cells, such as K562 cells, and allo-antibody-sensitized cells as target cells can be used to measure NKC and K-cell activity, respectively. Specific assays using CMV-infected target cells can measure one or more of these three effector cell types. By virtue of the different characteristics of these types of effectors, the specific cell types mediating cytotoxicity under different circumstances can be defined and the potential role of each cell type during various stages of infection elucidated. We have studied a number of different population groups to attempt to define abnormalities that enhanced susceptibility of some individuals to CMV infection.

As shown below following transplantation, prior to CMV infection, CMV-specific cytotoxic lymphocyte activity is low or absent. Early during infection a rise in CMV-specific cytotoxic lymphocyte activity occurs. The response is usually mediated, at least in part, by T cells which are HLA-restricted, they lyse only CMV-infected target cells with which they share HLA-A or B antigens in common (Solid Circles). Non-T cells, including natural killer cells and antibody-dependent killer cells may also mediate CMV-specific lysis. These cells are not HLA-restricted and may lyse CMV-infected cells which are either HLA-mismatched (Open Circles) or matched. After recovery from infection, HLA-restricted T cells are no longer detectable, but activity of non-restricted cells persists. NSA = not significant lysis.

Results of studies of bone marrow transplant (BMT) recipients which exemplify several features of the virus specific cytotoxic lymphocyte responses to CMV infection are shown in Figure 1. The results can be conveniently discussed in relation to three phases: preinfection, acute infection, and post-recovery. During the acute infection phase, cytotoxicity rises above the preinfection level and remains elevated for a period of time generally corresponding to the time of symptomatology. The cytotoxicity is frequently mediated by HLA-restricted Tc cells, in part or in total, during the acute phase, but is non-restricted at other times. Tc cell responses are, thus, only associated with acute infection.

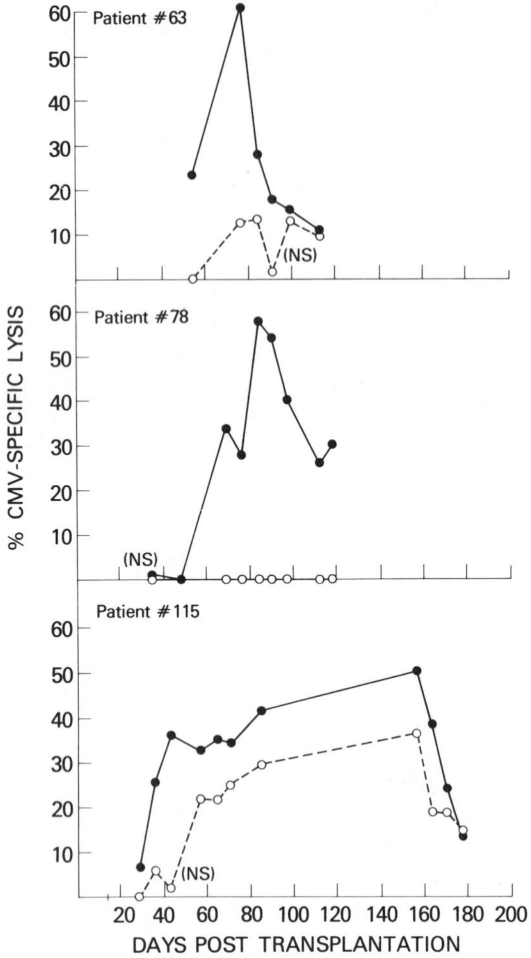

FIGURE 1. Different Patterns of Cytomegalovirus (CMV)-Specific Cytotoxic Lymphocyte Responses in Three Recipients of Bone Marrow Transplants who Survived CMV Infection.

In the early post-transplantation period BMT recipients have depressed or absent CMV-specific cytotoxicity compared to normal individuals, regardless of whether they or their donors were immune prior to transplantation. Non-restricted, NKC-mediated CMV-specific cytotoxicity is consistently demonstrable in peripheral blood of seronegative healthy volunteers, and cytotoxicity mediated by NKC and/or ADCC is found in healthy seropositive individuals (47). This abnormality in the BMT recipients may underly their susceptibility to develop infection by reactivation of latent virus from their own cells or from transplanted marrow or infused blood cells. Alternatively, the deficiency may relate to their inability to develop appropriate responses once infection develops.

In this acute infection phase, a significant rise in CMV-specific cytotoxicity occurs in the majority of BMT recipients. Although in most cases this response is comprised, at least in part, by Tc cells, nonrestricted, non-T cell responses can occur in recipients of marrow from seropositive donors and appear to have equivalent significance. In a prospective study of BMT recipients all 18 patients studied who survived CMV infection developed CMV-specific cytotoxic responses, whereas only two of 10 who died from infection had possible responses of a significantly lower level (42). Other factors such as CMV antibodies and lymphocyte blastogenic responses during infection, the presence of graft-versus-host disease, and diagnoses for which patients required transplantation did not correlate significantly with outcome of infection in these patients. Significant differences between survivors and non-survivors were noted in non-specific NKC and K cell activities, but these differences were less than for CMV-specific cytotoxic responses. Similar associations of absent cytotoxic responses with complicated or fatal infections in renal transplant recipients (48) and homosexuals with acquired immunodeficiency syndrome have been noted in preliminary reports (33). In contrast, cytotoxic responses resembling those of BMT recipients who survived infection have been noted in otherwise healthy volunteers (49). This consistent association of virus-specific cytotoxic responses with a favorable outcome clearly implicates this type of function in the process of recovery from CMV infection.

The association of depressed NKC activity with fatal and complicated infections could be significant for several reasons. NKC might contribute as an early defense mechanism which destroys virus-infected cells. However, the frequent association of deficient NKC activity and low or absent Tc cell responses may indicate that other activities required for adequate function of both cell types may be deficient. For example, we have found that depressed NKC activity of patients who eventually succumb to fatal infection can usually be markedly enhanced by interferon treeatment in-vitro, but that their lymphocytes fail to produce interferon when stimulated with Con A (50). In addition the defective responsiveness to Con A is of two types: in some cases lymphocyte proliferation is deficient while in others it is normal (a proposed interpretation of these findings

Nature of Infection		NKC		Concanavlin-A Response			Proposed Defect	
Asymptomatic or Self-Limited	Severe or Fatal	Activity	IFN Responsive	Proliferation	IFN Production	T_C Response	Lymphokines	Cellular Interactions
–	+	Decreased	–	–	–	–	IL-1 Production or Responsiveness	M → IL-1 → ?
–	+	Decreased	+	–	–	–	IL-2 Production or Responsiveness	NKC_P, T_P → ? IL-2
–	+	Decreased	+	+	–	–	IFN Production	NKC, T → IFN
+	–	Normal	+ /or –	+	+	+		NKC_A, T_C

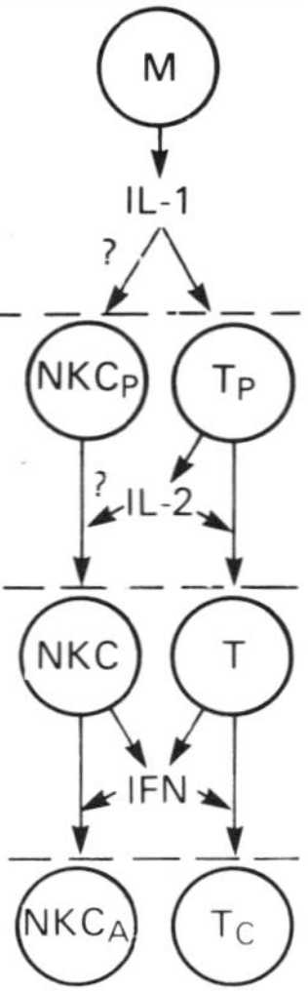

FIGURE 2. Cytotoxic Lymphocyte Responses in Cytomegalovirus Infections: Model for Interpretation of Deficient Responses and Associated Abnormalities. See text for discussion and abbreviations.

will be discussed below). The observations are also of interest in that they suggest a potential mechanism of action of exogenously administered interferon. Cheeseman, et al. reported that prophylactic treatment of renal transplant patients with interferon reduced the frequency of viremia and delayed the onset of CMV infection (51). Interferon administered in the presence of an endogenous production deficiency could inhibit latent virus reactivation either directly, or indirectly via NKC or K cell activation (52). Undoubtedly, there are different factors which account for deficient cytotoxic responses in various groups of patients, but even within the population of BMT recipients several different deficiencies may exist. A possible interpretation of the results we have obtained is summarized schematically in Figure 2.

BMT recipients who survive CMV infection develop Tc cell responses, have normal NKC activity which is usually augmented by IFN treatment in vitro (NKC_A), and their lymphocytes proliferate and produce IFN when stimulated with Con A. Patients with fatal infection do not develop Tc cell responses, have low NKC activity and their lymphocytes do not produce IFN. Since lymphocytes from some of these individuals proliferate in response to Con A, they must have a defect in effector cell differentiation subsequent to interleukin-2 (1L-2) dependent effects. Those whose lymphocytes do not proliferate may have a defect in 1L-2 production or responsiveness. Those who also lack IFN-responsive NKC precursors (NKCp) may have a defect at an earlier stage of the activation process if lymphokine activity is necessary for maturation of NKCp into normal NKC. Admittedly, these proposed defects are entirely speculative. If the speculations proved to be correct, however, it would be of interest to study immunotherapies using lymphokines which bypassed specific defects in effector cell differentiation. Through systematic study of responder cell and effector cell activities it should be possible to develop an understanding of the role of immune functions in virus infections and perhaps methods to alleviate severe virus diseases.

REFERENCES

1. Rubin, R.H., Russell, P.S., Levin, M., and Cohen, C. 1979. Summary of a workshop on cytomegalovirus infections during organ transplantation. J. Infect. Dis. 139:728.

2. Betts, R.F., Freeman, R.B., Douglas, R.G., and Talley, T.E. 1977. Clinical manifestations of renal allograft derived primary cytomegalovirus infection. Amer. J. Dis. Child. 131:759.
3. Neiman, P.E., Reeves, W., Ray, G., Flournoy, N., Lerner, K.G., Sale, G.E., and Thomas, E.D. 1977. A prospective analysis of interstitial pneumonia and opportunistic viral infection among recipients of allogeneic bone marrow grafts. J. Infect. Dis. 136:754.
4. Stagno, S., Reynolds, D.W., Tsiantos, A., Fuccilo, D.A., Long, W. and Alford, C.A. 1975. Comparative serial virologic and serologic studies of symptomatic and subclinical congenitally and natally acquired cytomegalovirus infections. J. Infect. Dis. 132:568.
5. Ballard, R.A., Drew, W.L., Hufnagle, K.G., and Riedel, P.A. 1979. Acquired cytomegalovirus infection in preterm infants. Am. J. Dis. Child. 133:482.
6. Selgrade, M.K., Ahmed, A., Sell, K.W., Gershwin, M.E., and Steinberg, A.D. 1976. Effect of murine cytomegalovirus on the in vitro response of T and B cells to mitogens. J. Immunol. 116:1459.
7. Starr, S.E., and Allison, A.C. 1977. Role of T lymphocytes in recovery from murine cytomegalovirus infection. Infect. Immun. 17:458.
8. Shellam, G.R., Allan, J.E., Papadimitriou, J.M., and Bancroft, G.J. 1981. Increased susceptibility to cytomegalovirus infection in beige mutant mice. Proc. Natl. Acad. Sci. 78:5104.
9. Bancroft, G.J., Shellam, G.R., and Chalmer, J.E. 1981. Genetic influences on the augmentation of natural killer (NK) cells during murine cytomegalovirus infection: correlation with patterns of resistance. J. Immunol. 126:988.
10. Merigan, T.C. 1981. Immunosuppression and herpesviruses. In The Human Herpesviruses. An Interdisciplinary Perspective. Edited by A.J. Nahmias, W.R. Dowdle and R.F. Schinazi. Elsevier, New York. p. 309.
11. Zaia, J.A., Leary, P.L., and Levin, M.J. 1978. Specificity of the blastogenic response of human mononuclear cells to herpesvirus antigens. Infect. Immun. 20:646.
12. Waner, J.L., and Budnick, J.E. 1977. Blastogenic response of human lymphocytes to human cytomegalovirus. Clin. Exp. Immunol. 30:44.
13. Levin, M.J., Rinaldo, C.R., Leary, P.L., Zaia, J.A., and Hirsch, M.S. 1979. Immune response to herpesvirus antigens in adults with acute cytomegalovirus mononucleosis. J. Infect. Dis. 140:851.

14. Linnemann, C.C., Kauffman, C.A., First, M.R., Schiff, G.M., and Phair, J.P. 1978. Cellular immune response to cytomegalovirus infections after renal transplantation. Infect. Immun. 22:176.
15. Meyers, J.D., Flournoy, N., and Thomas, E.D. 1980. Cytomegalovirus infection and specific cell-mediated immunity after marrow transplantation. J. Infect. Dis. 142:816.
16. Pass, R.F., Reynolds, D.W., Whelchel, J.D., Diethelm, A.G., and Alford, C.A. 1981. Impaired lymphocyte transformation response to cytomegalovirus and phytohemagglutinin in recipients of renal transplants: association with antithymocyte glovulin. J. Infect. Dis. 143:259.
17. Arvin, A.M., Pollard, R.B., Rasmussen, L.E., and Merigan, T.C. 1980. Cellular and humoral immunity in the pathogenesis of recurrent herpes viral infections in patients with lymphoma. J. Clin. Invest. 65:869.
18. Reynolds, D.W., Dean, P.H., Pass, R.F., and Alford, C.A. 1979. Specific cell-mediated immunity in children with congenital and neonatal cytomegalovirus infection and their mothers. J. Infect. Dis. 140:493.
19. Gehrz, R.C., Christianson, W.R., Linner, K.M., Conroy, M.M., McCue, S.A., and Balfour, H.H. 1981. Cytomegalovirus specific humoral and cellular immune responses in human pregnancy. J. Infect. Dis. 143:391.
20. ten Napel, C.H.H., and The, T.H. 1980. Acute cytomegalovirus infection and the host immune response. II. Relationship of suppressed in vitro lymphocyte reactivity to bacterial recall antigens and mitogens with the development of cytomegalovirus-induced lymphocyte reactivity. Clin. Exp. Immunol. 39:272.
21. Rand, K.H., Pollard, R.B., and Merigan, T.C. 1978. Increased pulmonary superinfections in cardiac transplant patients undergoing primary cytomegalovirus infection. N. Engl. J. Med. 298:951.
22. Hamilton, J., Overall, J.C., and Glasgow, L.A. 1976. Synergistic effect on mortality in mice with murine cytomegalovirus and Peudomonas aeruginosa, Staphylococcus aureus or Candida albicans infections. Infect. Immun. 14:982.
23. Hamilton, J., and Overall, J.C. 1978. Synergistic infection with murine cytomegalovirus and Pseudomonas aeruginosa in mice. J. Infect. Dis. 137:775.
24. Howard, R.J., Miller, J., and Najarian, J.S. 1974. Cytomegalovirus induced immune suppression. II. Cell-mediated immunity. Clin. Exp. Immunol. 18:119.

25. Carney, W.P., and Hirsch, M.S. 1981. Mechanisms of immunosuppression in cytomegalovirus mononucleosis. II. Virus-monocyte interactions. J. Infect. Dis. 144:47.
26. Gottlieb, M.S., Schroff, R., Schanker, H.M., Weisman, J.D., Fan, P.T., Wolf, R.A., and Saxon, A. 1981. Pneumocystis carinii pneumonia and mucosal candidiasis in previously healthy homosexual men: Evidence of a new acquired cellular immunodeficiency. N. Engl. J. Med. 305:1425.
27. Siegal, F.P., Lopez, C., Hammer, G.S., Brown, A.E., Kornfeld, S.J., Gold, J., Hassett, J., Hirschman, S.Z., Cunningham-Rundles, C., Adelsberg, R.B., Parham, D.M., Siegal, M., Cunningham-Rundles, S., and Armstrong, D. 1981. Severe acquired immunodefiency in male homosexuals manifested by chronic perianal ulcer-alive herpes simplex lesions. N. Engl. J. Med. 305:1439.
28. Booss, J., and Wheelock, E.F. 1977. Progressive inhibition of T cell function preceding clinical signs of cytomegalovirus infection in mice. J. Infect. Dis. 135:478.
29. Booss, J., and Wheelock, E.F. 1977. Progressive inhibition of T cell function preceding clinical signs of cytomegalovirus infection in mice. J. Infect. Dis. 135:478.
30. Rinaldo, C.R., Carney, W.P., Richter, B.S., Black, P.H., and Hirsch, M.S. 1980. Mechanisms of immunosuppression in cytomegaloviral mononucleosis. J. Infect. Dis. 141:488.
31. Rubin, R.H., Carney, W.P., Schooley, R.T., Colvin, R.B., Burton, R.C., Hoffman, R.A., Hansen, W.P., Cosimi, A.B., Russell, P.S., and Hirsch, M.S. 1981. The effect of infection on T lymphocyte subpopulations: A preliminary report. Int. J. Immunopharmac. 3:307.
32. Carney, W.P., Rubin, R.H., Hoffman, R.A., Hansen, W.P., Healey, K. and Hirsch, M.S. 1981. Analysis of T lymphocyte subsets in cytomegalovirus mononucleosis. J. Immunol. 126:2114.
33. Frederick, W., Masur, H., Rook, A., Mittal, K., Manischewitz, J., Jackson, L., Straus, S., and Quinnan, G.V. 1982. Immune functions during cytomegalovirus infection in immunodeficient male homosexuals. In Proceedings of the Seventh Cold Spring Harbor Meeting on Herpesviruses. (In press).
34. Oppenheim, J.J., and Schecter, B. 1980. Lymphocyte transformation. In Manual of Clinical Immunology. Edited by N.R. Rose, and H. Friedman. American Society for Microbiology. Washington, DC. p.233.
35. Interleukins and Lymphocyte Activation. 1982. Immunol. Rev. V. 63. Editor G. Moller, Munksgaard, Copenhagen.

36. Quinnan, G.V., Manischewitz, J.F., and Kirmani, N. 1982. Involvement of natural killer cells in the pathogenesis of murine cytomegalovirus interstitial pneumonitis and the immune response to infection. J. Gen. Virol. 58:173.
37. Quinnan, G.V., and Manischewitz, J.E. 1979. The role of natural killer cells and antibody-dependent cell-mediated cytotoxicity during murine cytomegalovirus infection. J. Exp. Med. 150:1549.
38. Quinnan, G.V., Manischewitz, J.E., and Ennis, F.A. 1978. Cytotoxic T lymphocyte response to murine cytomegalovirus infection. Nature (London) 273:541.
39. Quinnan, G.V., Manischewitz, J.E., and Ennis, F.A. 1980. Role of cytotoxic T lymphocytes in murine cytomegalovirus infection. J. Gen. Virol. 47:503.
40. Manischewitz, J.E., and Quinnan, G.V. 1980. Antiviral antibody dependent cell-mediated cytotoxicity during murine cytomegalovirus infection. Infect. Immun. 29:1050.
41. Quinnan, G.V., Kirmani, N., Esber, E., Saral, R., Manischewitz, J.F., Rogers, J.L., Rook, A.H., Santos, G.W., and Burns, W.H. 1981. HLA-restricted cytotoxic T lymphocyte and non-thymic cytotoxic lymphocyte responses to cytomegalovirus infection of bone marrow transplant recipients. J. Immunol. 126:2036.
42. Quinnan, G.V., Kirmani, N., Rook, A.H., Manischewitz, J.F., Jackson, L., Moreschi, G., Santos, G.W., Saral, R., and W.H. Burns. 1982. Cytotoxic T cells in cytomegalovirus infection: HLA-restricted T lymphocyte and non-T-lymphocyte cytotoxic responses correlate with recovery from cytomegalovirus infection in bone marrow transplant recipients. N. Engl. J. Med. 307:6.
43. Daisy, J.A., Tolpin, M.D., Quinnan, G.V., Rook, A.H., Levine, M., Mittal, K.K., Murphy, B.R., Clements, M.L., Mullinix, M.G., Kiley, S.C., and Ennis, F.A. 1981. Cytotoxic cellular immune responses during influenza A infection in human volunteers. In the Replication of Negative Strand Viruses. Edited by D.H.L. Bishop and R.W. Compans. Elsevier North Holland. New York. p.443-448.
44. Ennis, F.A., Rook, A.H., Yi-Hua, Q., Riley, D., Pratt, R., Potter, C.W., and Schild, G.C. 1981. HLA-restricted virus specific cytotoxic T lymphocyte responses to live and inactivated influenza vaccines. Lancet 2:887.
45. Misko, I.S., Moss, D.J., and Pope, J.H. 1980. HLA antigen related restriction of T lymphocyte cytotoxicity to Epstein-Barr virus. Proc. Natl. Acad. Sci. USA. 77:4247.
46. Kreth, H.W., Kress, L., Kress., H.G., Ott, H.F., and Eckert, G. 1982. Demonstration of primary cytotoxic T

cells in venous blood and cerebrospinal fluid of children with mumps meningitis. J. Immunol. 128:2411.

47. Kirmani, N., Ginn, R.K., Mittal, K.K., Manischewitz, J.F., and Quinnan, G.V. 1981. Cytomegalovirus-specific cytotoxicity mediated by non-T lymphocytes from peripheral blood of normal volunteers. Infect. Immun. 34:441.
48. Rook, A.H., Kirmani, N., Manischewitz, J.F., Jackson, L.B., Lee, B.B., Dantzler, T., Currier, C.B., and Quinnan, G.V. 1982. Cytomegalovirus specific and non-specific cytotoxic lymphocyte responses in renal transplant recipients. Kidney Int. 21:299.
49. Frederick, W., Rook, A.H., Delery, M., Epstein, J., Ramsey, K., Manischewitz, J.F., Jackson, L., and Quinnan, G.V. 1982. Comparison of virulence and immunogenicity of Towne strain and low-passage (Toledo-1 strain) isolate of human cytomegalovirus. In Proceedings of the 22nd Interscience Conference on Antimicrobial Agents and Chemotherapy. (In press).
50. Rook, A.H., Frederick, W.R.J., Burns, W.H., Kirmani, N., Jackson, L.B., Manischewitz, J.F., Saral, R., Santos, G.W., and Quinnan, G.V. Natural killer cell activity and interferon release predict survival from viral infection in bone marrow transplant recipients. Transpl. Proceed. (In press).
51. Cheeseman, S.H., Rubin, R.H., Stewart, J.A., Tolkoff-Rubin, N.E., Cosimi, A.B., Cantell, K., Gilbert, J., Winkle, S., Herrin, J.T., Black, P.H., Russell, P.S., and Hirsch, M.S. 1979. Controlled clinical trial of prophylactic human-leukocyte interferon in renal transplantation: effects on cytomegalovirus and herpes simplex virus infections. N. Engl. J. Med. 300:1345.
52. Herberman, R.B., Ortaldo, J.R., and Bonnard, G.D. 1979. Augmentation by interferon of human natural and antibody-dependent cell-mediated cytotoxicity. Nature (London) 277:221.

CHAPTER 17

THE PREVENTION OF CYTOMEGALOVIRUS DISEASE

S. A. Plotkin
H.M. Friedman
S. E. Starr
M. L. Smiley
R. G. Grossman
C. Barker

Departments of Pediatrics and Medicine
University of Pennsylvania
Philadelphia, Pennsylvania

INTRODUCTION

The prevention of cytomegalovirus (CMV) infection in humans is important for pediatrics, nephrology, oncology, cardiology, and many other aspects of medicine. CMV has risen in status from an exotic infection of the debilitated host to one of the more important viruses in human medicine. Approximately 1% of all infants are infected in utero, of which about 15-25% will have damage to the central nervous system, as evidenced by mental retardation, psychomotor difficulties, or auditory defects (1,2).

A central issue with regard to the possibility of protection by vaccine is whether or not damage to the CNS can occur as a result of recurrent maternal infection in an immune mother. Stagno et al (3) have recently published an important study of both primary and recurrent maternal infections. Among 3712 pregnancies there were 32 cases of congenital CMV infection, a rate of 0.86%. The rate of congenital CMV in infants born of initially seronegative women was 0.8% while for seropositive women it was 0.8%: assuming that 14% of seropositive women had active infection, it appears that 6% of their babies had congenital infection (4). In contrast, 52% of the infants born to mothers who seroconverted during pregnancy were congenitally infected. Five of 33 babies born after primary infection, but none of 27 babies born after recurrent infections were ill at birth.

ISBN 0-12-239980-3

The former group also excreted an average of 20 times more virus at birth than the aatter group. Thus natural maternal immunity was shown to be protective against fetal disease, but of only limited value against infection. Most symptomatic infants will show later neurologic or auditory problems (5). Inapparent primary infection may also lead to later disability (6,7).

Towne strain vaccine has been developed in the hopes of preventing primary infection, but tests in pregnant women are obviously difficult to perform. In order to test the safety and efficacy of Towne strain vaccine in a feasible manner, a trial was organized in renal transplant candidates (RTC). The rationale was that these patients suffer severe CMV infections in the post-transplantation period: vaccination might prevent or modify these infections. In addition, study of virus excretion after immunosuppression could tell us whether the vaccine virus was reactivated.

METHODS

The trial was performed by randomization of renal transplant candidates (RTC) according to a table of random numbers. Designated vaccine recipients were given 1ml. of Towne strain containing $10^{3.5}$ PFU, intramuscularly in the deltoid area. Designated placebo recipients were given 1ml. of reconstituted medium. Neither the patients nor the physician who followed the patients clinically knew the identity of the material administered.

The incolulated RTC were observed for at least eight weeks during which attemps were made to cultivate vaccine virus. After that they were transplanted whenever a kidney became available. Serum from the donors were tested for CMV antibodies except in the cases of a few cadaver donors from whom serum was unavailable. Specimens from the RTC were collected weekly after transplantation for as long as the patient was in the hospital and at the time of subsequent visits. Active surveillance for CMV disease was maintained for six months post-transplant, during which almost all CMV disease is likely to occur, but follow-up data were obtained up to the present time.

Serologic response to vaccination were measured by complement fixation (CF), anti-complementary immuno-fluorescence (ACIF), and neutralization (Nt).

Cell-mediated immune responses to immunization were measured by CMV-specific lymphocyte proliferation (8). Heparinized peripheral blood was obtained from RTC living in the Philadelphia area at the time of and eight weeks after immunization.

RESULTS

At the time of writing, 184 patients have been enrolled in the trial: 107 vaccinees and 77 placebo recipients. The vaccine was well tolerated from the clinical point of view, with no general reactions. More subtle pathology was sought by doing CBC's and chemistry tests on vaccinees (Table 1).

TABLE 1. Abnormal Responses Post-Vaccine or Placebo Among First 49 Patients#

	VACCINE	PLACEBO
Hematology	0/14	0/12
Liver Function	1/13	0/11
CMV Excretion	0/23	0/19
Local Reaction	13/28*	0/21

#Only subjects who were monitored closely with weekly bleeding. *13/14 seronegatives.

The results show that there was one patient with a very mild elevation of transaminase on one determination. Otherwise there was no evidence of systemic disturbance. On the other hand, local reactions to the vaccine were almost invariable in seronegatives. Seronegative recipients of the vaccine developed soreness and induration during the second week post-vaccination, which then disappeared after a median of 7 days. Whether the reaction represents dermal hypersensitivity or the local replication of the vaccine stain is unclear, but we have previously shown that CMV-specific lymphocyte proliferation appears at about the same time as the local reaction.

The following analyses are based on the first 65 patients, who have been followed at least six months post-transplant. However, the numbers do not always add up to 65 because the patients fell in different categories or because a particular measurement is incomplete.

The serologic responses in RTC were compared with data previously obtained in healthy normal subjects. As shown in Table 2, while 100% of normals responded with antibodies, there were two failures among 23 seronegative RTC who received vaccine. Moreover, geometric mean titers were lower in RTC than in normals. For example, GMT CF titers were 40%

of normal at the peak, which was eight weeks post-vaccination.

TABLE 2. Serologic Responses to CMV Vaccine

	Transplant Pts.	Normal Volunteers
Seronegatives	21/23 (91%)	25/25 (100%)
	CF-GMT=9.5	CF-GMT=24
Seropositives	0/9 (0%)	0/4(0%)

The neutralizing antibody responses of seronegative renal transplant candidates are shown in Table 3. Neutralizing antibodies were measured against Towne and AD169. In addition, patients from whom wild strain CMV was isolated after transplantation, had pre and post-vaccination sera tested against their own isolate. By 2 months post-vaccination 13/15 (87%) had developed neutralizing antibodies to Towne and at 3-6 months, 6/7 (86%) had antibodies detected. After Towne immunization, neutralizing antibody titers also developed to other CMV strains (AD169 and fresh clinical isolates), although the geometric mean titers and the percentage of patients producing antibodies were lower than to Towne virus. These latter observations support the findings (9,10) which indicate that strain variability exists as detected by neutralizing antibody assays. However it is worth emphasizing that pools of Towne, AD169 and fresh isolates that contain 100 PFU infections virus may contain differing amounts of non-infectious virus, which will influence the antibody levels measured in these assays.

TABLE 3. Neutralizing Antibody Responses In Seronegative RT Candidates

	1 Mo.	2 Mo.	3-6 Mo.
Towne	4/10	13/15	6/7
	2.3'	12.1	9.8
AD 169	1/9	7/14	3/6
	1.2'	2.6	2.5
CLINICAL ISOLATES*	0/4	5/7	2/2
	0+	4.9	11.3

'GMT: geometric mean titer

*Clinical isolates: Neutralizing antibody responses were measured pre and post-vaccination against CMV strains isolated from vaccinees after transplantation. Each vaccinee was tested for neutralizing antibodies against his own CMV strain.

At the time of renal transplantation, sixteen of nineteen (84%) patients had neutralizing antibodies to Towne virus, 9/15 (60%) to AD169, and 5/8 (63%) to fresh clinical isolates. These results indicate that at the time of transplantation most patients have detectable neutralizing antibodies to a variety of CMV strains. At present, we have too few patients to analyze whether the presence of neutralizing antibodies correlates with protection from CMV infection or disease. As more patients are enrolled the protective value of neutralizing antibodies can be evaluated.

Table 4 demonstrates the persistence of neutralizing antibodies in renal transplant candidates and normal patients. At 3-6 months, 6/7 (86%) of transplant candidates and 9/9 (100%) normal patients had neutralizing antibodies to Towne virus. By 12 months 9/10 (90%) normals had detectable antibodies. From these results it is apparent that normals develop antibodies earlier after vaccination (90% normals positive at 1 month vs. 40% transplant candidates) and that antibody titers are higher in normals than transplant candidates (GMT 27.5 vs. 12.1). These results are similar to our findings of CMI responses post-vaccination, that is, a blunting of the immune response in uremics compared with normals.

TABLE 4. Towne Neutralizing Antibody Responses in RTC and Normals

	1 Mo.	2 Mo.	3-6 Mos.	12 Mos
RT	4/10	13/15	6/7	N.T.*
	2.3'	12.1	9.8	
NORMALS	9/10	9/9	9/9	9/10
	13.9*	27.5	14.7	10.6

*N.T. not tested.
'GMT geometric mean titer.

The results of lymphocyte-proliferation tests are expressed as a stimulation index and are shown in Fig. 1. Sero-negative placebo recipients had low S.I.'s to Towne strain antigen before and after immuniation. The mean S.I. was 1.37 + .7. Two standard deviations above the mean gave a S.I. of 2.8. We therefore considered a S.I. of 2.8 or above as a positive response. Of 13 seronegative RTC who received vaccine nine developed positive responses, and four failed to respond. These results are similar to our previous observations (11) and are consistent with reports that some of these individuals have multiple deficits in immunity including impaired ability to develop cellular immune responses (12). In contrast as shown in Figure 1 eight out of eight normal volunteers developed positive lymphocyte proliferation responses. No significant changes in CMV-specific lymphocyte proliferation were noted in sero-positive individuals who received vaccine or placebo (data not shown).

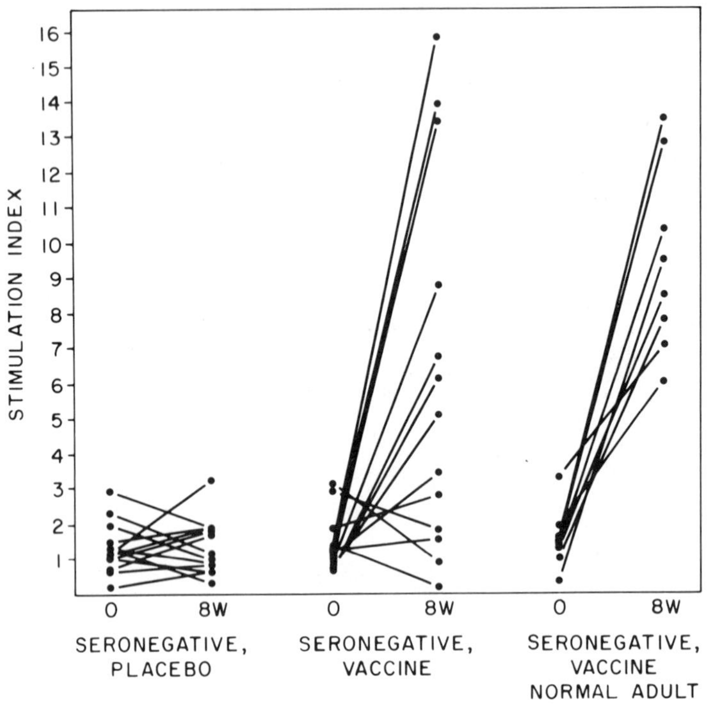

FIGURE 1. Lymphocyte stimulation responses to CMV antigen of seronegative placebo renal transplant candidates and seronegative vaccinated normal adults.

We have started to explore possible mechanisms involved in the failure of some vaccinees to develop CMV-specific proliferative responses. Since plasma from hemodialysis patients may inhibit lymphocyte proliferation (12) we compared proliferative responses when leukocytes were incubated in media containing autologous plasma to those when pooled homologous plasma was used. As shown in Fig. 2, of six seronegative RTC who were studied, only one had a positive proliferative response eight weeks after immunization when autologous plasma was used, while five had positive responses when pooled homologous plasma was used. In two instances the differences between autologous and pooled plasma were particularly striking. Thus, inhibitory effects of plasma provide a partial explanation for the impaired cellular responses to CMV noted in some of the renal transplant candidates.

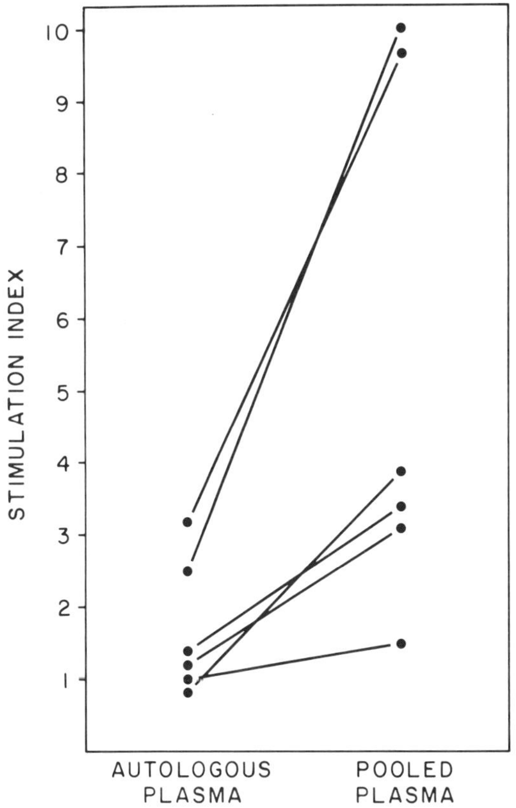

FIGURE 2. CMV-specific lymphocyte proliferation response eight weeks after immunization.

We have continued to obtain data on the proliferative responses of vaccinees to strains of CMV other than Towne as shown in Table 5. Renal transplant candidates (nos. 1-3) and normal volunteers (nos. 4-7) who responded to Towne antigen also responded to antigen prepared from Davis strain, which was selected because of its antigenic differences from Towne in kinetic neutralization tests (10).

TABLE 5. Strain-Specific Lymphocyte Proliferation Responses (Expressed as Stimulation Indexes) in Recipients of Towne Vaccine

		Antigens Tested							
	Weeks After			Wild Strains					
Vaccinee	Immun.	Towne	Davis	1	2	3	4	5	6
1	8	6.8[a]	5.7						
2	8	43.0	6.9						
3	8	8.8	20.4						
4	4	4.5	5.3						
5	4	8.4	12.7						
	8	14.0	5.5						
6	4	16.0	3.6						
	8	8.6	4.4						
7	2	6.8	10.0						
	4	16.8	28.6						
8	8	14.2				11.1	14.9	14.7	
9	4	28.1		ND	44.0	18.6	25.6	ND	32.1
	8	11.6		13.6	11.0	13.8	14.0	11.3	8.6
10	4	50.9		43.0	22.9	31.4	21.4	58.1	28.4
	8	10.6		17.0	17.6	12.9	6.9	9.1	8.7
11	4	29.8		31.5	23.2	17.2	23.2	5.6	28.5
	8	30.5		25.3	23.8	20.8	32.2	9.3	28.6
12	4	14.1		20.3	17.7	12.9	14.7	6.1	8.6
13	8	5.7		9.2	7.6	7.3	12.0	5.8	5.3
14	8	11.4		18.9	10.6	10.4	7.0	ND	6.0

[a]stimulation index

One immunized transplant candidate (no. 8) and six volunteers (nos. 9-14) were tested for their ability to respond to antigens prepared from several wild strains of CMV isolated from congenitally infected infants. As shown in Table 5 all responded to each of the antigens, and in most cases there were only minor differences in the magnitudes of the S.I.'s. These results confirm our earlier report that immunization with Towne some strain vaccine results in cellular reactivity in the proliferation assay to all CMV strains tested to date (11).

After transplantation lymphocyte proliferation responses were severely depressed for patients analyzed to date regardless of whether the patient was seropositive due to natural or vaccine-induced immunity. The following results were obtained for the indicated interval post transplantation: 0.2 mo, 2.3 ± 2.2 (n=12); 3-5 mo., 3.1 ± 3.5 (n=17); 6-9 mo., 3.4 ± 4.4 (n=20); 10-12 mo., 2.6 ±2.8 (n=12); 13-18 mo., 3.1 ± 3.3 (n=7); 19-24 mo., 3.7 ± 3.2 (n=5). These results should be compared to those for natural seropositive renal transplant candidates prior to transplantation: 13.4 ± 4.9 (n=26). There was no correlation in the transplanted patients between the magnitude of lymphocyte proliferation and the likelihood of developing CMV disease. Furthermore, transplanted individuals studied during CMV disease continued to have depressed proliferative responses. Several experiments were also done to compare responses in autologous plasma (shown above) with those obtained with pooled homologous plasma was used. In many instances higher responses were obtained with in homologous pooled plasma, however, the results with autologous plasma probably better reflect in-vivo circumstances.

Since lymphocyte proliferation measures only one aspect of cell-mediated immunity we are interested in using other assays, particularly cytotoxicity assays to assess cellular immunity to CMV. We recently developed an assay for natural killing of CMV infected target cells (13) and are in the process of preparing target cells to test for HLA-restricted T lymphocyte cytotoxicity.

Since CMV mononucleosis has been associated with immunosuppression and reversal of the T helper to T suppressor cell ratio we also used monoclonal antibodies to T lymphocyte subpopulations to study vaccinees immunized with Towne vaccine in order to determine whether similar changes occur. The results of this study, done in collaboration with Dr. Martin Hirsch of the Massachusetts General Hospital, are shown in Table 6. There were no changes in T lymphocyte subpopulations. These data provide further evidence that Towne vaccine is attenuated.

TABLE 6. %T Lympocyte Subsets in Recipients of CMV Vaccine and in CMV Mononucleosis Patients

Weeks post vaccin- ation	T Cells reactive with monoclonal antibodies (a)				
	OKT3	OKT4	OKT8	OKT4/OKT8 (b)	ConA responses CPM ± SEM (c)
0	75.7±8.7	47.5±9.2	29.5±7.7	1.8±0.9	180,322±11,254
1	78.3±6.0	46.0±6.3	20.9±4.6	2.3±0.6	166,893±23,153
2	77.3±6.9	46.2±5.9	24.7±5.6	2.0±0.8	156,979±19,710
3	66.6±10.6	43.6±5.8	23.6±12.1	2.1±0.7	161,817±19,710
4	72.5±8.6	43.7±6.1	22.9±8.3	2.2±1.0	154,285±30,903
6	70.1±5.4	42.7±7.6	27.4±8.1	1.7±0.8	148,444±27,677
8	78.3±6.0	52.6±5.9	18.5±3.6	2.9±0.9	111,545±19,041
Control donors	71.9±9.4	43.2±7.5	22.2±9.5	1.9±0.8	166,877±10,856
Acute CMV-Mononucle-osis	78.5±8.6	15.7±7.7	63.6±14.3	0.3±0.2	33.472±10,801

(a) Values represent the mean ± 1S.D for 6 immunized donors, 30 control donors and 17 acute CMV mononucleosis patients.

(b) The OKT4 to OKT8 ratios in acute CMV mononucleosis patients were significantly lower than ratios in immunized or control donors, $p<0.001$ (Student's t-test).

(c) ConA responses in acute CMV mononucleosis patients were significantly lower than those in immunized or control donors, $p<0.001$ (Student's t-test).

In order to evaluate the efficacy of Towne vaccine in RTC, a set of criteria for CMV disease that follows transplantation had to be developed. Since RTC suffer from a variety of problems aside from CMV infection, we started by defining a CMV illness as a febrile illness that occurred in relation to CMV infection (virus excretion or antibody rise). Then the various manifestations of illness were assigned scores depending on the significance of the problem (Table 7). The illnesses were scored by individuals who did not know whether the patients had received vaccine.

TABLE 7: Scoring System for CMV Disease*

	Mild Disease (1 point)	Mod Disease (2 points)	Severe Disease (3 points)
Fever >101 F (38.3 C) (oral or rectal)	2-4 days	5-20 days	>21 days
Lab abnormalities during febrile illness			
Leukopenia	< 4,000/mm^3		
Thrombocytopenia	<100,000/mm^3		
SGOT/PT	2x above baseline into abnormal range		
Pneumonia during febrile illness	infiltrate on x-ray	infiltrate plus symptoms	on respirator
CNS changes during febrile illness	lethargy	stupor/semi-coma	coma
Serum Creatinine changes during febrile illness baseline	2-4x above baseline (best Creatinine post-transplant)	>4x above baseline	nephrectomy or on permanent dialysis
Miscellaneous:			
			Superinfection-deep organ or blood stream infection-exclude UTI,HSV, VZV,EBV, Clinical Jaundice GI bleed
		Arthritis Muscle wasting (0 points for mylagias)	

Death - 4 points, in addition to other points accumulated by the patient.

*Disease which has onset on or after CMV disease, but during same hospitalization.

We have analyzed CMV infection (virus excretion or antibody rise) and disease (all types) after renal transplantation according to the CMV immune status of recipient and donor for the first 65 patients transplanted.

No seronegative patients (R-) who received kidneys from seronegative donors (D-), became ill. Except for 5 cases where the donor immune status is unknown, all CMV disease occurred in recipients who received kidneys from positive donors (D+). Thus, vaccine efficacy can best be judged in the R- D+ group, in which there are 20 patients: ten vaccinees and ten placebo recipients.

Of 10 R- placebo recipients who received a D+ kidney, 6 showed laboratory evidence of infection and all 6 had disease. Of 10 vaccinees who received a D+ kidney, 9 showed laboratory evidence of infection, among which 4 were asymptomatic and 5 had disease (Table 8).

Infection rates did not significantly differ between seronegative recipients (R-) who received vaccine and those who received placebo.

TABLE 8. CMV Infection and Disease in Seronegative Renal Transplant Recipients.

	Vaccine		Placebo	
Donor	Infection	Disease	Infection	Disease
Seroneg (D-)	0/12	0/12	0/8	0/8
Seropos (D+)	9/9	5/10	6/10	6/10

Vaccinees and placebo recipients both excreted virus if they were in the group that received a kidney from a seropositive donor (D+). Viruses recovered post-transplantation from vaccinees were examined by restriction endonuclease assays for similarity to the Towne vaccine strain.

At the time of writing 28 isolates obtained post transplant from 13 vaccinated RTC have been analyzed by R-E gels, using ECOR-1, Xba or BAMH-1. Figure 3 provides a photograph of a typical pattern. No isolate has been identical to the vaccine strain, although the pattern of the vaccine virus itself is well conserved over passage and from run to run. Six of the isolates, however, did show some medium molecular weight fragments that were similar to Towne, at least with ECOR-1 digestion. An example is isolate 1652. These isolates are being run after digestion with other endonucleases to see if the patterns are indeed similar to Towne. It should be mentioned, however, that these medium weight fragments are common to a great many CMV strains.

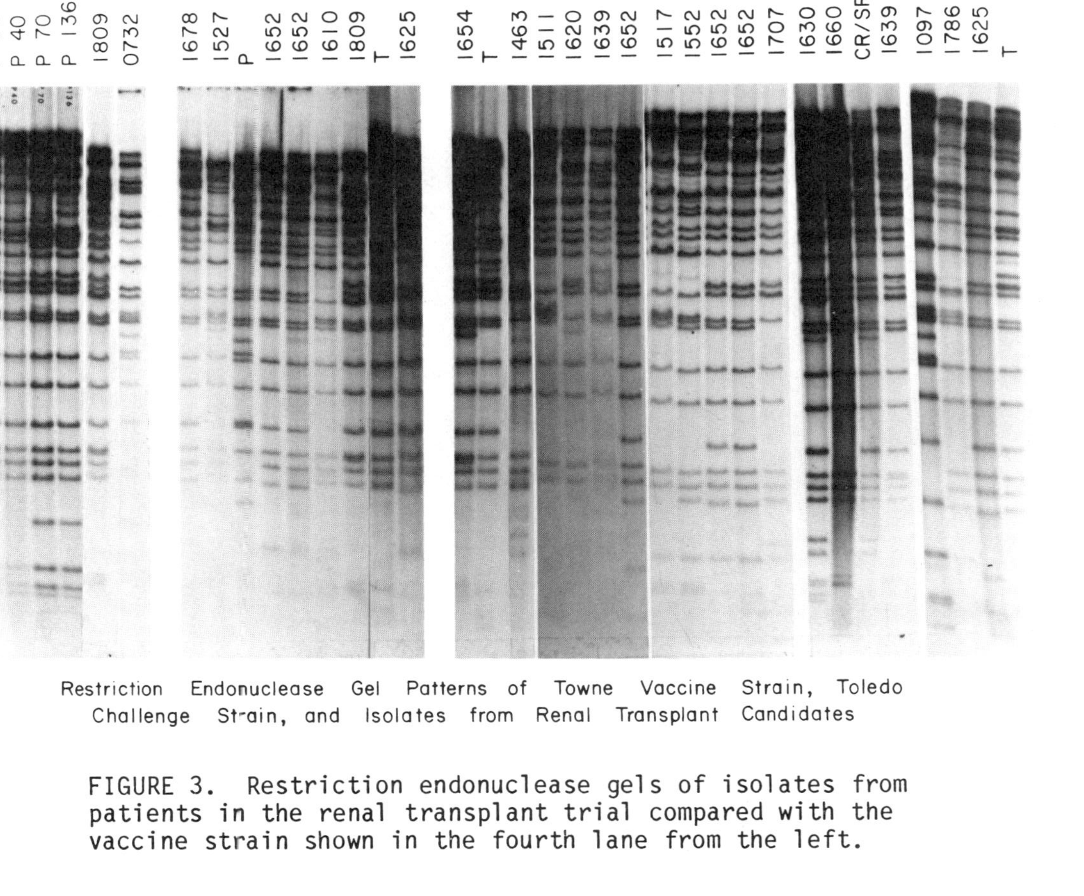

FIGURE 3. Restriction endonuclease gels of isolates from patients in the renal transplant trial compared with the vaccine strain shown in the fourth lane from the left.

Also interesting is the fact that not all of the viruses excreted after transplantation by the same patient were identical: two patients excreted viruses with different patterns from different sites. Examples are strains 1097 and 1132 from the same patients. It is possible that exogenous infection occurs with multiple strains.

The burden of evidence is thus against reactivation of the vaccine virus, in that immunosuppression failed to bring it out, and no post-transplant isolate was identical to Towne. The viruses isolated were presumably those that entered via that graft: however, it is still possible that the exogenous virus recombines with latent vaccine virus.

TABLE 9. Clinical Responses to CMV Infection in Seronegative Recipients Who Received Kidneys from Seropositive Donors According to Vaccine Status

	Vaccine (N=10)	Placebo (N=10)
Fever	5	6
Leukopenia	4	6
Thrombocytopenia	1	5
Abn. LFT	4	4
Pneumonia	0	1
CNS Symptoms	0	1
Creat. increase	3	5
Creat. 4x or more	0	4
Nephrectomy	0	2
Superinfections	0	2
Death	0	1

In Table 9 the actual clinical manifestations are tabulated. Vaccinees did not develop pneumonia, CNS symptoms, more than fourfold increases in creatinine, superinfections, or fatal episodes did not require nephrectomy and had less thrombocytopenia.

The illnesses that occurred are analyzed in Table 10 according to the scoring criteria in Table 7. Scores of 1-9 were termed mild to moderate and scores greater than 10 were termed severe. As defined by antibody responses and virus excretion one of the vaccinees and four of the placebo-inoculated did not receive a kidney carrying CMV. Of the remaining 6 RTC who received placebos 3 developed severe CMV disease and 3 mild CMV disease. Of the remaining 9 vaccinated RTC, 4 remained well, 5 had mild illness and none severe disease. This difference in clinical scores was just significant at the p=.05 level.

TABLE 10. Outcome According to Vaccine Status of CMV Challenge in Seronegative Transplant Patients who Received Kidneys from Seropositive Donors.

	Disease Score		
	0 No Disease	1-9 Mild Disease	>10 Severe Disease
Vaccine (N=10)	5 [d]	5 [a]	0
Placebo (N=10)	4 [e]	3 [b]	3 [c]

a=3, 4, 5, 5, 6 points
b=4, 6, 7 points
c=10, 12, 15 points
d=1 pt. not infected
e=4 pts. not infected

Persistence of immunity is incompletely assessed at this stage. Over the first two years, Nt antibodies to Towne strain had persisted well (Table 11). However, Nt antibodies against the heterologous AD-169 strain did not always persist, raising the possibility that immunity may be strain-specific. Lymphoproliferative assays were not helpful in evaluating immunity after transplantation, as transplantation was followed by prompt suppression of LP responses to CMV antigen, which persisted for many months. It should be noted that persistence of lymphoproliferation was found in normal vaccinees tested up to 28 months later.

TABLE 11. Persistence of Neut Ab Post Transplant in Patients Receiving Seronegative Kidneys.

		Titer >1:2 in Time in Months				
Virus	At Transplant	1-2	3-4	5-6	7-12	13-23
Towne	5/5	5/5	5/5	4/4	3/3	1/1
AD-169	4/5	3/5	4/5	1/4	1/3	1/1

A follow-up survey of the first 49 RTC for illness following the six-month period of susceptibility to CMV disease is summarized in Table 12. Noetworthy is the fact that no neoplasms have occurred in any patient in the trial, up to 39 months subsequent to being enrolled.

TABLE 12. 6-39 Month Follow-up of First 49 Patients Transplanted According to Vaccine Status

	Vaccine	Placebo
Functioning kidney	20	17
Mechanical Graft Failure	2	0
Nephrectomy	4	3
Death	1	2
Neoplasm	0	0

DISCUSSION

In order to judge vaccine initiatives, the protective value of natural immunity to CMV needs to be considered. Our present understanding can be summarized by the title of a recent editorial (4) "CMV Immunity Imperfect but Protective." Most clinically manifest CMV infections occur when cellular immunity is depressed or when the virus inoculum is large or acquired parenterally (14). The problems that occur in transplant patients appear to be largely related to their deficits in cellular immunity due to 1) underlying renal disease 2) chromic hemodialysis and 3) immunosuppressive therapy (15,16,17,18,19,12).

Humoral immunity may be of some protective value since as already discussed 1° infections tend to be more severe than 2° ones, despite the fact that CMI is depressed after transplantation. The post-transfusion syndrome is an example where immunity is partly protective against a large parenteral dose. Seronegative patients are more susceptible, but seropositive patients are also infected though usually asymptomatically (20). Transfusion transmitted disease also occurs in infants (21) and is less severe in those who have transplacentally acquired maternal antibodies despite the fact that such infants lack CMI (21,22). Also administration of CMV immune plasma to bone marrow transplant recipients significantly lowers the incidence of disease, but not of infection.

Congenital infection may be a special case of parenteral transmission, in that infection can take place in the presence of antibody, perhaps because of depression of cellular immunity in certain mothers (23,24). Nevertheless, as alluded to above, involvement of the central nervous system has been documented infrequently if at all in second infected siblings (25) or infants of seropositive women (3).

The actual cellular immune functions that are important in recovery from CMV are imperfectly understood. In several studies impaired specific lymphocyte proliferation to CMV antigens have been correlated with susceptibility to CMV disease. Recently assays for natural killing and putative HLA-restricted T lymphocyte killing of CMV-infected target cells have been described (13,26,27). The cells responsible for natural killing were shown to be natural killer (NK) cells, i.e., non-B, predominantly non-T, Fc receptor bearing cells (13). The cells responsible for HLA-restricted killing were predominately Fc receptor negative cells which rosetted with sheep RBC (27). Formal proof that they are T lymphocytes has not been presented. Quinnan et al (27) have shown that in bone marrow transplant patients infected with CMV the development of non-restricted and HLA-restricted cytotoxicity was associated with recovery while individuals who died of CMV disease failed to develop these cytotoxic responses.

In addition to the role of host immunity in modulating CMV infection, CMV infection may cause immunosuppression. Individuals with CMV mononucleosis have been shown to have suppressed lymphoproliferative responses to herpesvirus antigens (CMV, HSV, and VZV) (28) and to certain mitogens (pokeweed mitogen and concanavalin A) (29,30). Evidence has been presented suggesting that mitogen hyporesponsiveness may be mediated by adherent suppressor cells (29). Individuals with CMV mononucleosis also have an increased numbers of T suppressor cells and a reversal of the T helper to T suppressor cell ratio (31).

The results of the trial of Towne strain CMV vaccine in renal transplant candidates (RTC) should be evaluated in the light of the foregoing discussion of immunity. The target group for which the trial was designed suffers from several immunologic disabilities that mitigate the effect of immunization. First, the RTC are in a state of serologic and cellular hypo-responsiveness by virtue of their uremic state (32,33). Their responses to CMV vaccine are therefore inferior to those normal volunteers (discussed below). Second, immunosuppression at the time of transplantation results in depressed specific lymphocyte proliferation responses to CMV, whether the recipient has natural or vaccine-acquired immunity. Similar observations were made in a mouse CMV system (34) where steroids and antilymphocyte serum erased cellular immunity.

Nevertheless, these preliminary results suggest that the immunization of seronegatives conferred protection against severe disease, although infection and mild disease were not significantly reduced. Vaccine-immunity thus modified the extent of infection, either through antibody or through other mechanisms not yet understood.

SUMMARY

1. Towne strain vaccine is well tolerated with a local reaction being the only regularly observed sequel to vaccination.
2. The vaccine virus is not excreted by the vaccinee.
3. RTC do not respond to vaccine as do normals, and have lower serologic and cellular immune responses.
4. There is no evidence that the vaccine strain becomes latent in the vaccinee.
5. CMV infection that occurs in vaccinees transplanted with a D+ kidney may or may not result in illness but the illness is milder than that seen in similarly exposed placebo recipients.
6. Towne strain vaccine appear to prevent severe CMV disease.
7. Antibody data show persistence of immunity for at least the first six months post-vaccination.

Our general conclusion is that the Towne vaccine virus appears to be safe in the short term, does not establish latency, and protects the patients at risk of life-threatening disease. However, the evidence for the protective effect is based on numbers that are borderline for statistical significance at this assessment.

The reason for the vaccine's failure to prevent infection and mild disease probably resides in the suppression of cellular immunity attendant on transplantation. This profound suppression essentially ablates evidence of specific cellular immunity to CMV. It is therefore gratifying that the vaccine appeared to favorably influence susceptibility to severe CMV disease.

The importance of protection of this type is far from trivial. In our population 20 of 65 RTC (31%) were at risk for CMV dfisease (R-D+), and 3 of 10 unvaccinated had severe disease. If severe illnesses had occurred in vaccinees, there would have been 6 severe cases of 65 (9%). A vaccine that can prevent serious disease in 1 of 11 patients is not neglibible.

REFERENCES

1. Hanshaw JB: J Infect Dis 123:555, 1971.
2. Stagno S, Pass RF, Alford CA: Birth Defects 17:31, 1981.
3. Stagno S, Pass RF, Meyers ED, Henderson RE, Moore EG, Walton PD, Alford CA: New Engl J Med 306:945, 1982.
4. Medearis DN: New Engl J Med 306:985, 1982.
5. Pass RF, Stagno, S, Myers GJ, Alford CA: Pediatrics 66:758, 1980.
6. Hanshaw JB, Scheiner AP, Moxley AW, Gaev L, Abel V, Scheiner B: New Engl J Med 295:468, 1976.
7. Stagno S, Reynolds DW, Amos CS, Dahle AJ, McCollister FP, Mohindra I, Ermocilla R, Alford CA: Pediatrics 59:669, 1977.
8. Starr SE, Dalton B, Garrabrant T, Paucker K, Plotkin SA: Infect Immun 30:17, 1980.
9. Zablotney SL, Wentworth BB, Alexander ER: Am J Epidemiol 107:336, 1978.
10. Waner JL, Weller TH: Infect Immun 21:151, 1978.
11. Starr SE, Glazer JP, Friedman HM, Farquahar JD, Plotkin SA: J Infect Dis 143:585, 1981.
12. Goldblum SE, Reed WP; Ann Int Med 93:597, 1980.
13. Starr SE, Garrabrant T: Clin Exp Immunol 46:484, 1981.
14. Shore SL, Feorino PM: in The Human Herpesviruses: Nahmias AJ, Dowdle WR and Schinazi RF, editors, An Interdisciplinary Approach, Elsevier, New York, 1981, 267.
15. Linnemann CC, Jr, Kauffman CA, First MR, Schiff GM, Phair JP: Infect Immun 22:176, 1978.
16. Balfour HH, Jr, Slade MS, Kalis JM, Howard RJ, Simmons RL, Najarian JS: Surgery 81:487, 1977.
17. Rytel MW: Yale J Biol Med 49:63, 1976.
18. Lopez C, Simmons RL, Park BH, Najarian JS, Good RH: Clin Exp Immunol 16:565, 1974.
19. Haahr S, Moller-Larsen A, Andersen HK, Spencer ES: J Clin Microbiol 10:267, 1979.
20. Henle W, Henle G, Scriba M, Joyner CR, Harrison FS, Von Essen R, Paloheimo J, Klemola E: New Engl J Med 282:1068, 1970.
21. Ballard RA, Drew WL, Hufnagle KG, Reidel PA: Am J Dis Child 133:482, 1979.
22. Yeager AS, Grumet FC, Hafleigh EB, Arvin AM, Bradley JS, Prober CG: J Pediatr 98:2181, 1981.
23. Starr SE, Tolpin MD, Friedman HM, Paucker K, Plotkin SA: J Infect Dis 140:500, 1979.
24. Reynolds DW, Dean PH, Pass RH, Alford CA: J Infect Dis 140:493, 1979.

25. Plotkin SA: in Nahmias AJ and O'Reilly RJ, editors: Immunology of human infection. Part II: viruses and parasites; immunodiagnosis and prevention of infectious diseases, New York 1982, p.89.
26. Kirmani N, Ginn RK, Mittal KK, Manischewitz JE, Quinnan GV: Infect Immun 34:441, 1981.
27. Quinnan, GV, Jr, Kirmani N, Esber E, Saral R, Manischewitz JF, Rogers JL, Rook AH, Santos GW, Burns WH: J Immunol 126:2036, 1981.
28. Levin MJ, Rinaldo CR, Leary PL, Zaia JA, Hirsch MS: J Infect Dis 140:851, 1979.
29. Rinaldo CR, Jr, Carney WP, Richter BS, Black PH, Hirsch MS: J Infect Dis 141:488, 1980.
30. Rinaldo CR, Black PH, Hirsch MS: J Infect Dis 136:667, 1977.
31. Carney WP, Rubin RH, Hoffman RA, Hansen WP, Healey K, Hirsch MS: J Immunol 126:2114, 1981.
32. Holdsworth SR, Fitzgerald MC, Hosking CS, Atkins RC: Clin Exp Immunol 33:95, 1978.
33. Agatsuma Y, Fitzpatrick P, Baliah T, Kaul A, Kim P-K, Ogra PL: J Med Virol 4:147, 1979.
34. Howard RJ, Mattson IM, Balfour HH, Jr: Proc Soc Exp Biol Med 161:341, 1979.

V

OTHER VIRUSES

CHAPTER 18

CELLULAR IMMUNE RESPONSES AND EPSTEIN-BARR VIRUS

John L. Sullivan

Department of Pediatrics
University of Massachusetts Medical School
Worcester, Massachusetts

INTRODUCTION

In March of 1961, Dennis Burkitt gave a seminar entitled "The Commonest Children's Cancer in Tropical Africa" to the staff at Middlesex Hospital Medical School in London (reviewed in 1). During the seminar, Burkitt described the epidemiology of the lymphoma which today bears his name. Doctor M. Anthony Epstein attended this seminar and was intrigued by the possibility that this tumor might be associated with a vector-borne virus. Subsequent studies over the next three years by Epstein, Achong, and Barr resulted in the establishment of a Burkitt's lymphoma cell line (2). When examined by electron microscopy, this cell line was found to contain a previously unrecognized herpes virus, subsequently named Epstein-Barr Virus (EBV). Gertrude and Werner Henle, working at Children's Hospital in Philadelphia obtained the Burkitt's Lymphoma cell line and developed immunofluorescent assays to detect antibodies against EBV (3,4). They subsequently screened large populations of patients with a variety of diseases and demonstrated that EBV infection was common and occurred in children and adults. In 1968 the Henles made the critical observation that seroconversion to EBV occurred in a female laboratory technician (5) during the course of acute infectious mononucleosis. Furthermore, during her illness, an EBV carrying lymphoblastoid cell lines was established from peripheral leukocyte cultures. Subsequent seroepidemiologic studies have shown EBV to be a major cause of "mono syndrome" which is defined by Evans as an acute febrile illness of older children and young adults associated with an atypical lymphocytosis in the blood, lymphadenopathy

ISBN 0-12-239980-3

and splenomegaly (see 6). In this review, the cellular immunology and pathogenesis of infectious mononucleosis will be discussed. Recent studies of EBV infections in the immunodeficient host will be presented.

THE ORGANISM

Epstein-Barr Virus is a DNA virus and a member of the herpes virus family which also includes the following human viruses: herpes simplex, varicella zoster and cytomegalovirus. The viruses are antigenically related as seen by cross reactivity in immunofluorescent antibody tests. While antigenic diversity may exist, there is at present no evidence that antigenic variance is important clinically.

EBV has a very narrow host cell range and the B lymphocyte is at present the only known human cell in which virus replicates (7,8,9). Some investigators have also demonstrated infection of normal epithelial cells using molecular hybridization techniques (10). Like all other herpes viruses, EBV infection results in chronic latent infection which may be reactivated long after primary infection. The persistence of EBV infected B cells can be demonstrated by in vitro cell culture resulting in the outgrowth of a lymphoblastoid cell line containing the virus genome.

EBV is primarily a cell associated virus. Cell free virus can be found in the oropharyngeal secretions during the following acute infection (11). Virus has not been found in other secretions or excretions. The establishment of a virus genome positive B lymphoblastoid cell line from the peripheral blood is evidence for prior or current infection with EBV.

PATHOGENESIS AND HOST IMMUNE RESPONSE DURING INFECTIOUS MONONUCLEOSIS

While the complexities dealing with the pathogenesis and cellular immune responses to Epstein-Barr Virus infection are far from resolved, major advances have been made in our understanding of this host-parasite relationship in the past decade. These studies have resulted from intense interest kindled by the association of EBV with two human malignancies (African Burkitt's lymphoma and endemic nasopharyngeal carcinoma in China, see reference 12) and the rapid advances in the understanding of the human immune system. The major advances over the past decade in the understanding of host immune response to EBV can be summarized as follows:

1968 - Normal leukocytes can be infected in vitro by EBV (13).
1968–1974 - Development of serological techniques for detection of antibodies against EB Viral capsid, early, and nuclear antigens (3,4,14).
1974–1978 - Only B lymphocytes possess receptors for and are transformed by EBV (8,9,15).
1974–1975 - The majority of atypical lymphocytes in acute infectious mononucleosis are T lymphocytes (15).
1974–1975 - There is a marked depression of cell-mediated immunity (mitogen responsiveness, mixed leukocyte reaction, responses to soluble antigens) during the acute phase of infectious mononucleosis (16).
1974–1975 - Cytotoxic effector cells specific for EBV-infected cell lines are present in vivo during acute infectious mononucleosis (17,18,19).
1976 - Demonstration of antibody-dependent lymphocyte mediated cytotoxicity against cells expressing EBV antigens (20).
1977 - 1979 - EBV is a T-independent polyclonal activator of human B lymphocytes and stimulates the polyclonal secretion of immunoglobulins. The demonstration that suppressor T cells are activated during infectious mononucleosis and serve to suppress the polyclonal immunoglobulin secretion induced by EBV (21,22).
1978–1981 - The inability to demonstrate that cytotoxic T cells circulating in vivo during acute infectious mononucleosis show HLA-restricted lysis of target cells (23,24,25). However, it has been demonstrated that longterm T-cell mediated immunity in individuals with past EBV-infection as measured by regression of EBV-induced transformation does show HLA-antigen restriction (26,27) in accord with the Doherty-Zinkernagel model (28).
1979–1981 - The majority of atypical lymphocytes in the circulation during acute infectious mononucleosis belong to the non-T γ, Tμ subset (29). Further studies of these T cells have shown that they belong primarily to the T5/T8 subset as defined by a set of monoclonal antibodies which characterize T cell subsets in man (30,31). This T5 subset has been shown to express HLA-DR on the cell surface and can function as a suppressor cell in vitro, suppressing pokeweed mitogen driven immunoglobulin secretion by B lymphocytes (30). A cytotoxic/effector activity for this T5 subset found in acute infectious

mononucleosis has not been demonstrated (30).
1979-1980 - EBV superinfected lymphoblastoid cell lines are more susceptible to the cytotoxic reactivity of spontaneous natural killer (NK) cells in vitro (32). The in vitro outgrowth of EBV-infected lymphocytes can be inhibited by a population of T lymphocytes with properties suggestive of an NK cell (33).
1980 - Early in the first week of infectious mononucleosis up to 18% of B lymphocytes may be infected with EBV (34).
1981-1982 - The demonstration that EBV-specific cytotoxic T cells can be generated in vitro following stimulation of lymphocytes from seropositive individuals with EBV-infected B cells (35,36,37). These cytotoxic T cells belong to T8 cytotoxic/suppressor cell subset and show preferential cytotoxicity against HLA-matched target cells (35). These cytotoxic T cells can be cultured in the presence of T cell growth factors (38). Certain clones of cytotoxic T cells have demonstrated killing restricted to target cells expressing private HLA determinants while others show broad spectrum killing among allogeneic EBV-infected target cells (38).

Based on these observations of events which occur during acute infectious mononucleosis, a model of the host immune responses to EBV can be described. EBV infects the oropharynx, and replicates in B lymphocytes of the tonsillopharyngeal tissue. EBV-infected B lymphocytes disseminate throughout the lymphoid system and large numbers of EBV-infected B cells appear in the circulation. The EBV-infected B cells provoke an autologous mixed leukocyte reaction (MLR) resulting in the expansion of multiple T cell clones into atypical lymphocytes. Soluble factors induced by the autologous MLR expand clones of cytotoxic and suppressor T cells which belong to the T5 subset. It is postulated that the initial expansion of the T5 subset would favor cytotoxic clones induced by the large number of circulating EBV-infected B cells. The polyclonal T cell response would include alloreactive clones and HLA-restricted clones specific for EBV infected cells. The initial cytotoxic cells in the T5 subset is rapidly followed by the expansion of T suppressor cells also belonging to the T5 subset. The T suppressor cells are Ia positive and suppress the polyclonal immunoglobulin production stimulated by EBV infection of B lymphocytes. During the acute phase of infection longterm memory T cells are induced. These can be demonstrated as early as 2-3 weeks after infection (39). Memory T cells respond to EBV antigen in vitro to become cytotoxic cells which suppress outgrowth of EBV infected B cells. These memory T cells may limit EBV-induced B cell proliferation years after primary infection, during periods of EBV reactivation (26,27).

EBV infection and stimulation of T cells induces interferon which induces NK cell activity, which may be important in the elimination of EBV-infected B cells. Natural killer cell activity has been shown to be present during the acute phase of mononucleosis (18,40). Interferons have an inhibitory effect on the outgrowth of EBV-infected B lymphocytes in vitro (41), and interferon's effect on lymphoid cells during acute infectious mononucleosis has been described (42). A scheme of events occurring in the immune response of EBV is depicted in Figure 1, and these immunological reactions may cause symptoms of infectious mononucleosis (fever, pharyngitis, lymphadenopathy, splenomegaly, and malaise).

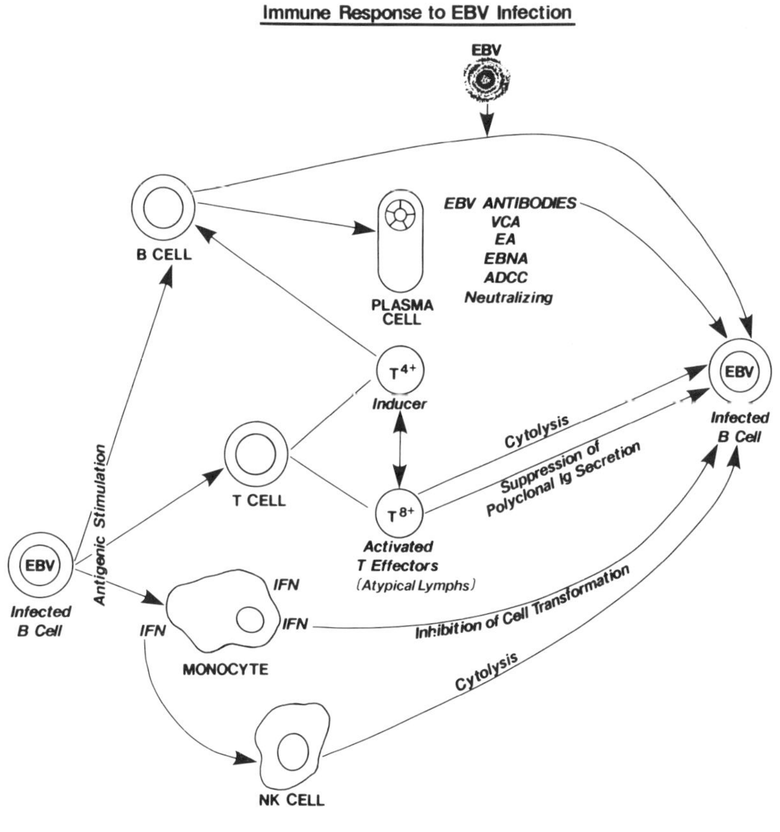

FIGURE 1. Schematic presentation of immunological events occurring during acute infectious mononucleosis. See text.

CELLULAR IMMUNODEFICIENCIES AND EBV X-LINKED LYMPHOPROLIFERATIVE SYNDROME

The importance of understanding the mechanisms responsible for control of EBV infection in man has been highlighted by the clinical observations made in the past six years. In 1974 and 1975, three families were described in which an X-linked immunodeficiency to Epstein-Barr Virus resulted in fatal infectious mononucleosis occurring in young male members of these kindreds (43,44,45). Intensive studies of these families with the X-linked proliferative (XLP) syndrome by Purtilo and his colleagues have demonstrated that in addition to fatal infectious mononucleosis, acquired immunodeficiency and lymphoproliferative disorders occur with a high frequency in males surviving their acute EBV infection (46). We have participated in the formation of a registry with the accumulation of approximately 100 cases of XLP (47). Our studies include family histories, review of medical records, and virological and immunological studies. In our evaluation of the phenotypic expression of the X-linked lymphoproliferative syndrome, we have observed that approximately 70% of affected males die with a fatal infectious mononucleosis syndrome. Of these individuals with fatal IM, approximately 15% demonstrate a lymphoproliferative disorder at autopsy. The lymphoproliferation has been classified on morphological criteria as immunoblastic sarcoma of B cells, Burkitt's lymphoma and other B cell non-Hodgkins lymphomas. Of those males who survive the initial encounter with EBV, virtually all will develop common varied immunodeficiency frequently characterized by recurrent infections and hypogammaglobulinemia. Lymphoproliferative disorders have occurred in approximately 20-40% of the surviving males.

We have prospectively studied immunological and virological events in a male infant with XLP who succumbed to primary Epstein-Barr Virus infection (48). The patient's brother died at age two years from infectious mononucleosis and immunoblastic sarcoma. At 18 months of age, the patient was found to have normal immunoglobulin levels, intact cell-mediated immunity and no antibodies to EBV. Two weeks prior to infection, the patient again was seronegative to EBV and had normal immunoglobulin levels. At age 26 months, he developed fever, lymphadenopathy and rash with atypical lymphocytosis. The diagnosis of acute EBV infection was made on the basis of Epstein-Barr nuclear antigen-positive cells in a lymph node biopsy and EBV-specific, IgM antibodies to viral capsid antigen. During the two week course of his infection, the patient was found to have normal T and B cell numbers and the decreased in vitro mitogen and antigen responses which are characteristic of acute EBV infection. Lymphocyte cytotoxicity studies showed marked cytotoxicity against EBV infected cells, spontaneous natural killer (NK) cell targets and cell lines resistant to NK cell activity. This vigorous cytotoxic activity was resistant to high dose prednisone therapy and the patient's downhill course terminated with fulminant liver failure. Marked necrosis and EBV-infected cells were found in all lymphoreticular organs at autopsy. DNA hybridization studies conducted on liver tissue obtained a post mortem demonstrated the presence of the EBV genome.

These studies suggest that males with the X-linked lymphoproliferative syndrome have a restricted immune deficiency which is initially limited to Epstein-Barr Virus. It appears that the more generalized immunodeficiency observed in males who survive their initial EBV infection is secondary to the effects of chronic Epstein-Barr Virus infection. An abnormal cytotoxic response during acute EBV infection in patients with XLP may result in a fatal infection with organ necrosis. Males who are fortunate enough to survive their initial EBV infection could become hypogammaglobulinemic because EBV-infected B cell clones are eliminated by the cytotoxic effector cells or clones of EBV-infected B cells are lost in a lytic viral cycle. The deficiency of T cell function and loss of NK cells in surviving males may occur secondarily to abnormal immunoregulation or to chronic infection resulting in dysfunction of effector cell clones. This secondary T and NK cell deficiency may then predispose those individuals to the lymphoproliferative effects of chronic Epstein-Barr Virus infection (47). Indeed, the occurrence of a polyclonal B cell lymphoma in a 4 year old girl during primary EBV infection suggests that subtle abnormalities in the regulation of the immune response during acute EBV infection may result in a fatal illness or the development of a malignant lymphoproliferative disorder (49).

PRIMARY IMMUNODEFICIENCY DISEASES

As a result of the description of the X-linked lymphoproliferative syndrome, Epstein-Barr Virus is now recognized as a potential cause of severe infections and lymphoproliferative disorders in immunodeficient individuals. In 1979 Borzy et al described three infants with severe combined immunodeficiency, in whom fatal lymphomas developed following thymus epithelium transplants

(50). The lymphomas were polyclonal immunoblastic sarcomas of B cells. Nine additional cases of malignancy have been reported in infants with severe combined immunodeficiency (51). Reece et al have reported that a polyclonal B cell lymphoma in a five year old child following a thymic epithelium graft contained Epstein-Barr Virus nuclear antigen (52). Further studies are needed to clarify the association between B cell lymphomas and EBV in infants with severe combined immunodeficiency, however, it seems certain that EBV-induced lymphoproliferative disorders will be recognized more frequently in these patients.

The relationship between EBV and the high risk of lymphorecticular malignancy (approximately 10%) in ataxia telangiectasia is presently under investigation. Chromosome 14 abnormalities identical to these observed in Burkitt's lymphomas (EBV and non-EBV associated) have been observed (53,54,55). Abnormal humoral-immune responses to EBV in patients with ataxia telangiectasia have been documented (56). In addition, deficient natural killer cell activity has been found in two patients with ataxia telangiectasia (57). Saemundsen et al have recently studied a B cell lymphoma in a patient with ataxia telangiectasia and demonstrated EBV genome in the malignant tissue (58). Interestingly, the patient in whom the malignant lymphoma developed had a normal antibody response to Epstein-Barr Virus.

RENAL TRANSPLANT RECIPIENTS

B cell lymphoproliferative disorders also occur in individuals with secondary immunodeficiencies. Approximately 6% of individuals receiving renal allografts develop malignancy (59). Immunoblastic sarcomas make up the majority of the lymphomas which occur. Hanto et al reported six renal transplant recipients who developed lymphoproliferative disorders following renal transplantation (60). Polyclonal B cell tumors were demonstrated to contain the EBV genome by the demonstration of EBV nuclear antigen and by DNA hybridization studies. It has been recognized that renal allograft recipients receiving the immunosuppressive agent Cyclosporin A may have an increased risk of malignant lymphoma development (61). Crawford et al have also demonstrated the presence of EBV genome in an immunoblastic sarcome which developed in a Cyclosporin treated renal allograft recipient (62). Cyclosporin has been shown to enhance the outgrowth of EBV-infected B lymphoblastoid cell lines in vitro (63). Renal transplant recipients receiving

Cyclosporin do not have memory T cells capable of causing regression of autologous EBV-infected B cell cultures (64).

SUMMARY

It is apparent from studies of normal individuals with infectious mononucleosis and immunodeficient individuals with Epstein-Barr Virus induced lymphoproliferative disorders that the immune responses to EBV are complex. Perturbations of normal immune mechanisms result in life threatening disease. It is likely that the lymphoproliferative syndromes observed in immunodeficient individuals are the result of defects at different levels of the immune response. Further studies of normal immunoregulation occurring during uncomplicated EBV-infection will define the specific effector cells and humoral factors responsible for recovery.

REFERENCES

1. Epstein,M.A., B.G.Achong. 1979. Discovery and General Biology of the virus in The Epstein-Barr Virus (Springer-Verlag, Heidelberg) pp.1-22.
2. Epstein,M.A., B.G. Achong,Y.M. Barr. 1964. Virus particles in cultured lymphoblasts from Burkitt's lymphoma. Lancet 1:702-703.
3. Henle,G. and W. Henle. 1966. Immunofluorescence in cells derived from Burkitt's lymphoma. J. Bacteriol. 91:1248-1256.
4. Henle,G., W. Henle, and G. Klein. 1971. Demonstration of two distinct components in the early antigen complex of Epstein-Barr virus infected cells. Int. J. Cancer. 8:272-282.
5. Henle,G., W.Henle,and V.Diehl. 1968. Relation of Burkitt's tumor-associated herpes-type virus to infectious mononucleosis. Proc. Natl. Acad. Sci. USA 59:94-97.
6. Evans,A.S. 1978. Infectious mononucleosis and related syndromes. Amer. J. Med. Sci. 176:325-339.
7. Jondal,M., G. Klein. 1973. Surface markers on human B and T lymphocytes. I. Presence of Epstein-Barr virus receptors on B lymphocytes. II. J. Exp. Med. 138:1365-1377.
8. Pattengale,P.K., R.W. Smith,P. Gerber. 1974. B cell characteristics of human peripheral and cord blood

lymphocytes transformed by Epstein-Barr virus. J. Natl. Cancer Inst. 52:1081-1086.
9. Bird,A.G., S. Britton,I.Ernberg, and K. Nilsson, 1981. Characteristics of Epstein-Barr virus activation of human B lymphocytes. J. Exp. Med. 154:832-839.
10. Lemon,S.M.,L.M. Hutt,J.E. Shaw, J.H. Li,J.S. Pagano. 1977. Replication of EBV in epithelial cells during infectious mononucleosis. Nature 268:268-270.
11. Miller,G., J.C. Niederman, and L.L. Andrews. 1973. Prolonged oropharyngeal excretion of Epstein-Barr virus after infectious mononucleosis, N. Engl. J. Med. 288:229-232.
12. Klein,G. 1975. The Epstein-Barr virus and neoplasia. New Engl. J. Med. 293:1353-1357.
13. Diehl,V., G. Henle,W. Henle,G. Kohn. 1968. Demonstration of a herpes group virus in cultures of peripheral leukocytes from patients with infectious mononucleosis. J. Virol. 2:663-669.
14. Reedman,B.M. and G. Klein. 1973. Cellular localization of an Epstein-Barr virus-associated complement-fixing antigen in producer and nonproducer lymphoblastoic cell lines. Int. J. Cancer 11:499-520.
15. Pattengale,P.K., R.W. Smith, and E. Perlin. 1974. Atypical lymphocytes in infectious mononucleosis: identification by multiple T and B lymphocyte markers. N. Engl. J. Med. 291:1145.
16. Mangi,R.J., J.C. Niederman,J.E. Kelleher, J.E. Dwyer,A.S. Evans and F.S. Kantor. 1974. Depression of cell-mediated immunity during acute infectious mononucleosis. N.Engl. J. Med. 291:1145.
17. Royston,I., J.L. Sullivan,P.O. Periman and E. Perlin. 1975. Cell-mediated immunity to Epstein-Barr virus-transformed lymphoblastoid cells in acute infectious mononucleosis. N. Engl. J. Med. 293:1159-1163.
18. Svedmyr,E., M. Jondal. 1975. Cytotoxic effector cells specific for B cell lines transformed by Epstein-Barr virus are present in patients with infectious mononucleosis. Proc. Natl. Acad. Sci. 72:1622-1626.
19. Hutt,L.M., Y.T. Huang,H.E. Discomb,J.S. Pagano. 1975. Enhanced destruction of lymphoid cell lines by peripheral blood leukocytes taken from patients with acute infectious mononucleosis. J. Immunol. 115:243-248.
20. Pearson,G.R., T.W.Orr. 1976. Antibody-dependent lymphocyte cytotoxicity against cells expressing Epstein-Barr virus antigens. J. Natl. Cancer Inst. 56:485-488.

21. Kirchner,H., G. Tosato,R.M. Blaese,S. Broder, and I.T. Magrath. 1979. Polyclonal immunoglobulin secretion by human B lymphocytes exposed to Epstein-Barr virus in vitro. J. Immunol. 122:1310-1313.
22. Tosato,G., I.T. Magrath,I. Koski,N. Dooley and M. Blaese. 1979. Activation of suppressor T cells during Epstein-Barr-virus-induced infectious mononucleosis. New Engl. J. Med. 301:1133-1137.
23. Bakacs,T., E. Svedmyr, and E. Klein. 1978. EBV-related cytotoxicity of Fc receptor negative T lymphocytes separated from the blood of infectious mononucleosis patients. Cancer Lett 4:185.
24. Lipinski,M., M.F. Fridman,T. Tursz,C. Vincent,D. Pious and M. Fellous. 1979. Absence of allogeneic restriction in human T-cell-mediated cytotoxicity to Epstein-Barr virus-infect ed target cells. J. Exp. Med. 150:1310-1322.
25. Seeley,J., E. Svedmyr, O. Weiland,G. Klein,E. Moller, E. Eriksson,K. Andersson, and L. Van der Waal. 1981. Epstein Barr virus selective T cells in infectious mononucleosis are not restricted to HLA-A and B antigens. J. Immunol. 127:293-300.
26. Rickinson,A.B., L.E. Wallace and M.A. Epstein. 1980. HLA-restricted T-cell recognition of Epstein-Barr virus-infected B cells. Nature 283:865-868.
27. Misko,I.S., D.J. Moss, J.H. Pope. 1980. HLA antigen-related restriction of T lymphocyte cytotoxicity to Epstein-Barr virus. Proc. Natl. Acad. Sci. 77:4247-4250.
28. Doherty,P.C., and R.M. Zinkernagel. 1974. T-cell mediated immunopathology in viral infections. Transplant. Rev. 19:89-120.
29. Haynes,B.F., R.T. Schooley,J.E. Grouse,C.R. Payling-Wright,R. Dolin and A.S. Fauci. 1979. Characterization of thymus-derived lymphocyte subsets in acute Epstein-Barr virus-induced infectious mononucleosis. J. Immunol. 122:699-702.
30. Reinherz,E.L., C. O'Brien,P. Rosenthal and S.F. Schlossman. 1980. Cellular basis for viral-induced immunodeficiency: Analysis by monoclonal antibodies. J. Immunol. 125:1269-1274.
31. DeWaele,M., C. Theilemans,B.K.G. Van Camp. 1981. Characterization of immunoregulatory T cells in Epstein-Barr virus-induced infectious mononucleosis by monoclonal antibodies. N. Engl. J. Med. 304:460-462.
32. Blazar, B., M. Patarroyo, E. Klein and G. Klein. 1980. Increased sensitivity of human lymphoid lines to natural killer cells after induction of the Epstein-Barr viral

cycle by superinfection or sodium butyrate. J. Exp. Med. 151:614-627.

33. Shope,T.C. and J. Kaplan. 1979. Inhibition of the in vitro outgrowth of Epstein-Barr virus-infected lymphocytes by T_G lymphocytes. J. Immunol. 123:2150-2155.
34. Robinson, J., D.Smith, and J. Niederman. 1980. Mitotic EBNA-positive lymphocytes in peripheral blood during infectious mononucleosis. Nature 287:334-335.
35. Tsoukas,C.D., R.I. Fox,S.F. Slovin,D.A. Carson,M. Pellegrino,S. F n P. Kung,J.H. Vaughn. 1981. T lymphocyte-mediated cytotoxicity against autologous EBV-genome bearing B cells. J. Immunol. 126:1742-1746.
36. Fakukowa,T., T. Hirano,N. Sakaguchi,T. Teraniski,I. Tsuyuguchi,N. Nagao,N. Naito,K. Yoshimura,Y. Okubo,H. Tohda,A.Oikawa. 1981. In vitro induction of HLA-restricted cytotoxic T lymphocytes against autologous Epstein-Barr virus transformed B lymphoblastoid cell lines. J. Immunol. 126:1697-1701.
37. Misko,I.S., R.G. Kane,J.H. Pope. 1982. Generation in vitro of HLA-restricted EB Virus-specific cytotoxic human T cells by autologous lymphoblastoid cell lines: The roles of previous EB Virus infection and fetal calf serum. Int. J. Cancer 29:41-48.
38. Tanaka,Y., K. Sugamura,Y. Hinuma. 1982. Heterogeneity of allogeneic restriction of human cytotoxic T cell clones specific for Epstein Barr Virus. J. Immunol. 128:1241-1245.
39. Schooley,R.T., B.F. Haynes,J. Grouse,C. Payling-Wright,A.S.Fauci, R. Dolin. 1981. Development of suppressor T lymphocytes for Epstein-Barr Virus induced B lymphocyte outgrowth during acute infectious mononucleosis: assessment by two quantitative systems. Blood 57:510-517.
40. Sullivan,J.L., K.S. Byron, F.E. Brewster, D.T.Purtilo. 1980. Deficient natural killer cell activity in the X-linked lymphoproproliferative syndrome. Science 543-545.
41. Thorley-Lawson,D. 1981. The Transformation of adult but not newborn human lymphocytes by Epstein Barr Virus and phytohemagglutin is inhibited by Interferon: The early suppression by T cells of Epstein Barr Infection is mediated by Interferon. J. Immunol. 126:829-833.
42. Schattner,W., D. Wallach,G. Merlin,T. Hahn,S. Levin,M. Revel. 1981. Assay of an Interferon-induced enzyme in white blood cells as a diagnostic aid in viral diseases. Lancet 2:500-502.

43. Bar,R.S., C.J. Delor,K.P. Clausen,P. Hurtubise,W. Henle,J.F. Hewetson. 1974. Fatal infectious mononucleosis in a family. New Engl. J. Med. 290:363-367.
44. Provisor,A.J., J.J. Iacuone, R.R. Chilcote, R.G. Neiburger, F.G. Crussi and R.L. Baehner. 1975. Acquired agammaglobulinemia after a lifethreatening illness with clinical and laboratory features of infectious mononucleosis in three related male children. New Engl. J. Med. 293:62-65.
45. Purtilo,D.T., J.P.Yang, C.K. Cassel,R. Harper,S.R. Stephenson, B.H. Landing,G.F.Vawter. 1975. X-linked recessive progressive combined variable immunodeficiency. Lancet i:935-940.
46. Purtilo,D.T., L. Paquin,D. DeFlorio,F. Virzi and R. Sakhuja. 1979. Immunodiagnosis and immunopathogenesis of the X-linked recessive lymphoproliferative syndrome. Seminars in Hematology 16:309-343.
47. Hamilton,J.K., L.A. Paquin,J.L. Sullivan, et al. 1980. X-linked lymphoproliferative syndrome registry report. J. Pediatr. 96:669-673.
48. Sullivan,J.L., K.S.Byron, F.E. Brewster,K. Sakamoto, J.E. Shaw and J.S. Pagano. 1982. Treatment of life threatening Epstein-Barr Virus infections with acyclovir. Am. J. Med. In press.
49. Robinson,J.E., N.Brown,W. Andiman et al. 1980. Diffuse polyclonal B-cell lymphoma during primary infection with Epstein-Barr Virus. New Engl. J. Med. 302:1293-1297.
50. Borzy,M.S., R. Hong, S.D. Horowitz, E.Gilbert, D.Kanfman, W. DeMendonca,V. Oxelius,M. Dictor, L. Pechman. 1979. Fatal lymphoma after transplantation of cultured thymus in children with combined immunodeficiency disease. New Engl. J. Med. 301:565-568.
51. Kersey,J.H., A.H. Filipowich,B.D. Spector, G.Frizerra. 1980. Lymphoma after thymus transplantation. New Engl. J. Med. 302:301.
52. Reece,E.R., J.G. Gartner,T.A. Seemayer,J.H. Joncas. 1980. Lymphoma after thymus transplantation. New Engl. J. Med. 302:302.
53. Hecht,F., B.K. McCaw, R.D. Koler. 1973. Ataxia-telangiectasia-clonal growth of translocation lymphocytes. New Engl. J. Med. 289:286-291.
54. Jean,P., C.L. Richer, M.M. Orlando, D.H. Luu, J.H. Joncas. 1979. Trnaslocation 8;14 in an ataxia telangiectasia-derived cell line. Nature. 277:56-57.
55. Zech,L., U. Haglund, K. Nilsson, G. Klein. 1976. Characteristic chromosomal abnormalities in biopsies and lymphoid-cell lines from patients with Burkitt and non-Burkitt lymphomas. Inter. J. Cancer 17:47-56.

56. Joncas,J., N. LaPointe, F. Gervaise,M. Leyritz. 1977. Unusual prevalence of Epstein-Barr virus early antigen (EBV-EA) antibodies in ataxia telangiectasia. J. Immunol. 119:1857-1879.
57. Lipinski, M., J.L. Virelizier, T. Tursz, C. Griscelli. 1980. Natural killer and killer cell activities in patients with primary immunodeficiencies or defects in immune interferon production. Eur. J. Immunol. 10:246-249.
58. Saemundsen,A.K., A.I. Berkel, W.Henle, G. Henle, M. Anvret, O. Sanal, F. Ersoy, M. Caglar, and G. Klein. 1981. Epstein-Barr virus carrying lymphoma in a patient with ataxia-telangiectasia. Brit. Med. J. i:425-427.
59. Penn, I. 1978. Malignancies associated with immunosuppressive or cytotoxic therapy. Surgery. 83:492-502.
60. Hanto,D.W., G. Frizzera, D.T.Purtilo, K. Sakamoto, J.L. Sullivan, A.K. Saemundsen, G. Klein, R.L. Simmons, J.S. Najarian. 1981. Clinical spectrum of lymphoproliferative disorders in renal transplant recipients and evidence for the role of the Epstein-Barr virus. Cancer Res. 41:4253-4261.
61. Bieber,C.P., B.A. Reitz, S.W. Jamieson. 1980. Malignant lymphoma in cyclosporin-A-treated allograft recipients. Lancet 1:43.
62. Crawford,D.H., J.A. Thomas, G.Janossy, P. Sweny,OnN. Fernando,J.F. Moorhead, J.H. Thompson. 1980. Epstein-Barr virus nuclear antigen positive lymphoma after cyclosporin A treatment in a patient with renal allograft. Lancet 1:1355-1356.
63. Bird, A.G., S.M.McLachan, S. Britton. 1981. Cyclosporin A promotes spontaneous outgrowth in vitro of Epstein-Barr virus-induced-B-cell lines. Nature 289:300-30.
64. Crawford, D.H., J.M.B. Edwards, P.Sweny, A.V. Hoffbrand, G.Janossy. 1981. Studies on longterm T cell mediated immunity to Epstein-Barr Virus in immunosuppressed renal allograft recipients. Int. J. Cancer 28:705-709.

CHAPTER 19

INDUCTION OF MEASLES VIRUS-SPECIFIC CYTOTOXIC T CELLS, NATURAL KILLER CELLS AND INTERFERON IN CULTURES OF HUMAN PERIPHERAL BLOOD LYMPHOCYTES FROM NORMAL VOLUNTEERS AND PATIENTS WITH MULTIPLE SCLEROSIS

Cornelis J. Lucas

Central Laboratory
Netherlands Red Cross Blood Transfusion Service
Laboratory of Experimental and Clinical Immunology
University of Amsterdam
Amsterdam, The Netherlands

Henry F. McFarland

Neuroimmunology Branch
National Institute of Neurological
and Communicative Diseases and Stroke
National Institutes of Health
Bethesda, Maryland

INTRODUCTION

The separation of what is referred to as cellular immunity and humoral immunity has become somewhat artificial. Both parts of the immune response use T helper cells in their regulatory circuits and there are indications that more places where they overlap exist. In addition, there is no a-priori higher sensitivity for example to influenza infections in T cell deficient patients, or agammaglobulinemic patients. This is likely to differ for different viruses but it still shows that the immune response has some built-in elasticity. One part may take over when the other part fails and this is likely to be the reason why experiments designed to localise viral defense mechanisms have so often yielded only equivocal results.

What do we currently understand cell mediated immunity to be? According to recent studies in the mouse immunization

ISBN 0-12-239980-3

with a virus causes stimulation of different subsets of T lymphocytes which can be defined by functional criteria (1). Four categories can be distinguished: (1) T lymphocytes that mediate a delayed type hypersensitivity response, (2) cytotoxic T lymphocytes, (3) T helper cells for T or B cell collaboration and (4) T suppressor lymphocytes (1). These cells are all thought to play a role in the regulation of an immune response and thus in the successful elimination of a virus. The examination of the individual T cell subpopulations is difficult even in the mouse and so far almost impossible in humans. In addition to the various effector or regulator cells in the immune response, humoral factors are produced which can act as antiviral factors (interferons) or as mediators between various cells (interleukins, chemotactic factors) (2,3). At present the relative roles of these various mechanisms are impossible to establish.

Since viruses are intracellularly replicating pathogens their elimination no doubt involves responses which may lead to the elimination of virus-infected cells. One such mechanism is T cell mediated cytotoxicity (4) but other cellular responses may also have important roles as viral defense mechanisms (5,6,7). Apart from cytotoxic T cells (CTL) there is evidence for three distinct classes of cytotoxic mechanisms: antibody-dependent cell-mediated cytotoxicity (ADCC), natural cytotoxicity (NK), and macrophage-mediated cytotoxicity. The importance of these processes in the killing of virus-infected cells is still unknown (5). Whether these mechanisms are in some way related to each other, for instance by common regulatory pathways, is also unknown at the moment.

The importance of cytotoxic T cells for in vivo elimination of viruses is indicated by experiments reported by Lin and Askonas (8). Monoclonal cytotoxic T cells specific for influenza A virus could protect mice against a challenge with influenza A, not with influenza B virus. Earlier experiments with other viruses, for instance Coxsackie B virus (9) failed to demonstrate a role for CTL, however, and it appears likely that the relative importance of protective mechanisms will vary with different viruses (10).

Which virus-specific T cell subsets can we study in humans? Cytotoxic T cells specific for influenza virus A and B (11), Epstein-Barr virus (12), cytomegalo virus (13), measles virus (14) and mumps virus (15) have been described. In addition T helper cells for the generation of influenza-specific CTL can be demonstrated (16) as well as helper T cells in the in vitro production of virus-specific antibodies (17). What is known about the relevance of the four mentioned cytotoxic mechanisms in humans? Evidence for the existence of cytotoxic T cells has been supplied by in vitro studies (8-12). Two studies suggest an important role for CTL in vivo. McMichael et al showed that individuals which were seronegative for influenza virus but who could generate influenza specific CTL in vitro were significantly better protected against challenge with live influenza vaccine than control individuals which could not generate CTL in vitro (18). In addition Quinnan et al showed a correlation between CTL levels and recovery from cytomegalo-virus episodes in recipients of bone marrow grafts (19 & chapter by Quinnan, this book). From the observation that CTL responses are specific for combinations of virus determinants and major histocompatibility determinants and that, for instance, the human HLA antigen B40 is never recognised in association with influenza A virus (20), a number of people, including these authors, would like to argue that the very presence of a polymorphic MHC is evidence for the biological importance of cytotoxic T cells (21,22).

Whether ADCC, NK or macrophage mediated lysis have in vivo counterparts and play a role in modulating viral infection remains to be demonstrated (15); the fact that NK-deficient Chediack-Higashi patients do not appear to have extraordinarilly great difficulties with virus infections suggests that NK might have a more important function elsewhere. However, Rager-Zisman and Bloom have presented a powerful case for NK cells in the control of persistent virus infections (6).

What is known about the immune response to measles virus? Good and Zak described a normal measles infection in agammaglobulinemic children (23) and from other clinical observations in immunodeficiency diseases in humans (24) it appears that recovery from measles is mediated by reactions requiring an intact T cell component of the response. In addition experiments with monkeys suggest control by T lymphocytes because anti-thymocyte globulin treated animals clear the virus more slowly. However, these animals also have impaired antibody production (25).

CELL-MEDIATED IMMUNITY TO MEASLES VIRUS

Several methods have been applied over the past years to demonstrate cell mediated immunity parameters. Lymphocyte transformation (stimulation of proliferation) studies have been reported (25-28). Although one study (29) was correlated with measles vaccination history the fundamental objection to be raised is that proliferation as such is not an effector-mechanism and, in addition, B lymphocytes have been shown to contribute to lymphocyte proliferation in vitro (30). Skin testing has been used to demonstrate delayed type hypersensitivity reactions with virus antigens. Although this method has given inconsistent results (31) it could provide valuable information. Ada and coworkers (1) have demonstrated a correlation between immunopathology and delayed type hypersensitivity. Thus it is important that this T cell subpopulation is studied. This has become more important, in the light of the possible connection between immunization with killed viruses and atypical responses to the wild virus later (see chapter by Karzon, this book). Migration-inhibition assays with measles virus have included false positive results, likely caused by virus-induced agglutination (32). Consequently experiments undertaken to establish the specificity of the migration reaction failed to show a correlation between inhibition and immunity to measles (32). Cell-mediated cytotoxicity assays will be described in more detail below.

ANTIBODY DEPENDENT CELL-MEDIATED CYTOTOXICITY

Lymphocytes with a receptor for the Fc portion of IgG can kill virus infected cells provided antibodies directed against the virus are present. Only 30% of the effector cells are T cells (34). There is not yet a unique cell surface determinant known. Whereas antibody dependent cell-mediated cytotoxicity (ADCC) is not a prominent mechanism in the mouse it is easily detected with human PBL (5). The cytotoxicity is not HLA restricted. Several authors have shown measles virus specific ADCC (35-40). Most of these studies employed lymphocytes from healthy individuals and all employed lymphocytes studied immediately after isolation from peripheral blood. From some studies it appears that the presence of antibodies is not always required (39); the possible presence of cytophilic antibodies sets these results apart from natural killing. In one study it was shown that monocytes contribute little if any to the observed killing (37). Unfortunately, the various studies on measles virus specific cellular cytotoxicity are somewhat difficult to compare since target cells of different origins were employed and it is our belief that the nature of a target cell plays a crucial role in the type of effector cell demonstrated. Galama et al (37) and Kreth et al (35) used virus infected, PHA-stimulated lymphocytes whereas the others used virus infected fibroblasts. The cytotoxic activity noted by Chiba et al using leukocytes from children 4 to 10 days after a measles infection is most likely an ADCC mediated killing (40). An in vivo role for ADCC has yet to be established. A recent study showed enhanced ADCC activities in PBL from multiple sclerosis patients (41), but the significance of this has not been determined.

NATURAL KILLING OF MEASLES VIRUS-INFECTED CELLS

Natural killing (NK) is the lysis of certain target cells (usually tumor cells) by non-immune leukocytes. After the observation by Santoli et al that interferon, induced or added, activates natural killer cells (42), this type of cytotoxic mechanism received more attention (6). Often it appears that NK is merely blamed for unexpected results but its importance might be underestimated. Ault and Weiner demonstrated NK activity by human peripheral blood mononuclear cells on measles virus-infected Hela cells (43). They showed a correlation between the killing of K562 cells and measles virus infected Hela cells and could conclude that measles virus renders a Hela cell susceptible to NK (43). Wright and Levy (44) in rather complicated experiments using measles virus-infected fibroblasts have reported both NK effector cells and HLA-restricted killer cells after in vitro restimulation of human peripheral blood mononuclear cells.

Since it appears likely that different effector cells might be responsible for the lysis of different types of cells (45,46) we investigated the question whether measles virus infected lymphocytes can be killed by natural killer cells. In an earlier report we had mentioned the possibility that non-HLA restricted killing which is sometimes observed might be mediated by NK (14). In a systematic study, however, with PBL from over thirty individuals we failed to observe NK activity on virus-infected lymphocytes. Two representative experiments are shown in Table 1.

Cultured lymphocytes, stimulated with allogeneic cells, influenza A virus or measles virus can kill K562 - the classical NK target cell - very efficiently. In no instance however, did these same effector cells significantly lyse virus infected lymphocytes, autologous or allogeneic. To analyse a possible relation between interferon induction and induction of NK cells in vitro, the titers of interferon in the supernatants of these cultures were measured and compared to levels of NK-mediated lysis of K562 cells. We could not establish a relationship between levels of interferon and levels of NK activity (Table 2, Figure 1). One donor, W6, had high levels of NK activity but had released no measurable amount of interferon.

TABLE 1. Induction of CTL and NK Activity in vitro. Absence of Lysis of Autologous, Virus-Infected Lymphocytes by NK Cells

Experiment 1 Effector cell	E:T	% specific lysis of: B21	B21-Influenza A	B-21-Measles	Allo	K562
B21 anti-	40	-4.8	-10.4	-7.6	4.4	20.2
	10	-4.0	- 6.1	-6.7	0.9	9.2
B21 anti influenza A	40	-4.2	24.9	13.9	13.6	38.5
	10	-4.7	18.5	4.4	5.6	15.0
B21 anti measles	40	-3.3	-6.8	12.7	9.1	45.9
	10	-5.4	-10.7	0.2	3.0	16.6
B21 anti allo	40	-4.7	1.7	5.2	72.0	29.1
	10	-3.9	-2.4	-2.8	39.0	13.8
Experiment 2		**B16**	**B16-influenza A**	**B16-Measles**	**Allo**	**K562**
B16 anti-	40	-8.2	-4.8	-7.5	-0.3	39.8
	10	-4.5	-3.6	-2.1	2.9	16.2
B16 anti influenza	40	-6.4	49.0	4.1	0.1	62.5
	10	-5.6	34.2	-0.5	0.0	40.1
B16 anti measles	40	-9.8	-1.6	6.4	-0.6	67.2
	10	-7.8	-5.9	2.5	-0.8	26.3
B16 anti allo	40	-2.5	0.5	2.1	50.3	60.6
	10	-4.4	-1.1	-4.7	29.6	27.2

On the other hand cells from donor G7 showed little NK activity despite the presence of a high titer of interferon in the culture supernatant (Table 2). It appears that the majority of the interferon activity is mediated by interferon gamma since no alpha interferon is detected by an elisa assay. We do not know however whether this method employing monoclonal anti-interferon alpha will detect all alpha subtypes. Experiments to extend these observations to include analysis of the killing of virus-infected fibroblasts are currently underway. The results so far, however, clearly indicate that NK do not play a role in the eradication of virus-infected lymphocytes. Secondly, these experiments show that interferon induction is not quantitatively correlated with generated NK activity and as will be described in a following paragraph, neither interferon induction nor NK activity are correlated with the generation of virus-specific, HLA-restricted cytotoxic T cells.

TABLE 2. Generation of Virus-Specific CTL and NK Cells and Induction of Interferon upon Exposure to Influenza A Virus or Measles Virus

Cells From Donor	Stimulated with:	Virus-Specific CTL	NK	INF bio-assay	INFα elisa
G5	-	±	-	-	-
G5	influenza A/HK	-	4.2	-	-
G5	measles virus	-	33.2	-	-
G7	-	-	-	-	-
G7	influenza A/HK	9.8	15.9	10-60	-
G7	measles virus	-	9.4	-	-
K18	-	-	-	-	-
K18	influenza A/HK	-	-	-	-
K18	measles virus	-	-	-	-
M4	-	-	-	-	-
M4	influenza A/HK	10.8	72.5	60	-
M4	measles virus	-	46.2	10-60	-
O3	-	-	-	-	-
O3	influenza A/HK	30.6	75.2	10-60	-
O3	measles virus	6.3	38.3	60	-
P3	-	-	-	-	-
P3	influenza A/HK	34.6	87.6	90	-
P3	measles virus	3.5	12.6	-	-
T8	-	-	16.5	-	-
T8	influenza A/HK	29.6	40.5	10-60	-
T8	measles virus	-	26.3	-	-
V2	-	-	-	-	-
V2	influenza A/HK	-	-	-	-
V2	measles virus	-	-	-	-
V3			16.9	-	-
V3	influenza A/HK	24.8	75.3	10-60	-
V3	measles virus	11.8	74.9	-	-
W6	-	-	22.8	-	-
W6	influenza A/HK	-	65.6	-	-
W6	measles virus	-	78.1	-	-
W10	-	-	-	-	-
W10	influenza A/HK	33.8	55.1	60	-
W10	measles	-	62.7	10-60	-
Z1	-	-	-	-	-
Z1	influenza A/HK	8.2	16.6	-	-
Z1	measles	12.5	37.6	-	-

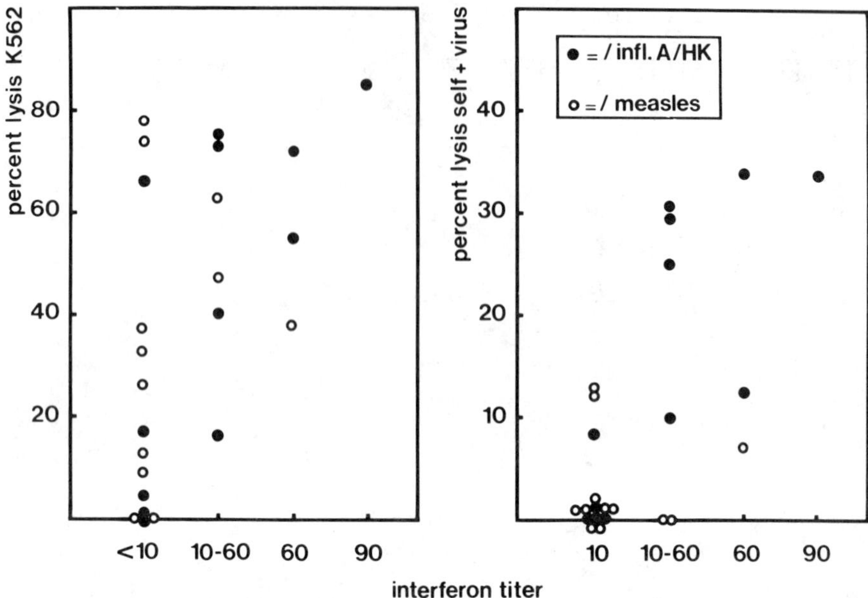

FIGURE 1. In one experiment cells from 12 donors were exposed to influenza virus or measles virus as described in ref. 14. Apart from influenza virus and measles virus specific CTL, natural killing and interferon levels were measured. NK was measured using K562 cells, interferon was titrated on wish cells using a challenge with VSV virus.

A function for NK activity in virus infections has yet to be shown. An intriguing relation between the genetics of resistance to hemopoietic grafts and susceptibility to Herpes viruses has been presented (47 and chapter by Lopez, this book).

CYTOTOXIC T CELLS SPECIFIC FOR MEASLES VIRUS

The first description of HLA-restricted T cell-mediated cytotoxicity against measles virus-infected cells was presented by Kreth et al (48) who used PBL of children with acute measles.

More recently we were able to generate HLA-restricted CTL specific for measles virus by in vitro stimulation (14). The effector cells were OKT3 and OKT8 positive, OKT4 negative and could be generated from highly purified T cell fractions (14). The frequency of donors from whose cells measles virus-specific CTL could be generated was however rather low. The most likely explanation is that in most healthy, adult individuals the size of the precursor CTL pool is too small to be augmented sufficiently by one in vitro stimulation although other explanations such as lack of help or excess suppression should not be discarded. McMichael (49) presented evidence that the size of the memory pool of influenza specific T cells remained sufficiently large for in vitro generation of CTL over a period of approximately 5 years after the last encounter of the antigen. Epstein-Barr virus specific CTL however appear demonstrable in most seropositive adults (50). We could generate measles specific CTL with PBL from a donor who recovered 2 months before from a severe case of atypical measles and from one SSPE patient (Table 3) which suggests that recent or active exposure to measles antigens facilitates CTL generation in vitro. Sethi et al could culture measles virus specific CTL-lines out of PBL from all 8 seropositive donors tested indicating that precursors of measles specific CTL are present in most individuals albeit in small numbers (51).

McFarland, McFarlin and co-workers, as part of an ongoing study of multiple sclerosis in twins (52) investigated the proliferative response to measles. In 3 our of 30 sets of twins, discordant for MS, the effected twin showed a proliferative response to measles virus much higher than the normal twin (52). Two of these sets of twins were tested for the generation of measles virus specific CTL in vitro. In both cases the effected twin did generate measles virus specific CTL. Control cultures showed that both sets of twins showed similar responses to influenza virus and allogeneic cells (Tables 4 & 5). From experiments in which from one twin (M15 and R9) cells were mixed no evidence was obtained for suppression by the non-responder nor for delivery of help from the responder.

TABLE 3. Generation of Measles Specific CTL in Cultures of Lymphocytes from a Patient with Atypical Measles and a Patient with SSPE

Donor	Stimulated in vitro with	E:T	% lysis of target cell: autologous noninfected	autologous measles-infec.	mismatched measles-infec.
B23	-	40	nt	-1.4	nt
B23	measles virus	40	-9.4	29.9	6.9*
B23		10	3.2	22.7	3.3
		4	1.0	7.2	1.6
EK	-	40	-5.4	-3.1	nt
EK	measles virus	40	-4.2	21.8	nt
		10	-5.4	12.5	nt
		4	-5.5	10.6	nt

*Mean lysis on 4 mismatched target cells
B23: Atypical measles. HLA serotype: A1, A23; B49, B51
EK: Subacute sclerosing pan encephalitis (SSPE) patient

TABLE 4. Measles Virus Specific CTL Generated in Cultures of Lymphocytes from a Set of Monozygotic Twins, Discordant for Multiple Sclerosis

HLA		% lysis of target cell: J2-measles A2,B40	M20 measles A2, B40	W6 measles A3,A23,B14,B35
Effector	E:T			
J2 anti nothing	40	-1.4	nt	nt
J2 anti measles	40	-3.9	12.7	10.2
	10	-2.8	7.8	2.8
M20 anti nothing	40	nt	2.9	nt
M20 anti measles	40	28.7	37.8	12.0
	10	15.7	21.9	-0.3
W6 anti measles	40	2.3	17.3	66.2
	10	2.9	10.4	32.0

Note: This is set no. 1 in reference 52
M20 is patient

TABLE 5. Measles Virus Specific CTL Generated in Cultures of Lymphocytes from a Set of Dizygotic Twins Discordant for Multiple Sclerosis

		% lysis of				
		Self	Self Measles	Self Influenza	Allo	HLA Mismatched Measles
Effector	E:T					
R9 anti nothing	10	nt	5.0	3.9	-0.4	nt
R9 anti A/HK		7.3	nt	48.7	nt	nt
R9 anti measles		-1.4	10.1	3.8	nt	4.0*
R9 anti allo		2.8		18.6	21.1	nt
M15 anti nothing		nt	11.7	-2.3	-0.3	nt
M15 anti A/HK		7.7	nt	36.2	nt	nt
M15 anti measles		3.1	28.0	3.9	nt	12.5*
M15 anti allo		6.3		11.3	29.6	nt

*: mean of 5
M15 is patient
This is set no. 2 in reference 52

Subsequently, two alternative approaches were taken in an attempt to increase the number of cytotoxic T cells generated in vitro. Interleukin 2 (IL-2) was added as a source of helper signals but did not turn a non-responder into a responder. The second approach was to restimulate the stimulated lymphocytes. Optimal restimulation conditions were found at day 9. The second culture period was 4 days but it is possible that individual donors might show different optimal periods for the first and second tissue culture period.

The cytotoxic activity of effector cells generated after a second in vitro stimulation are shown in Figure 2. The combined results of a series of experiments shows that the number of responders (individuals whose PBL can be made to generate measles virus-specific CTL in vitro) could thus be increased to at least 7 out of 31 healthy donors (another 7 giving equivocal results). The five MS patients tested so far were all positive. One experiment in which 4 healthy donors and 4 MS patients were tested is shown in Table 6. One donor, S12, shows a small extent of lysis on HLA mismatched cells, one donor (B20) did not generate CTL; from 6 donors measles virus-specific, HLA restricted CTL were generated; only donor H10 and S12 released interferon during the second in vitro culture period. All donors generated NK activity which might be lower in the MS patients (mean lysis

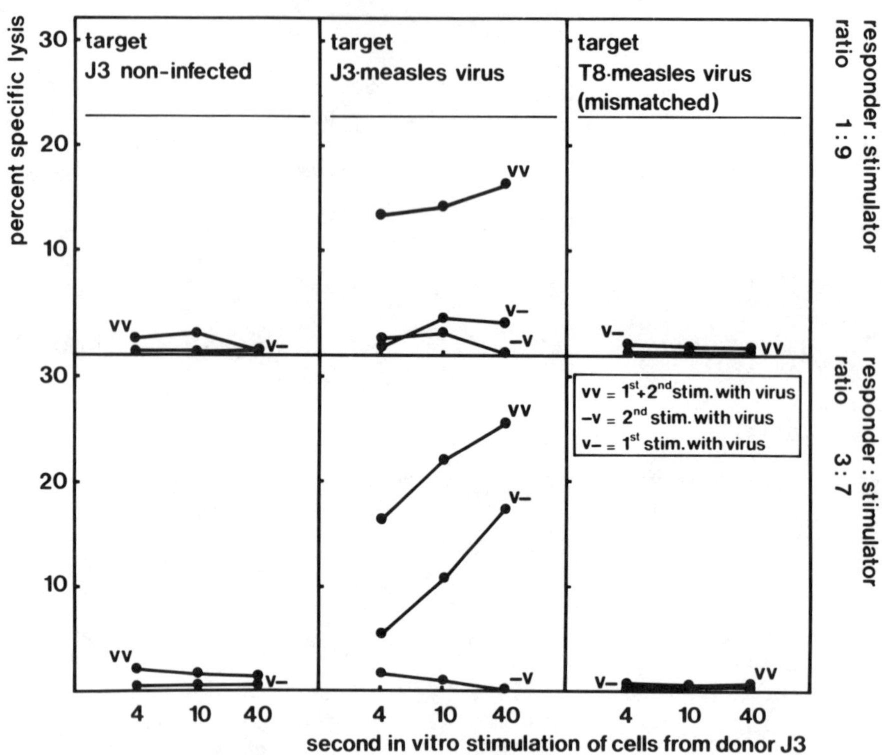

FIGURE 2. Cells from donor J3 were after a first in vitro culture of 9 days with measles virus restimulated with infected, irradiated cells from donor J3 in the ratio of 10^6 responder cells and 9 X 10^6 stimulator cells (top row) or 3 X 10^6 responder cells and 7 X 10^6 stimulator cells (bottom row).

of K562 target cells 32.7% at 40:1 effector:target and 50.8% for the controls).

TABLE 6. Panel Study. Generation of Measles Immune CTL by Two In Vitro Stimulations

	% lysis of measles infected TARGETS from donor:							
	B20	H5	H10	K22	M4	S12	V3	Z1
Effector								
B20	-*	nt	nt	nt	nt	nt	nt	nt
HLA shared:	auto							
H5	-	27.2	-	-	-	-	-	8.0
HLA shared:	no	auto	no	no	B14	no	no	A28
H10	-	7.6	29.1	17.8	10.5	6.6	-	24.5
HLA shared:	no	no	auto	B7	no	A2	no	B55
K22	nt	-	20.3	15.2	nt	12.6	nt	14.5
HLA shared:		no	B7	auto		no		no
M4	nt	8.3	-	-	28.4	30.8	-	9.9
HLA shared:		B14	no	A3	auto	B35	no	no
S12	nt	13.7	19.8	8.1	25.0	35.1	17.8	18.7
HLA shared		no	A2	no	B35	auto	no	B40
V3	nt	nt	-	nt	-	-	15.8	9.3
HLA shared:			no		no	no	auto	no
Z1	nt	nt	nt	nt	nt	nt	1.6	32.7
HLA shared:							no	auto

* - = <5%

Although for the individual case of donor S12 it appears that high levels of NK did correlate with some kill on mismatched target cells, overall this seems not to be true. More patients, at different stages of the disease, will need to be tested before any firm conclusions can be made.

COMPARISON OF CTL INDUCTION, NK INDUCTION AND INTERFERON INDUCTION

From Table 2 it is evident that NK levels are not always high when high levels of interferon are generated in vitro by exposure of PBL to measles virus. This was also not true for CTL generation and interferon induction (Figure 1; Table 7).

TABLE 7. Generation of Measles-specific CTL, NK Cells and Induction of Interferon

Measles-stimulated cells from donor	E:T	% Lysis of self-measles	% Lysis of mismatched measles	% Lysis of K562	IFN
B20	40	0	nt	30.2	<10
	10	0		11.5	
H5	40	27.2	2.0	25.5	<10
	10	18.1	0.1	10.7	
H10	40	29.1	6.0	53.6	0-60
	10	25.3	3.0	23.6	
K22	40	27.9	8.9	33.5	<10
	10	20.3	6.0	15.7	
M4	40	28.4	7.5	53.5	<10
	10	22.8	3.9	27.1	
S12	40	35.1	13.2	65.8	60
	10	27.5	9.2	39.0	
V3	40	15.8	5.9	43.2	<10
	10	13.9	2.7	33.0	
Z1	40	32.7	1.6	28.7	<10
	10	27.5	0.6	11.4	

From our limited study with PBL from multiple sclerosis patients it appears that, if anything, they respond better to measles antigens than either their healthy twins or healthy control individuals. In several studies it has been shown that levels of NK cells are low in MS patients (53,56). It remains to be investigated whether the lower NK and possibly higher measles specific CTL precursor levels are related to each other.

Askonas recently demonstrated release of interferon during the actual lysis of target cells by CTL (57). Ennis and co-workers observed a high release of gamma interferon when lymphocytes were incubated with influenza virus infected stimulator cells (58). It appears that a systemic study of the relations between and the regulation of induction of interferon and cytotoxic T cells will provide better insights in the importance of these components of a virus-specific immune response (59).

SUMMARY AND CONCLUSION

Four cytotoxic mechanisms by which virus-infected cells may be eradicated have been described: T cell-mediated cytotoxicity, antibody dependent cell mediated cytotoxicity, natural cytotoxicity and macrophage mediated cytotoxicity.

The relative contributions of each of these in measles infection - if any - are still unknown. Their intra-relationship is also unknown. Recent developments in the study of various effector cells and their regulation will provide valuable information.

Of these cytotoxic mechanisms only the first three are discussed here. The study of cytotoxic T cells, an important subset of T lymphocytes which is subject to regulation by other T cells, has only recently become possible. Measles virus specific cytotoxic T cells can be demonstrated albeit in a small number of adult, healthy volunteers. In vitro generation of cytotoxic T cells results concomittantly in the generation of NK cells which however do not kill measles virus infected lymphocytes. Interferon induction takes place as well. The data so far appear to indicate that levels of cytotoxic T cells, NK cells and interferon are not related, suggesting that all have their own regulatory mechanisms.

In an attempt to demonstrate measles virus specific CTL in a larger number of individuals, the cultures were restimulated after an initial period of 9 days. This procedure resulted in successful generation of measles immune CTL in cultures of PBL from 7 out of 31 healthy volunteers (7 others being equivocal) and in 5 out of 5 cultures of PBL from multiple sclerosis patients.

ACKNOWLEDGEMENTS

We thank Pammy Treep-van Leeuwen and Liz Boone for excellent technical assistance. Dr. Huub Schellekens and co-workers were of great help by performing the interferon titrations.

REFERENCES

1. Ada, G.L., Leung,K.N. & Ertl,H. Imm. Rev. 58:5, 1981.
2. Waksman,B.H.: in Cohen,S., Pick,E., Oppenheim,J.J. (eds). The Biology of the lymphokines, Ac. Press,N.Y. 1979. P.585-615.

3. Mims,C.A. The pathogenesis of infectious disease. Ac.Press. N.Y. 1977.
4. McMichael,A.J. Springer Sem. Immunopathol. 3:3-22, 1982.
5. Sissons,J.G.P. & Oldstone,M.B.A. J. of Inf. Dis. 142:114,1980.
6. Rager-Zisman,B. & Bloom, B.R. Natural killer cells in resistance to virus-infected cells. Springer Sem. Immunopathol. 4:397-414,1980.
7. Welsh,R.M. Antiviral Res. 1:5, 1981.
8. Lin,Y.L., Askonas,B.A. J.Exp. Med. 154:225,1981.
9. Wong,C.Y., Woodruff,J.J. & Woodruff,J.F. J. Immunol. 118:1159,1977.
10. Hirsch,R.L. Immunol. 43:81,1981.
11. Biddison,W.E., Shaw,S. & Nelson,D.L. J. Immunol. 122:660,1979.
12. Moss,D.J., Wallace,L.E., Rickinson,A.B. & Epstein,M.A. Eur. J. Imm. 11:686,1981.
13. Quinnan,G.V.Jr., Kirmani,N., Esber,E., Saral,R., Manischewitz,J.F., Rogers,J.L., Rook,A.H., Santos,G.W. & Burns,W.H. J. Immunol. 126:2036,1981.
14. Lucas,C.J., Biddison,W.E., Nelson,D.L. & Shaw,S. Infect. Immun. 1982. 38:226,1982
15. Kreth,H.W., Kress,L., Kress,H.G., Ott,H.F. & Eckert,G. J. Immunol. 128:2411,1982.
16. Biddison,W.E., Sharrow,S.O. & Shearer,G.M. J. Immunol. 127:487,1981.
17. Yarchoan,R., Biddison,W.E. & Nelson,D.L. J.Clin.Immunol. 2:118,1982.
18. McMichael,A.J. (This book).
19. Quinnan,G.V.jr., Kirmani,N., Rook,A.H., Manischewitz,J.F., Jackson,L., Moreschi,G., Santos,G.W., Saral,R. & Burns,W.H. New Engl. J. Med. 307:7,1982.
20. Biddison,W.E. J.Clin.Immunol. 2:1,1982.
21. Bodmer,W.F. Tissue Antigens 17:9,1981.
22. Dausset,J. Science 213:1469,1981.
23. Good,R.A. & Zak,S.J. Pediatrics 18:109,1956.
24. Nahurias,A.J., Griffith,D. Salsbury,C. & Yoshida, K. J.A.M.A. 201:729,1967.
25. Hicks,J.T., Sullivan,J.L. & Albrecht,P. J.Immunol. 119:1452,1977.
26. McFarland,H.F., Pedone,C.A., Mingioli,E.S. & McFarlin,D.E. J.Immunol. 125:221,1980.
27. Ilonen,J., Lanning,M., Herva,E. & Salmi,A. Scand. J. Immunol. 12:383,1980.
28. Cunningham-Runkles,S., Dupont,B., Posner,J.B., Hansen,J.A. & Good,R.A. Lancet II. 1204,1975.
29. Kreeftenberg,J.G. & Loggen,H.G. Cell Immunol. 33:443,1977.

30. Astaldi,G.C.B., Wright,E.P., Willems,Ch., Zeijlemaker,W.P. & Janssen,M.C. J.Immunol. 128:2539,1982.
31. Valdimarsson,H., Agnarsdottir,G. & Lachmann,P.J. Proc. Roy. Soc.Med. 67:1125,1974.
32. Utermohen,V., Levine,J. & Ginsparg,M. Clin.Immunol., Immunopathol. 9:248,1978.
33. Nordel,H.J., Froland,S.S., Vandvik,B. & Norrby,E. Scand. J. Immunol. 5:969,1976.
34. Oers,M.H.J. van, Zeijlemaker,W.P. & Schellekens,P. Th.A. Eur.J.Immunol. 7:143, 1977.
35. Kreth,H.W. & Meulen,V. ter. J.Immunol. 118:291,1977.
36. Perrin,L.H., Tishon,A. & Oldstone,M.B.A. J.Immunol. 118:282-290,1977.
37. Galama,J.M.D., Vos,A. & Lucas,C.J. Cellul. Immunol. 48:296, 1979.
38. Whittle,M.C. & Werblinska, J.Clin. Exp. Immunol. 42:136,1980.
39. Ewan,P.W. & Lackmann,P.J. Clin. Exp. Immunol. 30:22,1977.
40. Chiba,S., Yamanaka,T., Nakao,T. Tohoku J. Exp. Med. 112:285, 1974.
41. Merrill,J.E., Wahlin,B., Siden,A. & Perlmann,P. J. Immunol. 128:1728,1982.
42. Trinchieri,G., Santoli,D., Dec,R.R. & Knowles,B.B. J. Exp. Med. 147:1299,1978.
43. Ault,K.A. & Weiner,H.L. J. Immunol. 122:2611,1979.
44. Wright,L.L. & Levy,N.L. J.Immunol. 122:2379,1979.
45. Koszinowski,U. & Ertl,H. J. of Immunogenetics 4:107,1977.
46. Dubey,D.P., Stannton,D., Azocar,J., Stux, S., Essex,M. & Yunis,E.J. Clin. Immunol. Immunopath. 23:215,1982.
47. Lopez,C. (This Book).
48. Kreth,H.W., Meulen,V. ter, & Eckert,G. Med.Microbiol. Immunol. 165:203,1979.
49. McMichael,A.J. Personal Communication.
50. Wallace,L.E., Rickinson,A.B., Rowe,M., Moss,D.J., Allen,D.J. & Epstein,M.A. Cellul. Immunol. 67:129,1982.
51. Sethi,K.K., Stroehmann,I. & Brnadis,H. Infect. Immun. 36:657,1982.
52. Greenstein,J.I. & McFarland,H.F. Clinics in Immunology and Allergy (in press).
53. Benczur,M., Petranyi,G.G., Palffy,G., Varga,M., Falas,M., Kotsy,B., Folders,I. & Hollan,S.R. Clin. Exp. Immunol. 39:657,1980.
54. Hauser,S.J., Ault,M.J., Levin,J., Garovoy,M.R. & Weiner,H.L. J. Immunol. 127:1114, 1981.
55. Neighbour,P.A., Grayzel, A.I. & Miller,A.E. Clin. Exp. Immunol. 49:11,1982.
56. Merrill,J.E., Jondal,M., Seeley,J., Ullberg,M. & Siden,A. Clin. Exp. Immunol. 47:419,1982.

57. Morris,A.G., Lin,Y.L. & Askonas,B.A. Nature 295:150,1982.
58. Ennis,F.A. & Meager,A. J.Exp. Med. 154:1279,1981.
59. Torres,B.A., Farrar,W.L. & Johnson,H.M. J. Immunol. 128:2217,1982.

CHAPTER 20

IMMUNOPATHOLOGY OF DENGUE HEMORRHAGIC FEVER: NEW PERSPECTIVES

Philip K. Russell

Walter Reed Army Institute for Research
Washington, District of Columbia

INTRODUCTION

Our current concepts of the pathogenesis of Dengue Hemorrhagic Fever/Dengue Shock Syndrome are derived from studies of the epidemiology of the disease, clinical investigation of patients, laboratory studies of the biology of viruses and studies of the immune response they elicit in man and experimental animals. From a multitude of studies done by many scientists since the disease was first recognized in the Philippines in 1954, a useful but still imperfect understanding of the disease has been derived. In this paper I will discuss some recent studies and some recent epidemiologic events which I believe provide some additional insight into the problem of pathogenesis and the nature of the immunopathologic mechanisms involved.

A brief review of the clinical picture and the pathophysiology will help focus on the critical areas where current explanations are inadequate or lacking.

The typical case of DHF/DSS goes through a febrile period which averages five days during which time fever, malaise, anorexia, nausea, vomiting are prominent symptoms and a macular or petechial rash is usually present. The second, much more serious phase, is marked by vascular collapse, shock and a bleeding diathesis which may be severe. The shock is due to a loss of plasma from the circulating blood volume accompanied by hemoconcentration. The cause of the increased vascular permeability which allows the plasma to escape is the most perplexing and probably the most important unanswered question in this disease. I postulated several years ago that a chemical mediator must be involved because of the rapid onset, rapid reversal and lack of destructive lesions or inflammation in the vessels.

ISBN 0-12-239980-3

Two other important aspects are a profound thrombocytopenia occurring slightly before or concommitant with the shock and an impressive activation of both pathways of complement system also occuring just before the onset of shock. Some degree of disseminated intravascular coagulation is usually present also. Explaining the immunopathology of DHF/DSS requires answering questions relating to the causes of: vascular permeability, thrombocytopenia, complement consumption, disseminated intravascular coagulation.

EPIDEMIOLOGICAL STUDIES

Central to discussions of the causes of DHF/DSS have been disagreements about the importance of second dengue infections versus primary dengue infections. Several studies done in the hyperendemic areas in Southeast Asia point to a much higher risk from a second infection in indigenous children. The epidemiologic events in Cuba between 1978 and 1981 provide some very important data on this point. Cuba was dengue-free from 1947 until 1977 at which time Dengue-1 virus was introduced probably from Africa via Jamaica. A massive epidemic of classic dengue fever occurred with no evidence of DHF/DSS. The Cuban government reported 553,132 casses between 1977 and 1980. One estimate of the total number of infections was five million; no deaths were reported. The prevalence of dengue-1 antibody in Cuba in 1981 was estimated at 45 percent.

In May 1981 Dengue-2 virus appeared. The origin of the virus is as yet unknown. Dengue-2 was endemic elsewhere in the Caribbean as well as in Africa and Asia at the time. It is of some note that a dengue-2 virus with a fingerprint similar to an African strain was isolated in Jamaica shortly after the Cuban epidemic.

Over 344,203 cases occurred in a five month period. This was a rapidly developing epidemic which put a tremendous load on the patient care system.

Full blown DHF/DSS was seen in adults and children. Over 116,000 cases were hospitalized and 168 deaths occurred in spite of what appeared to be excellent medical treatment. The clinical, laboratory and pathologic manifestations reported by Cuban investigators were the same as seen in Southeast Asian children. This "experiment of nature" provides strong reinforcement for the concept that a prior dengue infection markedly increases the risk of serious disease when the second infection occurs. Clearly, dengue-2 following shortly after dengue-1 is a dangerous situation. It is of interest to note that recent prospective studies done by Dr. Donald Burke in Bangkok school children also point to dengue-2 as an especially dangerous virus when it occurs in a child previously infected with another serotype.

IMMUNE ENHANCEMENT

Another aspect of recent dengue research related to the DHF problem is the emerging information on immune enhancement. The infection enhancing effect of non-neutralizing dengue antibody is readily demonstrated in vivo with polyclonal human or animal antisera and cells bearing FC receptors. Several laboratories have been studying the phenomenon using monoclonal antibodies against dengue and other flaviviruses and some interesting facts are emerging which most probably are pertinent to the DHF pathogenesis problem. At Walter Reed we have investigated the biological activity of a series of antidengue monoclones and have related infection enhancement activity with other properties of the antibody. Mouse monoclones of isotypes IgG 1, 2a and 2b can have enhancing ability. Infection enhancement activity of an antibody appears to be related to the physical position of the antigenic determinant or epitope on the glycoprotein. There are multiple epitopes on dengue viruses which can be involved in the enhancement. Some of the epitopes are shared with all flaviviruses (i.e. they are genus specific), some are shared within the dengue complex but not with other flaviviruses and some are shared between two members of the dengue complex. There is disagreement in the literature about enhancement involving serotype specific antibodies. Enhancement by type specific monoclones can be demonstrated in mouse cell lines but not in human monocytes or the U-939 human histiocyte derived cell line.

The potential exists for infection with one dengue serotype to give rise to multiple antibody clones directed at several different determinants which can enhance infection by other dengue viruses which share the same determinants on the envelope glycoprotein. These enhancing antibodies may or may not have other types of activity such as neutralization or hemagglutination inhibition or complement fixation. These antibodies which have both neutralization and enhancing activity may have enhancement titers one thousand fold higher than the neutralization titer.

Enhancibility of dengue viruses seems to vary widely between serotypes. Dengue-2 virus appears to be most readily enhanced by a variety of polyclonal and monoclonal antibodies, on the other hand, dengue-4 virus is not enhanced by some antibodies that react with dengue-4 and do enhance dengue-2. In our laboratory we have not yet convincingly demonstrated enhancement with dengue-4.

Exactly how this relates to the pathogenesis of DHF remains to be shown but it seems highly likely that the ability of some dengue viruses to stimulate the production of multiple clones that enhance heterologous serotypes and the varying ability of dengue viruses to be enhanced may be very important in determining the outcome of a dengue infection. Qualitative and quantitative differences may be involved in determining which sequence of dengue infections is the most dangerous. The fact that dengue-2 appears to be the most readily enhanced in vitro fits with the epidemiologic perception that dengue-2 virus is an especially dangerous virus in a second infection. Quantitative differences may explain why antibody to other flaviviruses (e.g. YF vaccination) does not appear to predispose to DHF although enhancement can be demonstrated in vitro.

One field study which I believe demonstrates the role of enhancing antibody in DHF/DSS was conducted in Bangkok by Burke, Kliks, Nisalak and Nimantya. They focused on the peak of severe DHF/DSS which occurs in infants 6 to 9 months old. These cases of DHF/DSS are often very severe and are due to primary infections. They studied 13 infants with DHF/DSS and related the decay of maternal antibody levels to the time of onset of severe disease. To summarize their findings, they found that antibody dependent enhancement titers in maternal sera were two to fifteen fold higher than neutralization titers. As the level of maternal IG in the infant drops, neutralizing activity disappears first (median 6 months) and enhancing activity persists two or three months longer.

Using measured maternal antibody levels and assuming a half life to 30 days they found that the cases in this series occurred after neutralizing activity of the infant's sera disappeared and infection enhancing antibody was still present. The authors conclude that these data support the conclusion that infection enhancing antibody is important in the pathogenesis of the disease in these children. This interpretation appears very sound. It is noteworthy that these cases were all due to dengue-2 viruses.

The accumulating epidemiologic information on the increased risk of second infections in children and adults, the studies on the role of maternal antibody in infants and the emerging information on the infection enhancement phenomenon in vitro all point toward an important role of infection enhancing antibody in the pathogenesis of disease.

If infection enhancing antibodies play a major role in producing DHF/DSS then the risk to an individual experiencing a second dengue infection would be determined by the following factors: (1) The antigenic configuration of the first infecting virus and the numbers of epitopes on the virus which may stimulate the production of enhancing antibody clones.

(2) The response of the individual to those epitopes which probably varies widely between individuals and is under genetic control. (3) The antigenic configuration of the second infecting virus and the numbers of epitopes in common with the first virus to which the individual responded and which will result in enhancement when antibody attaches.

Consideration of these factors leads to the conclusion that both viral and human genetics play significant roles. Future epidemiologic and immunologic studies should be able to assess risk to individuals based on investigation of the antibody response to the primary infection.

DENGUE VIRUSES

Another factor in the complex equation we are trying to solve relates to the viruses themselves. Studies of molecular biology especially oligonucleotide analysis are producing impressive and somewhat surprising information on the extent of genetic variation among viruses of the same serotype. Analysis of dengue-1 strains in our laboratory and analysis of dengue-2 strains by Trent and Monath at the CDC, Ft. Collins, Colorado, have demonstrated major differences between strains of different geographic origin and between strains from the same area isolated at different times. RNA fingerprints of different strains of the same type may differ by as much as 80 percent of large oligonucleotides or 20 percent of the total RNA genome. So far the differences seen correlate only with geography and time. No correlation has been related to disease severity or any in vitro virulence marker or immune enhancement. Nonetheless, it is clear that dengue viruses are heterogenous and the genomic differences may possibly be related to expression of epitopes important in infection enhancement by heterologous antibody. This is a very complex issue but worth pursuing through further studies of infection enhancement and genetic variation of the viruses.

SUMMARY

The role of cells of the monocyte-macrophage series appears to be significant in the pathogenesis of DHF/DSS in view of their role in supporting dengue virus replication and of their involvement in the supporting dengue virus replication and of their involvement in the infection enhancement phenomenon. Isolation of dengue viruses from circulating mononuclear leukocytes and detection of dengue antigen in macrophages in tissue from patients combined with the demonstration of the susceptibility to infection of glass adherent peripheral blood monocytes has led to wide acceptance of the view that monocyte-macrophages are the predominant site of replication in human dengue infections. Enhancing antibody certainly would be expected to increase the numbers of infected macrophages in vivo as it does in vitro. This leads to the question of whether the role of these cells in DHF/DSS is merely to produce more virus and viral antigen or whether these infected cells produce products which directly produce the end effects, i.e. vascular permeability, DIC and thrombocytopenia. These infected macrophages may be responding to (1) the virus infection, (2) stimulation by virus-antibody complexes, (3) immunologic attack by antibody complement and/or cytotoxic lymphocytes because they express viral antigen on their surface and become target cells.

Infected macrophages under these conditions may release sufficient tissue factor and plasminogen activator to activate the clotting mechanism. This seems to be a reasonable explanation for the DIC which occurs although direct experimental evidence is lacking.

It has been postulated by Halstead that infected macrophages release mediators such as prostaglandins which act directly on the vascular endothelium to produce the vascular permeability. This may occur but there is no direct evidence for the close cell to cell interaction usually needed for macrophages to affect other cells. It appears more likely that the effect on the vascular endothelium is produced principally through the action of complement and production of anaphylotoxins $C3_2$ and $C5_2$. The fact that the degree of complement activation correlates with disease severity is consistent with this interpretation.

There are several possible mechanisms all of which may contribute: (1) release of viral antigens which form immune complexes in the serum, (2) expression of antigens on the macrophage surface which react with antibody and complement, and (3) release of proteinase or other substances which activate the alternate pathway. Previous studies showed significant variation in the extent of activation of the classical and alternate pathways of complement activation. The relative importance of the various mechanisms of complement activation varies from case to case. It seems probably that direct activation by a macrophage factor may be a more important mechanism in primary infection such as infants where antibody levels are low initially whereas in the usual secondary infection case where antibody levels are high early in the diseases antibody mediated activation may play a bigger role.

The role of lymphocytes in the immunopathology of DHF is more difficult to define. The importance of lymphocyte action in clearing virus infection is well recognized with many viruses and certainly the action of specifically activated cells and K cells will be shown to play a role in clearing dengue infections. The possible relationship between lymphocytes, macrophages, the dengue virus and complement presents an incredibly complex series of interactions involving multiple mediators. Given the present paucity of specific knowledge it seems premature to try to evaluate the real importance of the possible interaction mechanism(s). This may be one of the most rewarding areas for future research.

CHAPTER 21

IMMUNE RESPONSES TO HUMAN GASTROENTERITIS VIRUSES: NORWALK VIRUS AND ROTAVIRUS

Neil R. Blacklow

George Cukor

Division of Infectious Diseases
University of Massachusetts Medical School
Worcester, Massachusetts

BACKGROUND

Acute viral gastroenteritis is an extremely common illness that affects all age groups and occurs in both epidemic and endemic forms (1). It is second in frequency only to the common cold among illnesses affecting United States families under epidemiological surveillance. It is also responsible for some of the common travelers' diarrhea encountered in Latin America, Africa, and Asia. The illness varies in its clinical presentation, but in general it is self limited, begins with an explosive onset, and consists of varying combinations of diarrhea, nausea, vomiting, low grade fever, abdominal cramps, headache, anorexia, myalgia and malaise. It can be severe, indeed fatal, in the elderly, infant, debilitated or malnourished patient.

Viral gastroenteritis occurs primarily in two epidemiologically distinct clinical forms (1). One entity is characteristically epidemic and is responsible for family and community-wide outbreaks of gastroenteritis among older children and adults. The older medical literature gives a variety of descriptive labels to this one to two day illness, such as winter vomiting disease, epidemic collapse, viral diarrhea, epidemic diarrhea and vomiting, and acute infectious nonbacterial gastroenteritis. In recent years, a newly discovered agent, Norwalk virus, has been shown to be responsible for about one-third of these disease outbreaks in the United States. Other Norwalk-like viruses have also been discovered such as Hawaii agent and W agent, and although

ISBN 0-12-239980-3

they have not yet been studied epidemiologically, they are likely to be responsible for many more epidemic cases of this illness.

The second clinical entity is usually sporadic and occasionally epidemic and it occurs predominantly in infants and young children (1). This form of illness typically produces severe diarrhea that commonly lasts for five to eight days and is usually accompanied by fever and vomiting. Rotavirus, which was discovered during the 1970's, is responsible for approximately one half of the cases of this clinical entity world-wide requiring hospitalization. Although the major target of rotavirus is the very young, it can produce clinical disease in adults but the infection is most commonly subclinical in this age group.

Despite the frequency of viral gastroenteritis syndromes, the etiology of these illnesses remained obscure until the 1970's. Our understanding of the cause of viral gastroenteritis was initially advanced when gastroenteritis was transmitted to healthy adult volunteers by the oral administration of bacteria-free, toxin-free stool filtrates derived from several outbreaks of the disease. These studies led to the discovery of the first major group of agents responsible for viral diarrhea, the Norwalk-like viruses (2,3) which are of uncertain classification. The prototype Norwalk virus, which is currently noncytopathic in vitro and not disease producing for experimental animals, was subsequently visualized in infectious stool filtrates and partially characterized as a 27nm small particle of definable density by immune electron microscopy (IEM) and ultracentrifugation (4). Other Norwalk-like viruses, such as Hawaii and Ditchling viruses, have been uncovered by similar techniques; these two agents appear to form (with Norwalk virus) three immunologically distinct agents based on IEM studies (1). Both the Norwalk and Hawaii agents produce a mucosal lesion of the proximal human small intestine, the likely site for replication of these viruses (5,6). This lesion is accompanied by transient small intestinal malabsorption, and also by delayed gastric emptying despite normal gastric morphology and secretory function (7).

A radioimmunoassay (RIA) technique has been developed for the detection of Norwalk virus in diarrheal stools and for quantitation of antibody to the agent (8,9). It relies upon clinical materials derived from human volunteer studies since it has not been possible to prepare hyperimmune animal serum to the virus. The RIA procedure has been used to demonstrate the epidemiologic importance of Norwalk virus in various parts of the world, including its involvement in waterborne, foodborne, nursing home, and school and community outbreaks of acute gastroenteritis (10-16). The virus has also been associated with cases of travelers' diarrhea (17,18).

During the mid-1970's, a second viral gastroenteritis pathogen of man was identified and is now known to be a major cause of diarrhea in infants and young children (19-21). This pathogen, the 70nm rotavirus, has been easily identified by routine electron microscopy in stool filtrates derived from ill individuals (22). Serologic assay techniques have been developed for this agent and can detect antibodies in human sera (22,23). In addition, rotavirus has been identified in diarrheal feces by immunologic assays such as RIA or enzyme-linked immunosorbent assay (ELISA) techniques (24-26). Available laboratory techniques have readily permitted in vitro study of the biologic properties of rotavirus and have shown that it possesses double stranded segmented RNA. The etiologic role of rotavirus in diarrheal illness has been demonstrated in many parts of the world, and in addition to pediatric and family settings has also been associated with diarrhea experienced by adults including travelers (18,27-35). Recently, human rotavirus has been cultivated in cell culture by incorporating low concentrations of trypsin into the culture medium (36,37). At least three and perhaps as many as five serotypes of human rotavirus exist (38,39).

During the past few years, several other agents of viral gastroenteritis have been described, including enteric adenovirus, calcivirus, enteric coronavirus, and astrovirus (1). The medical importance of these agents is currently not known, in contrast to Norwalk virus and rotavirus.

IMMUNE RESPONSE TO NORWALK VIRUS

Epidemiological Data. Epidemiological data indicate that 50 to 75% of adults worldwide possess serum RIA antibody to Norwalk virus. Serum antibody prevalence levels rise during adolescence in the U.S. (9), implying that infection is uncommon during early childhood. However, in less developed and tropical areas of the world, antibody to Norwalk virus is acquired at an earlier age (about 4 to 6 years old) (10-11). In the United States, limited epidemiological studies of Norwalk virus infection among families indicates that the agent is an uncommon cause of illness among infants and is a relatively infrequent cause of endemic diarrhea (40).

HUMAN VOLUNTEER STUDIES

Most of our understanding of the clinical immunity to Norwalk virus derives from human volunteer studies. A striking unusual pattern of clinical immunity has been seen in these volunteers (9,41) and this pattern fails to fit immunologic concepts traditionally associated with common human viral illnesses. Only about half of the subjects inoculated with Norwalk virus develop gastroenteritis. Although serum RIA and IEM antibody levels rise after Norwalk illness, these responses appear to reflect infection in susceptible persons and not to have a protective role, because illness commonly occurs in the presence of serum antibody. In contrast, volunteers who resist illness usually have low to absent serum antibody levels before and after exposure to the virus. Findings similar to those found in serum have also been noted with antibody levels in duodenal fluids (9,42). Paradoxically, then, the presence of antibody to the virus and the ability to generate it constitute risk factors for this illness.

When 12 volunteers were inoculated with Norwalk virus and then rechallenged 27 to 42 months later, precisely the same 6 volunteers who became ill on the initial challenge again became ill on rechallenge (41). Antibody responses occurred, usually from baselines of pre-challenge antibody. Those 6 volunteers who were clinically well on the first challenge remained unaffected on the second. Antibody responses were usually absent, and pre-challenge antibody was for the most part absent. Interestingly, short-term resistance to Norwalk illness has been noted in that most previously ill volunteers who were rechallenged 4 to 14 weeks later remained well (9,41-43).

It is not known whether this unusual pattern of clinical immunity to Norwalk virus occurs with natural infection. However, there is a suggestion that this may be the case. Familial clusters of susceptibility and resistance to the virus have been described in a waterborne disease outbreak in which similar degrees of exposure to the virus for different families were shown epidemiologically (14).

The reason for the pattern of clinical immunity to Norwalk virus is unknown. Speculation has centered on whether there may be a genetic susceptibility to infection in certain individuals. Perhaps they possess a receptor site on their small intestinal epithelial cells that is lacking for the "immune" individuals. In this regard, a limited number of ill and well volunteers have been studied for the histocompatibility loci A, B and D and no differences have been found.

Another potential explanation for the Norwalk pattern of clinical immunity is that repetitive exposures to the virus are necessary to generate eventual immune responses as well as concomitant illness. This hypothesis implies that the adult volunteers who remain well are not "primed" and have had fewer naturally occurring exposures to the virus during their lifetimes than those who develop illness. It is certainly clear from the volunteer studies that clinical resistance to Norwalk virus is not longstanding for the known susceptible person, and it may be that repetitive bouts of illness due to this virus occur in some individuals during their lifetimes.

The serum IgM response to Norwalk virus has been studied in volunteers (44). An IgM response has occurred in subjects who became ill, whether or not prechallenge total serum antibody was present. The peak IgM response occurred at about two weeks after illness but IgM was detectable in lower titers for up to 21 weeks following infection. On long-term rechallenge, volunteers who were previously ill and had produced IgM antibody again became ill and a secondary IgM response, greater than the first, was seen. Non-ill, challenged volunteers, as well as previously ill volunteers on short term rechallenge, usually failed to generate an IgM response, whether or not they had an IgG response. It seems clear that virus-specific IgM is not necessarily indicative of primary infection with Norwalk virus in as much as reinfection produces an enhancement of the IgM response. Furthermore, Norwalk-specific IgM responses appear not be associated with subclinical illness. IgM testing has yet to be performed for naturally occurring Norwalk disease outbreaks.

PROSPECTS FOR IMMUNOPROPHYLAXIS

Based on what has been learned about the clinical immunity to Norwalk virus, prospects for immunoprophylaxis appear dim. Inasmuch as ill individuals can develop disease again 27 to 42 months later, the use of a vaccine for producing long lasting immunity seems improbable. Perhaps short-term immunity could conceivably be produced by vaccination for individuals at a high risk of short term exposure, such as travelers. However, the technology for producing a vaccine for Norwalk virus is essentially undeveloped, since the agent has yet to be cultivated in vitro and it is also shed in relatively low titers in feces. The noncultivatable nature of the virus, as well as the lack of animal disease models for its study, also has precluded for the present an assessment of cell-mediated immune responses to infection.

IMMUNE RESPONSE TO ROTAVIRUS

The prime factors involved in the clinical immunity to rotavirus infection have yet to be determined conclusively. Current evidence indicates potentially important protective roles for substances in breast milk, antibodies in serum including IgM, and locally produced intestinal tract antibodies. Reported studies, however, need to be analysed carefully since different serologic techniques have been employed, most of which measure responses to the rotavirus group-specific antigen; few studies have measured serotype-specific neutralizing antibody responses since human rotavirus has only recently been cultivated in cell culture. In addition only limited information has been gathered from studies of adult human volunteers infected with rotavirus.

EPIDEMIOLOGICAL DATA

Epidemiological data provide some important clues to the clinical immunity to rotavirus infection (45). First, individuals in the 6 to 24 month old age group are those who are most susceptible to clinical illness with rotavirus infection (1,21). Younger infants are most commonly infected asymptomatically. Second, most individuals show serological evidence of having been infected with rotavirus by the third year of life (21,23). Third, adult contacts of ill children are often infected with rotavirus but usually their infection is asymptomatic (34). Finally, sequential rotavirus illnesses in a limited number of individual children have been demonstrated but the second infection has always been due to a different rotavirus serotype (45,46). Currently, at least three and perhaps as many as five rotavirus serotypes are known, based on classification using viral neutralization techniques (38,39). All serotypes appear to produce indistinguishable epidemiological patterns of clinical illness. It certainly seems clear that prior illness in a young child with one rotaviral serotype does not protect against subsequent clinical disease due to a second serotype.

ROLE OF BREAST MILK

It is generally accepted that breast feeding reduces the incidence and mortality of infantile gastroenteritis (47). In regard to the rotavirus component of this syndrome, clinical studies in newborn babies in nurseries have shown that breast milk fed babies are less often infected with rotavirus and if infected excrete less virus than formula fed newborns (48,49). However, breast feeding does not always protect newborns from rotavirus diarrhea (50). Furthermore, when young children were followed prospectively from birth for a mean period of 16.3 months, breast feeding did not appear to be statistically significant in providing protection against rotavirus infection during this longer period of surveillance (51) (39% breast fed infected versus 55% not breast fed infected). Perhaps larger studies may show clinical significance.

Human breast milk contains secretory IgA antibody to rotavirus (52,53). Antibody levels are highest in colostrum but also persist in most milk specimens for up to 24 months of lactation. However, it is not known whether this specific antirotavirus secretory IgA (11S) is responsible for the clinical effect of breast milk that has been shown to date. One study indicates that rotavirus specific 9S IgA and IgG in breast milk do not protect against infection in newborns (54). In this study, it was suggested that perhaps rotavirus neutralizing antibodies in breast milk not detected by the authors' ELISA techniques could conceivably prove protective. In addition, it is also possible that other antiviral factors in breast milk may be important in providing clinical protection to newborns against rotavirus. For example, breast milk is rich in cellular components, and virus-specific cell-mediated immune responses including antibody-dependent cytotoxic responses may be important (49,55). Furthermore, "nonspecific" antiviral properties of milk have been reported (56,57).

Another consideration in assessing the mechanism of clinical efficacy of breast feeding in areas of poor hygiene is that breast fed infants can be expected to receive less enteric pathogens via contaminated food and water than their formula fed counterparts (55). In addition, the amount of breast feeding done by the individual mother may vary greatly and needs to be controlled for in clinical studies. Animal rotavirus models also exist, showing a beneficial effect of milk, but these models need to be interpreted with the realization that maternal antibody doesn't cross the placenta in young calves and pigs, unlike man, and that maternal antibody reaches the offspring only via colostrum (55).

ROLE OF SERUM ANTIBODY

Clinical studies of naturally occuring human rotavirus infection clearly reveal that infantile gastroenteritis can develop in the presence of serum antibody to the groupspecific antigen common to rotaviruses (21). Also, reinfection in adults occurs in the presence of this serum antibody (34). Maternally acquired serum ELISA or FA antibody (not serotype-specific) also fails to protect against rotavirus infection in newborns (51,54).

However, these studies do not take into consideration serotype-specific neutralizing antibodies in serum. It is possible that serum antibody may play a role in clinical protection against rotavirus when serotype-specific antibodies are examined instead of antibodies to the viral group specific antigen. One clue that antibody in serum may play a role in clinical protection comes from a prospective seroepidemiological study of children in Bangladesh (58). In this study, subjects with high titers of preexisting CF (group-specific) antibody less frequently developed a subsequent titer rise than did subjects with lower titers.

The pattern of serum IgM antibody response to rotavirus infection differs for symptomatic children and adults. Rotavirus-specific IgM is found in the acute sera of children by 5 days or later after onset of illness (59), initially in the absence of antirotavirus IgG and IgA (60). In adults with travelers' diarrhea associated with rotavirus reinfection, no antirotavirus IgM responses were seen even though virus-specific serum IgG and IgA responses were observed (61).

HUMAN VOLUNTEER STUDIES

Role of Intestinal Antibody. A few adult human volunteers have been infected with human rotavirus. One preliminary report revealed that the prime correlate of resistance to illness with one stain of rotavirus was the presence of local intestinal IgA antibody to this viral strain (45). In contrast, presence of local IgA antibody to a second strain of rotavirus failed to correlate with resistance to rotavirus challenge with the first strain. It should also be noted that in naturally occurring rotaviral diarrhea in children, most fecal specimens recovered during the acute and convalescent phases of illness have been shown to contain secretory IgA antibody to rotavirus (60).

More recent volunteer studies reveal that the relationship of prechallenge local intestinal fluid rotavirus neutralizing activity to clinical resistance is less clearcut than originally suggested (62). There is, however, a tendency for volunteers possessing pre-existing higher levels of intestinal fluid neutralizing activity to develop less illness than those with lower levels. Most importantly, these later studies have clearly shown a strong correlation of pre-existing high levels of serum neutralizing antibody to type-specific rotavirus with resistance to diarrhea and fecal shedding of the virus (62).

CONCLUSIONS, AND PROSPECTS FOR IMMUNOPROPHYLAXIS

What conclusions may be drawn from the studies to date of factors involved in the clinical immunity to rotavirus infection, and what are the prospects for immunoprophylaxis? An analysis of reported studies reveals that different serologic techniques have been employed in various investigations of serum and breast milk antibodies to rotavirus. Usually, these reports have analysed antibodies against the group-specific antigen common to rotavirus strains and have not taken into consideration serotype-specific neutralizing responses. One should anticipate that future studies will be reported on correlates of clinical resistance with serotype-specific responses, now that human rotavirus has been cultivated in vitro. The ability to grow this virus will also likely lead to the technology necessary for an assessment of cell mediated immune responses to rotaviral infection, an area which has yet to be explored.

Various approaches to the development of a vaccine against rotavirus may be considered, while the clinical correlates of immunity are being worked out and the definitive classification of viral serotypes is being performed. First, it is possible that a live attenuated vaccine for oral administration can be produced using cell culture adapted human rotavirus which can then be analysed for virulence characteristics based on analysis of its genetic composition (36,37,63). Second, a live attenuated recombinant virus could be prepared possessing genes mixed from an animal rotavirus and the human virus so that necessary characteristics of immunogenicity and lack of pathogenicity are attained (45, 63). Third, recombinant DNA technology could be utilized to prepare sufficient quantities of the viral protein that induces presumably protective neutralizing antibodies so that the viral protein could be used as an immunogen (64). In this regard, the genes responsible for neutralization specificity appear to have been defined in the segmented RNA-containing genome of human rotavirus (65). Finally, the experience of Jenner with cowpox could be exploited with the use of an animal rotavirus as an immunogen. Although it is uncertain as to the kind of immunity that might be conferred with such a potential vaccine, it is intriguing to contemplate the fact that calves infected in utero with calf rotavirus are protected against subsequent experimental challenge with either human rotavirus or the homologous virus (66), both of which are normally pathogenic experimentally for the calf.

REFERENCES

1. Blacklow, N.R. and Cukor, G.: Viral gastroenteritis. New Eng. J. Med. 304:397-406,1981.
2. Dolin R., Blacklow,N.R., DuPont, H. et al: Transmission of acute infectious nonbacterial gastroenteritis by oral administration of stool filtrates. J. Infect. Dis. 123:307-312, 1971.
3. Dolin, R., Blacklow, N.R., DuPont, H. et al: Biological properties of Norwalk agent of acute infectious nonbacterial gastroenteritis. Proc. Soc. Exp. Biol. & Med. 140:578-583, 1972.
4. Kapikian,A.Z., Wyatt,R.G., Dolin,R. et al: Visualization by immune electron microscopy of a 27nm particle associated with acute infectious nonbacterial gastroenteritis. J. Virol. 10:1075-1081, 1972.
5. Schreiber,D.S., Blacklow,N.R., Trier, J.S.: The mucosal lesion of the proximal small intestine in acute infectious nonbacterial gastroenteritis. New Eng. J. Med. 288:1318-1323, 1973.
6. Schreiber,D.S., Blacklow,N.R., Trier,J.S.: Small intestinal lesion induced by Hawaii agent acute infectious nonbacterial gastroenteritis. J. Inf. Dis. 129:705-708, 1974.
7. Meeroff, J.C., Schreiber,D.S., Trier,J.S. and Blacklow,N.R.: Abnormal gastric motor function in viral gastroenteritis. Ann. Int. Med. 22:370-373, 1980.
8. Greenberg,H.B., Wyatt,R.G., Valdesuso,J. et al: Solid-phase microtiter radioimmunoassay for detection of the Norwalk strain of acute nonbacterial, epidemic gastroenteritis virus and its antibodies. J. Med. Virol. 2:97:-108, 1978.

9. Blacklow,N.R., Cukor,G., Bedigian, M.K. et al: Immune response and prevalence of antibody to Norwalk enteritis virus as determined by radioimmunoassay. J. Clin.Micro. 10:903-909, 1979.
10. Greenberg,H.B., Valdesuso, J., Kapikian, A.Z. et al: Prevalence of antibody to the Norwalk virus in various countries. Infect. & Immun. 26:270-273, 1979.
11. Cukor,G., Blacklow,N.R., Echeverria, P., Bedigian,M.K., Puruggan,H. and Basaca-Sevilla, V.: Comparative study of the acquisition of antibody to Norwalk virus in pediatric populations. Inf. & Immunity 29:822-823, 1980.
12. Greenberg,H.B., Valdesuso,J., Yolken,R.H. et al: Role of Norwalk virus in outbreaks of non-bacterial gastroenteritis J.Inf.Dis. 139:564-568, 1979.
13. Taylor,J.W., Gary,G.W. and Greenberg,H.B.: Norwalk-related gastroenteritis due to contaminated drinking water. Amer.J.Epid. 114:584-592, 1981.
14. Koopman,J.S., Eckert,E.A., Greenberg,H.B. et al: Norwalk virus enteric illness acquired by swimming exposure: Amer.J.Epid. 115:173-177, 1982.
15. Gunn,R.A., Terranova,W.A., Greenberg,H.B. et al: Norwalk virus gastroenteritis aboard a cruise ship: An outbreak of five consecutive cruises. Am.J.Epid.112:820-827, 1980.
16. Griffin,M.R., Surowiec,J.J., McCloskey,D.I., Capuano,B., Pierzynski, B., Quinn,M., Wojnarski, R., Parkin, W.E., Greenberg, H., and Gary G.W.: Foodborne Norwalk virus. Amer.J.Epid. 115:178-184, 1982.
17. Keswick,B.H., Blacklow,N.R., Cukor, G., DuPont,H.L. and Vollet, J.J. Norwalk virus and rotavirus in travellers' diarrhea in Mexico. The Lancet 1:109-110, 1982.
18. Echeverria,P., Blacklow,N.R., Sanford,L.B. and Cukor,G.: Travelers' diarrhea among American Peace Corps volunteers in rural Thailand. J. Inf. Dis. 143:767-771, 1981.
19. Bishop,R.F., Davidson, G.P., Holmes,I.H., et al: Detection of a new virus by electron microscopy of fecal extracts from children with acute gastroenteritis. Lancet 1:149:-151, 1974.
20. Flewett,T.H., Bryden,A.S., Davies,H. et al: Relation between viruses from acute gastroenteritis of children and newborn calves. Lancet 2:61-63, 1974.
21. Kapikian,A.Z., Kim,H.W., Wyatt,R.G. et al: Human reovirus-like agent as the major pathogen associated with "winter" gastroenteritis in hospitalized infants and young children. New Eng. J. Med. 294: 965-972, 1976.
22. Kapikian,A.Z., Kim, H.W., Wyatt,R.G., et al: Reovirus-like agent in stools: association with infantile diarrhea and development of serologic tests. Science 185:1049-1053, 1974.

23. Blacklow,N.R., Echeverria, P., Smith,D.H.: Serologic studies with reovirus-like enteritis agent. Infect.Imm. 13:1563-1566, 1976.
24. Kalica,A.R., Purcell,R.H., Sereno,M.M. et al: A microtiter solid phase radioimmunoassay for detection of the human reovirus-like agent in stools. J. Immunol. 118:1275-1279, 1977.
25. Cukor,G., Berry,M.K., and Blacklow,N.R.: Simplified radioimmunoassay for detection of human rotavirus in stools. J.Inf.Dis. 138:906-910, 1978.
26. Yolken,R.H., Kim,H.W., Clem,T. et al: Enzyme-linked immunosorbent assay (ELISA) for detection of human reovirus-like agent of infantile gastroenteritis. Lancet 2:263-267, 1977.
27. Echeverria,P., Ho,M.T., Blacklow,N.R. et al: Relative importance of viruses and bacteria in the etiology of pediatric diarrhea in Taiwan. J.Inf.Dis. 136:383, 1977.
28. Echeverria,P., Blacklow,N.R., Vollet,J.J. et al: Reovirus-like agent and enterotoxigenic Escherichia coli infections in pediatric diarrhea in the Philippines. J.Inf.Dis. 138:326, 1978.
29. Echeverria,P., Hodge,F.A., Blacklow,N.R. et al: Travelers' diarrhea among United States Marines in South Korea. Amer.J.Epid. 108:68, 1978.
30. Echeverria,P., Ramirez,G., Blacklow,N.R. et al: Travelers' diarrhea among United States Army troops in South Korea. J.Inf. Dis. 139:215, 1979.
31. Echeverria,P., Blacklow,N.R., Vollet,J.J. et al: Etiology of gastroenteritis among Americans living in the Philippines. Am.J.Epid. 109:493,1979.
32. vonBonsdorff,C.H., Hovi,T., Makela,P.: Rotavirus infections in adults in association with acute gastroenteritis. J.Med.Virol. 2:21, 1978.
33. Bolivar,R., Conklin,R.H. Vollett,J.J. et al: Rotavirus in travelers' diarrhea: Study of an adult student population in Mexico. J.Inf.Dis. 137:325-327, 1978.
34. Wenman,W.M., Hinde,D., Feltham,S. et al: Rotavirus infection in adults: results of a prospective family study. New Eng.J. Med. 301:303-306, 1979.
35. Cubitt,W.D. and Holzel,H.: An outbreak of rotavirus infection in a longstay ward of a geriatric hospital. J.Clin.Path. 33:306-308, 1980.
36. Sato,K., Inaba,Y., Shinozaki,T. et al: Isolation of human rotavirus in cell cultures. Arch.Virol. 69:155-160, 1981.
37. Urasawa,T., Urasawa,S. and Taniguchi,K.: Sequential passages of human rotavirus in MA-104 cells. Microbiol. Immunol. 25:1025-1035, 1981.

38. Beards,G.M., Pilford,J.M., Thouless,M.E. and Flewett,T.H.: Rotavirus serotypes by serum neutralization. J.Med.Virol. 5:231-237,1980.
39. Urasawa,S., Urasawa, T. and Taniguchi,K.: Three human rotavirus serotypes demonstrated by plaque neutralization of isolated strains. Infection and Immunity, 38:781-784, 1982.
40. Pickering,L.K., Blacklow,N.R., DuPont,H.L. and Cukor,G.: Diarrhea due to Norwalk virus in families. J.Inf.Dis., 146:116-117, 1982.
41. Parrino,T.A., Schreiber,D.S., Trier,J.S., Kapikian,A.Z., Blacklow,N.R.: Clinical immunity in acute gastroenteritis caused by Norwalk agent. New Eng. J. Med. 297:86-89, 1977.
42. Greenberg,H.B., Wyatt,R.G., Kalica,A.R., Yolken,R.H., Black,R., Kapikian,A.Z. and Chanock,R.M.: New insights in viral gastroenteritis. In Perspectives in Virology XI, Ed. Pollard,M., Alan,R. Liss Inc., New York, 1981.
43. Blacklow,N.R., Dolin,R., Fedson,D.S. et al: Acute infectious nonbacterial gastroenteritis: etiology and pathogenesis. Ann.Int.Med. 76:993-1008, 1972.
44. Cukor,G., Nowak,N.A., and Blacklow,N.R.: Immunoglobulin M responses to the Norwalk virus of gastroenteritis. Infection and Immunity, 37:463-468, 1982.
45. Kapikian,A.Z., Wyatt,R.G., Greenberg,H.B., Kalica,A.R., Kim,H.W., Brandt,C.D., Rodriguez,W.J., Parrott,R.H. and Chanock,R.M.: Approaches to immunization of infants and young children against gastroenteritis due to rotaviruses. Rev. Inf.Dis. 2:459-469, 1980.
46. Wyatt,R.G., Yolken,R.H., Urrutia,J.J., Mata,L., Greenberg,H.B., Chanock,R.M. and Kapikian,A.Z.: Diarrhea associated with rotavirus in rural Guatemala: A longitudinal study of 24 infants and young children Am.J.Trop.Med.Hyg. 28:325-328, 1979.
47. Schoub,B.D., Prozesky,O.W., Lecatsas,G. and Oosthiuzen,R.: The role of breastfeeding in the prevention of rotavirus infection. J.Med.Microbiol. 11:25-31, 1977.
48. Chrystie,I.L., Totterdell,B.M. and Banatvala,J.E.: Asymptomatic endemic rotavirus infections in the newborn. The Lancet 2:1176-1178, 1978.
49. McLean,B.S. and Holmes,I.H.: Effects of antibodies, trypsin, and trypsin inhibitor on susceptibility of neonates to rotavirus infection. J.Clin.Micro. 13:22-29, 1981.
50. Bishop,R.F., Cameron,D.J.S., Veenstra,A.A. and Barnes,G.L.: Diarrhea and rotavirus infection associated

with differing regimens for postnatal care of newborn babies. J.Clin.Micro. 9:525-529, 1979.

51. Gurwith,M., Wenman,W., Hinde,D., Feltham,S. and Greenberg,H.: A prospective study of rotavirus infection in infants and young children. J.Inf.Dis. 144:218-224, 1981.
52. Yolken,R.H., Wyatt,R.G., Mata,L., Urrutia,J.J., Garcia,B., Chanock,R.M. and Kapikian,A.Z.: Secretory antibody directed against rotavirus in human milk: measurement by means of enzyme-linked immunosorbent assay. J.Ped. 93:916-921, 1978.
53. Cukor,G., Blacklow,N.R., Capozza,F.E., Panjvani,Z.F., and Bednarek,F.: Persistence of antibodies to rotavirus in human milk. J.Clin.Micro. 9:93-96, 1979.
54. Totterdell,B.M., Chrystie,I.L. and Banatvala,J.E.: Cord blood and breast milk antibodies in neonatal rotavirus infection. Brit., Med. J. 1:828-836, 1980.
55. Editorial: The how of breast milk and infection. The Lancet 1:1192-1193, 1981.
56. Welsh,J.K. and May,J.T.: Anti-infective properties of breast milk. J.Ped. 94:1-9, 1979.
57. Matthews,T.H.J., Nair, C.D.G., Lawrence,M.K. and Tyrrell,D.A.J.: An antiviral activity in milk of possible clinical importance. The Lancet 2:1387-1389, 1976.
58. Sack,D.A., Gilman,R.H., Kapikian,A.Z. and Aziz,K.M.S.: Seroepidemiology of rotavirus infection in rural Bangladesh. J.Clin.Micro. 11:530-532, 1980.
59. Yolken,R.H., Wyatt,R.G., Kim, H.W., Kapikian,A.Z. and Chanock,R.M.: Immunological response to infection with human reovirus-like agent: Measurement of anti-human reovirus-like agent immunoglobulin G and M levels by the method of enzyme-linked immunosorbent assay. Infection and Immunity 19:540-546, 1978.
60. Riepenhoff-Talty,M., Bogger-Goren,S., Li,P., Carmody,P.J., Barrett,H.J. and Ogra, P.L.: Development of serum and intestinal antibody response to rotavirus after naturally acquired rotavirus infection in man. J.Med.Virol. 8:215-222, 1981.
61. Sheridan,J.F., Aurelian,L., Barbour,G., Santosham,M., Sack,R.B. and Ryder,R.W.: Travelers' diarrhea associated with rotavirus infection: Analysis of virus-specific immunoblobulin classes. Infection and Immunity 31:419-429, 1981.
62. Kapikian,A.Z., Wyatt,R.G., Levine,M.M., Yolken,R.H., VanKirk,D.H., Dolin,R., Greenberg,H.B. and Chanock,R.M.: Oral administration of a human rotavirus to volunteers: Induction of illness and correlates of resistance. J.Inf.Dis., In Press.

63. Greenberg,H.B., Kalica,A.R., Wyatt,R.G., Jones,R.W., Kapikian,A.Z. and Chanock,R.M.: Rescue of noncultivatable human rotavirus by gene reassortment during mixed infection with ts mutants of a cultivatable bovine rotavirus. Proc.Natl.Acad.Sci. U.S.A. 78:420-424, 1981.
64. Editorial: Towards a rotavirus vaccine. The Lancet 2:619-620, 1981.
65. Kalica,A.R., Greenberg,H.B., Wyatt, R.G., Flores,J., Sereno,M.M., Kapikian,A.Z. and Chanock,R.M.: Genes of human (strain Wa) and bovine (strain UK) rotaviruses that code for neutralization and subgroup antigens. Virol. 112:385-390, 1981.
66. Wyatt,R.G., Mebus,C.A., Yolken,R.H., Kalica,A.R., James,H.D., Kapikian,A.Z. and Chanock,R.M.: Rotaviral immunity in gnotobiotic calves: heterologous resistance to human virus induced by bovine virus. Science 203:548-550, 1979.

CHAPTER 22

MONOCLONAL ANTIBODIES TO POLIOVIRUS

Geoffrey C. Schild, Morag Ferguson, Philip D. Minor, Moses Spitz and David I. Magrath

National Institute for Biological Standards & Control
Holly Hill
Hampstead
London
England

SUMMARY

Monoclonal antibodies to poliovirus type 3 strains have been used for the antigenic characterization of infectious poliovirus (D antigen) particles and noninfectious, empty particles (C antigen). The antibodies could be divided into 3 groups which exhibited: a) exclusive reactivity with D antigen, b) exclusive reactivity with C antigen or, c) common reactivity with both D and C antigen. Thus, in addition to possessing unique determinants, the D and C antigen particles of poliovirus type 3 appear to share one or more common antigenic determinants. All monoclonal antibodies which bound to the determinant(s) common to D and C antigen neutralised a wide range of type 3 poliovirus strains. Only 12 of the 19 antibodies with Dantigen specificity and, unexpectedly, one of the 24 C antigen specific antibodies had virus neutralizing activity.

Several D specific monoclonal antibodies which neutralised only Sabin vaccine strains of poliovirus 3 and vaccine derived viruses but not wild viruses were identified.

The antibodies were also tested for their ability to react with isolated poliovirus capsid proteins (VP1, VP2, VP3 and VP4) in immunoblot techniques. Six of the 51 antibodies tested bound to the isolated virus proteins, 5 with VP1 and one with VP3. All 6 antibodies which reacted in this test were non-neutralising and C antigen specific. None of the 20 antibodies of D and C or D specificity which possessed virus neutralising properties reacted in the immunoblot test.

ISBN 0-12-239980-3

Nevertheless, evidence is available that the majority of these antibodies are directed against VP1 (see reference 4). These findings suggest that the antigentic determinants of the poliovirus capsid which are involved in neutralisation are specified largely by the 3 dimensional tertiary or quarternary conformation of the capsid proteins.

INTRODUCTION

Despite the availability of much detailed information on the replication, assembly and structure of poliovirus, there is little specific information on the antigenic composition of the virus (1). Historically, the examination of the polio virus progeny in tissue culture fluid harvests has revealed the presence of two major populations of particles sedimenting at 155S (infectious particles) and 80S (non-infectious empty particles) respectively (2,3) which are antigenically distinct and have been designated as D antigen and C antigen respectively (3). Several approaches have been made in attempts to locate and identify the antigenic sites responsible for neutralization and the induction of neutralizing antibodies. Minor et al (4) recently showed that antigenic mutants of poliovirus type 3 selected for resistance to individual monoclonal antibodies had point mutations clustered in a short sequence of RNA coding for a region of VP1 eight amino-acids in length. In some studies low titres of neutralizing antibody have been obtained following immunisation of animals with purified polypeptides VP1, VP3 and VP4 (5,6,7). We have produced 51 hybridoma rat and mouse cell lines secreting monoclonal antibodies to type 3 poliovirus and describe here their use in studies of the antigenic determinants present on infectious and empty poliovirus particles. Some of the studies described in this brief paper have been reported in detail elsewhere (Ferguson, M. et al, Amer. J. Epidem., in press, 1983).

METHODS

Cell lines secreting monoclonal antibody to type 3 poliovirus were prepared by fusion of rat spleen cells with rat Y_3Ag1.2.3 cells or by fusion of Balb/c mouse spleen cells with P3x63Ag cells (8). Fusions were carried out with spleen lymphocytes of animals immunised with purified type 3 poliovirus and received two inoculations approximately 28 and 3 days prior to fusion or just one inoculation 3-4 days prior to fusion.

Assays of virus neutralisating antibody were carried out on Hep 2 C cell cultures by the method of Domok and Magrath (9). The challenge dose of poliovirus was 100 $TCID_{50}$.

The antigen blocking technique used was a modification of an autoradiographic single radial diffusion (SRD) method described previously by Schild et al (10). Antibodies for assay were mixed with ^{35}S methionine radioactively labelled 155S D antigen or 80S C antigen peaks of poliovirus particles from sucrose gradients. Where the antibodies react, the poliovirus particles are rendered nondiffusable in agarose gels, thus reducing the diameter of the zone produced when antigen is mixed with phosphate buffered saline (11). The blocking titre of serum is taken as the limiting dilution which reduces the autoradiographic SRD zone by approximately 50%.

Virus polypeptides from purified virus were resolved in polyacrylamide gels after treatment with 5DS and reducing agents at 100°C. Immunoblot experiments were carried out by the methods described by Thorpe et al (12).

EXPERIMENTAL RESULTS

Monoclonal antibodies from 51 independent hybridoma cell lines have been characterised and the results are reported here; 41 were prepared by fusion of mouse spleen cells and 10 by fusion of rat spleen cells. The antibodies were tested for reactivity in antigen blocking tests with poliovirus type 3 D and C antigens, eight bound to both antigens, i.e. they were C and D antigen reactive, 19 bound uniquely to D antigen and 24 uniquely to C antigen particles. Thus, the poliovirus particles appeared to express three distinct types of antigenic determinants, which were specific to D antigen, specific to C antigen or shared between C and D antigen.

Each antibody was assayed for virus neutralising activity. All antibodies (Table 1) which bound to the shared D and C determinant had high titres of neutralising activity but only 12 of the D specific and one C specific antibody neutralised virus infectivity. This neutralising activity was type specific.

The neutralising monoclonal antibodies were tested against a range of type 3 viruses the genetic composition of which had been characterised by TI-oliognucleotide maps (4). Some monoclonal antibodies reacted broadly with a wide range of wild and vaccine related viruses, where as others were highly specific for Sabin vaccine virus and closely related strains (Table 2). NIBp 132 and NIBp 134 reacted with almost

TABLE 1. Virus Neutralizing Activity of Monoclonal Antibodies to Poliovirus 3

Poliovirus Particle (D+C)* specificity of antibody*	No. of antibodies tested**	No. of antibodies with virus neutralising activity at stated titres***				
		<10	$10^1<10^2$	$10^2<10^3$	$10^3<10^4$	$<10^4$
D+C cross reactive	8	0	0	3	0	5
D specific	19	7	8	3	0	1
C specific	24	23	0	0	1	0
All	51	30	8	6	1	6

*Based on autoradiographic immuno-diffusion assays, reference 11.

**Each antibody was obtained from an independent hybridoma clone in fusions involving the lymphocytes of mice or rats immunised with poliovirus type 3 strains, reference 8.

***Dilution of antibody just neutralizing 100 tissue culture infectious doses 50% of virus in microtitre assays.

TABLE 2. Poliovirus Type 3 Strain Specificity of Neutralizing Monoclonal Antibodies

Virus Strains	Monoclonal Antibody: Neutralisation titre against stated virus.			
	NIBp 132	NIBp 134	NIBp 138	NIBp 165
Type 3 strains with Sabin-like maps:				
Sabin Vaccine Strain	360	4100	64	256
106	360	10000	90	256
116	180	>30000	20	45
119	256	3600	32	181
122	256	>60000	45	90
131	128	41000	8	256
285/UK/74	90	10000	11	32
5229/UK/74	128	10000	45	128
11340/UK/74	362	>30000	128	720
Leon/USA/39*	512	1400	<5	56
Type 3 strains with non-Sabin-like maps:				
Saukett/USA/50 (COP)	90	900	<4	<4
30/USA/52	<4	<4	<4	<4
190/USA/52	64	10000	<4	<4
715/India/58	180	10000	<4	<4
6/UK/62	<4	<4	<4	<4
476/UK/62	<4	<4	<4	<4
10/USA/52	16	640	<4	<4
77689/USA/53	22	90	<4	<4
Type 1 Mahoney/USA/41	<4	<4	<4	<4
Type 2 MEF/USA/42	<4	<4	<4	<4

*Leon/USA/39 is the 'wild' progenitor strain of Sabin type 3 vaccine virus.

all strains tested whereas NIBp 138 and 165 only neutralised strains which gave TI-oligonucleotide maps showing that they were genetically closely related to Sabin type 3 vaccine virus. NIBp 138 did not react with Leon/USA/39, the vaccine progenitor strain which has a Tl-oligonucleotide map identical to that of Sabin virus.

The reactivity of all the monoclonal antibodies with electrophoretically separated poliovirus capsid proteins was investigated. Of the 27 antibodies which were D antigen specific, or D and C antigen reactive, including the 20 antibodies which neutralised virus infectivity and the 7 antibodies which reacted with D antigen in antigen blocking tests but were not neutralizing, none reacted with the denatured polypeptides of VP1, V2, VP3 or VP4. However, six of the twenty-four C antigen specific antibodies bound to denatured proteins, 5 to VP1 and one to VP3. These six antibodies were also tested against types 1 and 2 poliovirus and the results shown in Table 3. NIBp 196 and NIBp 203 bound to the VP1 of type 2 and 3 but not type 1, but NIBp 176 reacted with VP3 of all 3 types. Cross reactivity also observed with NIBp 196 and NIBp 203 in antigen blocking tests with type 2 antigens but not type 1.

CONCLUSION

Our data from antigen blocking tests show that infectious and empty particles possess a shared antigenic determinant in addition to unique determinants on each particle. All antibodies directed against the shared determinant had high titres of neutralising activity. However, only 12 of the D specific antibodies neutralised virus infectivity indicating that although monoclonal antibodies bind to D antigen, specific epitopes are important for virus neutralisation. The neutralisation of virus by a C specific antibody is unexpected as this antibody does not bind to infectious virus in antigen blocking tests. Its mechanism of neutralisation is being investigated further.

In general, antibodies directed against the shared D and C determinant had a high titre of neutralising activity against a wide range of viruses. Some D specific antibodies also neutralise to high titre whereas other react to low titre with a narrow range of strains. NIBp 138 and NIBp 165 only neutralise strains with TI-oligonucleotide maps related to that Sabin type 3 virus and do not react with strains unrelated to Sabin virus.

These vaccine-specific antibodies have considerable potential value for routine use in identifying poliovirus 3

TABLE 3. Polypeptide Specificity of Non-neutralising, C Antigen Specific Monoclonal Antibodies

Monoclonal Antibody	C Antigen Blocking	Immunoblot Reactivity			Type 3 C Antigen Blocking	Immunoblot Reactivity			Type 2 C Antigen Blocking	Type 1 Immunoblot Reactivity		
		VP1	VP2	VP3		VP1	VP2	VP3		VP1	VP2	VP3
N1By 25-2-11	50	+	–	–	<10	–	–	–	<10	–	–	–
N1By 25-4-4	50	+	–	–	<10	–	–	–	<10	–	–	–
N1Bp 118	30	+	–	–	<10	–	–	–	<10	–	–	–
N1Bp 196	300	+	–	–	100	+	–	–	<10	–	–	–
N1Bp 203	300	+	–	–	100	+	–	–	<10	–	–	–
N1Bp 176	300	–	–	+	<10	–	–	+	<10	–	–	–

isolates as being derived from Sabin vaccine. However, reaction of viruses with monoclonal antibodies was not correlated with neurovirulence. The vaccine-specific monoclonal antibodies reacted with several fully neurovirulent isolated including 119, 106 and 116 which were isolated from cases of paralytic poliomyelitis temporally associated with the administration of Sabin vaccine and therefore thought to be vaccine derived.

Immunoblot experiments showed that none of the antibodies which neutralised virus infectivity bound to the denatured virus polypeptides VP1, VP2, VP3 or VP4, suggesting that many of the antigenic sites present on the infectious particle, including those responsible for virus neutralisation are structurally complex and dependent on tertiary or quaternary conformation of the virus capsid proteins, rather than being specified simply by amino acid sequences. Nevertheless, evidence has been obtained (4) that the neutralizing monoclonal antibodies react with an antigenic site present on the major capsid protein VP1.

Antigenic determinants common to type 1, 2 and 3 polio virus have been shown to exist on VP1 using antigen blocking and immunoblot experiments (12) and also on VP1, VP2, VP3 in immunoprecipitation studies (13). However, only 2 of the C specific antibodies possessed antigen blocking activity with type 2 but not type 1 C antigen suggesting that there is greater homology between certain regions of types 2 and 3 than types 1 and 3. NIBp 176, which is directed against VP 3, cross-reacts in immunoblot experiments but not in antigen blocking tests indicating that the amino acid sequence against which it is directed must be masked or in a different conformation in types 1 and 2.

These findings formed a valuable basis for further work (4) (14) leading to the precise identification of a major antigenic site for virus neutralization containing an 8 amino acid sequence of VP1 approximately one third of its length from the N terminu.

REFERENCES

1. Putnak,J.R., and Phillips,B.A. Picornaviral structure and assembly. Microbiol. Rev. 45:287-315, 1981.
2. Minor,P.D., Schild,G.C., Wood,J.M. and Dandawate,C.N. The preparation of specific immune sera against type 3 poliovirus D-antigen and C-antigen, and the demonstration of two C-antigenic components in vaccine strain populations. J.Gen.Virol. 51:147-156, 1980.
3. Mayer,M.M., Rapp,H.J., Roizman,B., Klein,S.W.,

Cowan,K.M., Lukery,D., Schwerdt,C.E., Schaffer,F.L. and Charney,J.J. The purification of poliomyelitis virus as studied by complement fixation. J.Immunol. 78:435-455, 1957.

4. Minor,P.D., Schild,G.C., Bootman,J., Evans,D.M.A., Ferguson,M., Reeve,P., Spitz,M., Stanway,G., Cann,A.J., Hauptmann,R., Clarke,L.D., Mountford,R.C., Almond,J.W. Location and primary structure of a major antigenic site for poliovirus neutralisation. Nature. 301:674-679, 1983.
5. Blondel,B., Crainic, R. and Horodniceanu,F. Le polypeptide structural VP1 du poliovirus type 1 induit des anticorps neutralisants. C.R. Acad.Sci. Paris, 294:91-94, 1982.
6. Chow,M. and Baltimore,D. Isolated poliovirus capsid protein VP1 induces a neutralising response in rats. Proc. Natl. Acad. Sci. USA, 79:7518-7521, 1982.
7. Emini,E.A., Dorner,A.J., Dorner,L.F., Jameson,B.A. and Wimmer,E. Identification of a poliovirus neutralisation epitope through use of neutralising antiserum raised against a purified structural protein. Virology 124:144-151, 1983.
8. Minor,P.D., Schild,G.C., Ferguson,M., Mackay,A., Magrath,D.I., John,A., Yates,P.J. and Spitz,M. Genetic and antigenic variation in type 3 polioviruses: characterisation of strains by monoclonal antibodies and T1 oligonucleotide mapping. J. Gen. Virol. 61:167-176, 1982.
9. Domok, I. and Magrath,D.I. Guide to poliovirus isolation and serological techniques for poliomyelitis surveillance. WHO Publication No. 46, 1979.
10. Schild,G.C., Wood,J.M., Minor,P.D., Dandawate,C.N. and Magrath,D.I. Immunoassay of poliovirus antigens by single-radial-diffusion: development and characteristics of a sensitive autoradiographic zone size enhancement (ZE) technique. J.Gen.Virol. 51:157-170, 1980.
11. Ferguson,M., Qi Yi-Hua, Minor,P.D., Magrath,D.I., Spitz,M., Schild,G.C. Monoclonal antibodies specific for the Sabin vaccine strain of poliovirus. Lancet ii 122-124, 1982.
12. Thorpe,R., Minor,P.D., Mackay,A., Schild,G.C. and Spitz,M. Immunochemical studies of polioviruses: identification of immunoreactive virus capsid polypeptides. J.Gen.Virol. 63:487-492, 1982.
13. Blondel,B., Crainic,R., Akacem,O., Bruneau,P., Girard,M. and Hordniceanu,F. Evidence for common intertypic antigenic determinants on poliovirus capsid polypeptides. Virology 123:461-463, 1982.
14. Evans,D.M.A., Minor,P.D., Schild,G.C. and Almard, S.W., 1983. Submitted for publication.

INDEX

D

E

F

G

H

I